Editors

ASIF M. ILYAS
SHITAL N. PARIKH
SAQIB REHMAN
GILES R. SCUDERI
FELASFA M. WODAJO

ORTHOPEDIC CLINICS OF NORTH AMERICA

www.orthopedic.theclinics.com

January 2016 • Volume 47 • Number 1

ELSEVIER

1600 John F. Kennedy Boulevard • Suite 1800 • Philadelphia, Pennsylvania, 19103-2899.

http://www.orthopedic.theclinics.com

ORTHOPEDIC CLINICS OF NORTH AMERICA Volume 47, Number 1
January 2016 ISSN 0030-5898, ISBN-13: 978-0-323-41460-9

Editor: Jennifer Flynn-Briggs
Developmental Editor: Kristen Helm

Orthopedic Clinics of North America (ISSN 0030-5898) is published quarterly by Elsevier Inc., 360 Park Avenue South, New York, NY 10010-1710. Months of issue are January, April, July, and October. Business and Editorial Offices: 1600 John F. Kennedy Blvd., Suite 1800, Philadelphia, PA 19103-2899. Customer Service Office: 3251 Riverport Lane, Maryland Heights, MO 63043. Periodicals postage paid at New York, NY and additional mailing offices. Subscription prices are $310.00 per year for (US individuals), $653.00 per year for (US institutions), $365.00 per year (Canadian individuals), $797.00 per year (Canadian institutions), $450.00 per year (international individuals), $797.00 per year (international institutions), $100.00 per year (US students), $220.00 per year (Canadian and international students). Foreign air speed delivery is included in all *Clinics* subscription prices. All prices are subject to change without notice. **POSTMASTER:** Send change of address to *Orthopedic Clinics of North America*, **Elsevier Health Sciences Division, Subscription Customer Service, 3251 Riverport Lane, Maryland Heights, MO 63043. Customer Service (orders, claims, online, change of address): Elsevier Health Sciences Division, Subscription Customer Service, 3251 Riverport Lane, Maryland Heights, MO 63043. Tel: 1-800-654-2452 (U.S. and Canada); 314-447-8871 (outside U.S. and Canada). Fax: 314-447-8029. E-mail:** journalscustomerservice-usa@elsevier. com **(for print support);** journalsonlinesupport-usa@elsevier.com **(for online support).**

Reprints. For copies of 100 or more, of articles in this publication, please contact the Commercial Reprints Department, Elsevier Inc., 360 Park Avenue South, New York, NY 10010-1710. Tel.: 212-633-3874; Fax: 212-633-3820; E-mail: reprints@elsevier. com.

Orthopedic Clinics of North America is covered in *MEDLINE/PubMed (Index Medicus)*, *Cinahl*, *Excerpta Medica*, and *Cumulative Index to Nursing and Allied Health Literature*.

PROGRAM OBJECTIVE
Orthopedic Clinics of North America offers clinical review articles on the most cutting-edge technologies and techniques in the field, including adult reconstruction, the upper extremity, pediatrics, trauma, oncology, and sports medicine.

TARGET AUDIENCE
Practicing orthopedic surgeons, orthopedic residents, and other healthcare professionals who specialize in orthopedic technologies and techniques for adult reconstruction, the upper extremity, pediatrics, trauma, oncology, and sports medicine.

LEARNING OBJECTIVES
Upon completion of this activity, participants will be able to:
1. Review the diagnosis and revision of infections following joint arthroplasty.
2. Discuss management options for traumas to the lower extremity, such as distal femur fractures and patellar fractures.
3. Recognize developing treatments for injuries of the upper extremity, including biceps ruptures, traumatic amputations, and open fractures of the hand.

ACCREDITATION
The Elsevier Office of Continuing Medical Education (EOCME) is accredited by the Accreditation Council for Continuing Medical Education (ACCME) to provide continuing medical education for physicians.

The EOCME designates this enduring material for a maximum of 15 *AMA PRA Category 1 Credit*(s)™. Physicians should claim only the credit commensurate with the extent of their participation in the activity.

All other health care professionals requesting continuing education credit for this enduring material will be issued a certificate of participation.

DISCLOSURE OF CONFLICTS OF INTEREST
The EOCME assesses conflict of interest with its instructors, faculty, planners, and other individuals who are in a position to control the content of CME activities. All relevant conflicts of interest that are identified are thoroughly vetted by EOCME for fair balance, scientific objectivity, and patient care recommendations. EOCME is committed to providing its learners with CME activities that promote improvements or quality in healthcare and not a specific proprietary business or a commercial interest.

The planning committee, staff, authors and editors listed below have identified no financial relationships or relationships to products or devices they or their spouse/life partner have with commercial interest related to the content of this CME activity:
Megan E. Anderson, MD; Odion Binitie, MD; Daniel J. Blizzard, MD, MS; Michael P. Bolognesi, MD; Edward S. Chang, MD; Roger Cornwall, MD; William C. Eward, DVM, MD; Jennifer Flynn-Briggs; Anjali Fortna; John R. Fowler, MD; Anup K. Gangavalli, MD; Thorsten A. Gehrke, MD; Nicholas J. Greco, MD; Dustin Greenhill, MD; John S. Groundland, MD; Alexander Hahn, BS; Christopher Haydel, MD; Colin C. Heinle, MD; John G. Horneff, MD; Stephen M. Howell, MD; Jason E. Hsu, MD; Ronald Huang, MD; Jerry I. Huang, MD; Maury L. Hull, PhD; Asif M. Ilyas, MD; John D. Jennings, MD; Rafael Kakazu, MD; Colin D. Kennedy, MD; Constantinos Ketonis, MD, PhD; Kevin Kruse, MD; Kevin J. Little, MD; Marios G. Lykissas, MD; Moiz I. Manaqibwala, MD; Laura Matsen Ko, MD; Michael P. McClincy, MD; Christopher Myer, MD; Alexander J. Nedopil, MD; Brian T. Nickel, MD; Chinenye O. Nwachuku, MD; Shital N. Parikh, MD, FACS; Santha Priya; Saqib Rehman, MD; Thorsten M. Seyler, MD, PhD; Faseeh Shahab, MBBS; Mark K. Solarz, MD; Laura E. Stoll, MD; Megan Suermann; Joseph J. Thoder, MD; Mohan S. Tripathi, MD; Jacob E. Tulipan, MD; Julia D. Visgauss, MD; Michael M. Vosbikian, MD; Felasfa M. Wodajo, MD; Lewis G. Zirkle, MD; Shahabuddin, MBBS, FCPS (Ortho).

The planning committee, staff, authors and editors listed below have identified financial relationships or relationships to products or devices they or their spouse/life partner have with commercial interest related to the content of this CME activity:
Michael T. Archdeacon, MD, MSE is on the speakers' bureau for Stryker and AO North America, is consultant/advisor for Stryker, and receives royalties/patents from Stryker and The Wyanoke Group.
James P. Bradley, MD receives royalties/patents from Arthrex, Inc.
Brian E. Brigman, MD, PhD is a consultant/advisor for Musculoskeletal Transplant Foundation and Plexxikon.
Mark R. Brinker, MD receives royalties/patents from Zimmer Inc.
Albert O. Gee, MD is a consultant/advisor for, with roylaties/patents from, MedBridge Inc.
Jess H. Lonner, MD is a consultant/advisor for Zimmer Inc.; Biomet, Inc.; Blue Belt Technologies; and CD Diagnostics, Inc, has stock owenership in Blue Belt Technologies and CD Diagnostics, Inc, research support from Zimmer Inc.; Biomet, Inc.; and royalties/patents from Zimmer Inc; Biomet, Inc.; and Blue Belt Technologies.
Daniel P. O'Connor, PhD is a consultant/advisor for Nimbic, Inc. and royalties/patents for The Wyanoke Group.
Javad Parvizi, MD, FRCS is a consultant/advisor for The Journal of Arthroplasty; Philadelphia Orthopaedic Society; Eastern Orthopedic Association; 3M, The Journal of Bone and Joint Surgery; The Bone and Joint Journal; Muller Foundation; Zimmer Inc.; ConvaTec Inc.; TissueGene, Inc.; CeramTec; Medtronic; Ethicon US, LLC; PainReform Ltd.; has research support from National Institutes of Health; Orthopaedic Research and Education Foundation; Stryker; Zimmer Inc.; 3M; CeramTec; DePuy

Sythes; Pfizer Inc.; and Medtronic, and receives royalties/patents from Elsevier B.V.; Wolters Kluwer; The Wyanoke Group; JP Medical Ltd.; and Data Trace Publishing Company.

Giles R. Scuderi, MD is on the speakers' bureau for Zimmer Inc; Medtronic; ConvaTec Inc.; and Pacira Pharmaceuticals, is a consultant/advisor for Zimmer Inc. and Merz, Inc., and has research support from Pacira Pharmaceuticals.

Alfred J. Tria Jr, MD is on the speakers' bureau for Pacira Pharmaceuticals, is a consultant/advisor for Smith & Nephew and Medtronic, and receives royalties/patents from Smith & Nephew.

Akos Zahar, MD is on the speakers' bureau for Waldemar LINK GmbH & Co. KG.

UNAPPROVED/OFF-LABEL USE DISCLOSURE

The EOCME requires CME faculty to disclose to the participants:

1. When products or procedures being discussed are off-label, unlabelled, experimental, and/or investigational (not US Food and Drug Administration [FDA] approved); and
2. Any limitations on the information presented, such as data that are preliminary or that represent ongoing research, interim analyses, and/or unsupported opinions. Faculty may discuss information about pharmaceutical agents that is outside of FDA-approved labelling. This information is intended solely for CME and is not intended to promote off-label use of these medications. If you have any questions, contact the medical affairs department of the manufacturer for the most recent prescribing information.

TO ENROLL

To enroll in the *Orthopedic Clinics of North America* Continuing Medical Education program, call customer service at 1-800-654-2452 or sign up online at http://www.theclinics.com/home/cme. The CME program is available to subscribers for an additional annual fee of USD 215.

METHOD OF PARTICIPATION

In order to claim credit, participants must complete the following:

1. Complete enrolment as indicated above.
2. Read the activity.
3. Complete the CME Test and Evaluation. Participants must achieve a score of 70% on the test. All CME Tests and Evaluations must be completed online.

CME INQUIRIES/SPECIAL NEEDS

For all CME inquiries or special needs, please contact elsevierCME@elsevier.com.

Contributors

EDITORS

ASIF M. ILYAS, MD – *Upper Extremity*
Program Director of Hand Surgery
Fellowship, Rothman Institute; Associate
Professor of Orthopaedic Surgery, Jefferson
Medical College, Philadelphia, Pennsylvania

SHITAL N. PARIKH, MD, FACS – *Pediatrics*
Pediatric Orthopaedics and Sports Trauma,
Associate Professor of Orthopaedic Surgery,
Cincinnati Children's Hospital Medical Center,
University of Cincinnati School of Medicine,
Cincinnati, Ohio

SAQIB REHMAN, MD – *Trauma*
Director of Orthopaedic Trauma,
Associate Professor, Department of
Orthopaedic Surgery and Sports Medicine,
School of Medicine, Temple University
Hospital, Temple University, Philadelphia,
Pennsylvania

GILES R. SCUDERI, MD – *Adult
Reconstruction*
Vice President, Orthopedic Service Line,
Northshore Long Island Jewish Health System;
Fellowship Director, Adult Knee
Reconstruction Lenox Hill Hospital, New York,
New York

FELASFA M. WODAJO, MD – *Oncology*
Musculoskeletal Tumor Surgery, Inova Fairfax
Hospital, Fairfax, Virginia; Associate Professor,
Orthopedic Surgery, VCU School of Medicine,
Inova Campus; Assistant Professor,
Orthopedic Surgery, Georgetown University
Hospital, Arlington, Virginia

AUTHORS

MEGAN E. ANDERSON, MD
Department of Orthopaedic Surgery,
Boston Children's Hospital and Beth Israel
Deaconess Medical Center; Assistant
Professor, Harvard Medical School, Boston,
Massachusetts

MICHAEL T. ARCHDEACON, MD, MSE
Department of Orthopaedic Surgery, University
of Cincinnati Academic Health Center,
Cincinnati, Ohio

ODION BINITIE, MD
Assistant Member, Department of Sarcoma,
H. Lee Moffitt Cancer Center; Assistant
Professor, Department of Orthopedics and
Sports Medicine, University of South Florida,
Tampa, Florida

DANIEL J. BLIZZARD, MD, MS
Department of Orthopaedic Surgery, Duke
University Medical Center, Durham, North
Carolina

MICHAEL P. BOLOGNESI, MD
Department of Orthopaedic Surgery, Duke
University Medical Center, Durham, North
Carolina

JAMES P. BRADLEY, MD
Professor, Department of Orthopaedic
Surgery, University of Pittsburgh Medical
Center, Pittsburgh, Pennsylvania

BRIAN E. BRIGMAN, MD, PhD
Division of Orthopaedic Oncology, Duke
Cancer Institute, Durham, North Carolina

MARK R. BRINKER, MD
Director of Acute and Reconstructive Trauma, Director of the Center for Problem Fractures, and Limb Restoration, Fondren Orthopedic Group LLP, Texas Orthopedic Hospital; Clinical Professor, Department of Orthopaedic Surgery, The University of Texas Medical School at Houston, Houston, Texas

EDWARD S. CHANG, MD
Assistant Professor, Department of Orthopaedic Surgery, Sports Medicine Institute at Inova Medical Group, Inova Health System, Fairfax, Virginia

ROGER CORNWALL, MD
Division of Pediatric Orthopaedics, Department of Orthopaedic Surgery, Cincinnati Children's Hospital Medical Center, University of Cincinnati School of Medicine, Cincinnati, Ohio

WILLIAM C. EWARD, DVM, MD
Division of Orthopaedic Oncology, Duke Cancer Institute, Durham, North Carolina

JOHN R. FOWLER, MD
Assistant Professor, Department of Orthopaedics, University of Pittsburgh, Pittsburgh, Pennsylvania

ANUP K. GANGAVALLI, MD
Department of Orthopaedic Surgery, St. Luke's University Health Network, Bethlehem, Pennsylvania

ALBERT O. GEE, MD
Assistant Professor, Department of Orthopaedics and Sports Medicine, University of Washington, Seattle, Washington

THORSTEN A. GEHRKE, MD
Professor of Orthopedics, Medical Director, HELIOS ENDO Klinik Hamburg, Hamburg, Germany

NICHOLAS J. GRECO, MD
Resident, Department of Orthopaedic Surgery, University of Pittsburgh Medical Center, Pittsburgh, Pennsylvania

DUSTIN GREENHILL, MD
Department of Orthopaedic Surgery and Sports Medicine, Temple University Hospital, Philadelphia, Pennsylvania

JOHN S. GROUNDLAND, MD
Department of Orthopedics and Sports Medicine, University of South Florida, Tampa, Florida

ALEXANDER HAHN, BS
Department of Orthopedic Surgery and Sports Medicine, Temple University School of Medicine, Philadelphia, Pennsylvania

CHRISTOPHER HAYDEL, MD
Department of Orthopaedic Surgery and Sports Medicine, Temple University Hospital, Philadelphia, Pennsylvania

COLIN C. HEINLE, MD
Department of Orthopaedic Surgery, Rutgers-Robert Wood Johnson Medical School, New Brunswick, New Jersey

JOHN G. HORNEFF, MD
Resident, Department of Orthopaedic Surgery, University of Pennsylvania, Philadelphia, Pennsylvania

STEPHEN M. HOWELL, MD
Department of Biomedical Engineering, University of California, Davis, Sacramento, California

JASON E. HSU, MD
Assistant Professor, Department of Orthopaedics and Sports Medicine, University of Washington, Seattle, Washington

JERRY I. HUANG, MD
Associate Professor, Program Director, UW Combined Hand Fellowship, Department of Orthopaedics and Sports Medicine, University of Washington Medical Center, Seattle, Washington

RONALD HUANG, MD
Resident, Orthopaedic Surgery, Thomas Jefferson University Hospital, Philadelphia, Pennsylvania

MAURY L. HULL, PhD
Department of Mechanical Engineering, University of California, Davis, Sacramento, California

ASIF M. ILYAS, MD
Program Director of Hand Surgery
Fellowship, Rothman Institute; Associate
Professor of Orthopaedic Surgery, Jefferson
Medical College, Philadelphia, Pennsylvania

JOHN D. JENNINGS, MD
Department of Orthopaedics and Sports
Medicine, Temple University Hospital,
Philadelphia, Pennsylvania

RAFAEL KAKAZU, MD
Department of Orthopaedic Surgery, University
of Cincinnati Academic Health Center,
Cincinnati, Ohio

COLIN D. KENNEDY, MD
Resident Physician, Department of
Orthopaedics and Sports Medicine, University
of Washington Medical Center, Seattle,
Washington

CONSTANTINOS KETONIS, MD, PhD
Resident, Orthopaedic Surgery, Thomas
Jefferson University Hospital, Philadelphia,
Pennsylvania

KEVIN KRUSE, MD
Department of Orthopaedics, University of
Pittsburgh, Pittsburgh, Pennsylvania

KEVIN J. LITTLE, MD
Division of Pediatric Orthopaedics,
Department of Orthopaedic Surgery, Cincinnati
Children's Hospital Medical Center, University
of Cincinnati School of Medicine, Cincinnati,
Ohio

JESS H. LONNER, MD
Attending Orthopedic Surgeon, Rothman
Institute; Associate Professor of Orthopedic
Surgery, Thomas Jefferson University,
Philadelphia, Pennsylvania

MARIOS G. LYKISSAS, MD
Department of Orthopaedic Surgery,
University of Ioannina School of Medicine,
Ioannina, Greece

MOIZ I. MANAQIBWALA, MD
Department of Orthopaedic Surgery,
Rutgers-Robert Wood Johnson Medical
School, New Brunswick, New Jersey

LAURA MATSEN KO, MD
Rothman Institute, Thomas Jefferson
University, Seattle, Washington

MICHAEL P. McCLINCY, MD
Resident, Department of Orthopaedic Surgery,
University of Pittsburgh Medical Center,
Pittsburgh, Pennsylvania

CHRISTOPHER MYER, MD
Department of Orthopaedics, University of
Pittsburgh, Pittsburgh, Pennsylvania

ALEXANDER J. NEDOPIL, MD
Department of Orthopaedics, University of
California, Davis, Sacramento, California

BRIAN T. NICKEL, MD
Department of Orthopaedic Surgery, Duke
University Medical Center, Durham, North
Carolina

CHINENYE O. NWACHUKU, MD
Department of Orthopaedic Surgery, St. Luke's
University Health Network, Bethlehem,
Pennsylvania

DANIEL P. O'CONNOR, PhD
Associate Professor, Department of Health and
Human Performance, University of Houston,
Houston, Texas

SHITAL N. PARIKH, MD, FACS
Pediatric Orthopaedics and Sports Trauma,
Associate Professor of Orthopaedic Surgery,
Cincinnati Children's Hospital Medical Center,
University of Cincinnati School of Medicine,
Cincinnati, Ohio

JAVAD PARVIZI, MD, FRCS
James Edwards Professor of
Orthopaedic Surgery, Sidney Kimmel
School of Medicine, Rothman Institute,
Thomas Jefferson University, Philadelphia,
Pennsylvania

SAQIB REHMAN, MD
Director of Orthopaedic Trauma, Associate
Professor, Department of Orthopaedic Surgery
and Sports Medicine, School of Medicine,
Temple University Hospital, Temple University,
Philadelphia, Pennsylvania

THORSTEN M. SEYLER, MD, PhD
Department of Orthopaedic Surgery, Duke University Medical Center, Durham, North Carolina

FASEEH SHAHAB, MBBS
Resident, Rehman Medical Institute, Peshawar, Pakistan

SHAHABUDDIN, MBBS, FCPS (Ortho)
Professor and Chair, Department of Orthopaedics and Traumatology, Lady Reading Hospital, Peshawar, Pakistan

MARK K. SOLARZ, MD
Resident, Department of Orthopaedics and Sports Medicine, Temple University Hospital, Philadelphia, Pennsylvania

LAURA E. STOLL, MD
Resident, Department of Orthopaedics and Sports Medicine, University of Washington Medical Center, Seattle, Washington

JOSEPH J. THODER, MD
John W. Lachman Professor and Director of Hand Surgery, Department of Orthopaedics and Sports Medicine, Temple University Hospital, Philadelphia, Pennsylvania

ALFRED J. TRIA Jr, MD
Department of Orthopaedic Surgery, The Orthopaedic Center of New Jersey, St. Peter's University Hospital, Somerset, New Jersey

MOHAN S. TRIPATHI, MD
Department of Orthopaedic Surgery, Rutgers-Robert Wood Johnson Medical School, New Brunswick, New Jersey

JACOB E. TULIPAN, MD
Department of Orthopaedic Surgery, Thomas Jefferson University, Philadelphia, Pennsylvania

JULIA D. VISGAUSS, MD
Department of Orthopaedic Surgery, Duke University, Durham, North Carolina

MICHAEL M. VOSBIKIAN, MD
Fellow, Hand and Microvascular Surgery, Harvard–Beth Israel Deaconess Medical Center, Boston, Massachusetts

AKOS ZAHAR, MD
Consultant Orthopedic Surgeon, HELIOS ENDO Klinik Hamburg, Hamburg, Germany

LEWIS G. ZIRKLE, MD
Founder and President, SIGN Fracture Care International, Richland, Washington

Contents

Adult Reconstruction

a high degree of accuracy of implant positioning and soft tissue balance are required to optimize durability and implant survivorship. First-generation robotic technology improved implant position compared with conventional methods. This article reviews the next-generation robotic technology, an image-free handheld robotic sculpting tool, which offers an alternative method for optimizing implant positioning and soft tissue balance without the need for preoperative computed tomography scans and with price points that make it suitable for use in outpatient surgery centers.

Internal and external malrotation of the femoral and tibial components is associated with poor function after total knee arthroplasty (TKA). We determined the degree of malrotation for both components in kinematically aligned TKA and whether this malrotation compromised function. Seventy-one patients (mean age 68 years) were followed after TKA. Malrotation was measured. Simple regression determined the association between malrotation and function. Even though the range of malrotation of the tibial component can be greater than that of the femoral component, the malrotation of the femoral and tibial components bounded by the ranges reported in this study is compatible with a well-functioning TKA.

Total knee arthroplasty (TKA) for the obese patient entails more preoperative comorbidities and complications, and shorter longevity. This article is a retrospective review comparing longevity of the constrained implant with a standard prosthesis. Patient-specific data, Knee Society Scores, complications, and revisions were recorded and compared. No statistical differences were found. The constrained condylar knee for obese patients improves the intramedullary alignment of the prosthesis and supports the surrounding soft tissues. The clinical results are similar to a standard implant in the nonobese with similar longevity at midterm follow-up.

Trauma

Surgical Implant Generation Network (SIGN) was founded 15 years ago to create equality of fracture care throughout the world. This is done by education and supply of the appropriate implants and instruments to implement the education. SIGN implants have been used in 150,000 long bone fractures in developing countries. The same implants and instruments are used to provide intramedullary nail interlocking

for each instability pattern. Existing classification systems do not include the entire spectrum of patellar instability patterns. The aim of this article is to review the nomenclature and existing patellar instability classification systems and analyze the different patterns into a comprehensive system.

Physicians who specialize in pediatric orthopedics and hand surgery frequently encounter congenital hand abnormalities, despite their relative rarity. The treating physician should be aware of the associated syndromes and malformations that may, in some cases, be fatal if not recognized and treated appropriately. Although these congenital disorders have a wide variability, their treatment principles are similar in that the physician should promote functional use and cosmesis for the hand. This article discusses syndactyly, preaxial polydactyly and post-axial polydactyly, and the hypoplastic thumb.

Upper Extremity

Recurrent tears after rotator cuff repair are common. Postoperative rehabilitation after rotator cuff repair is a modifiable factor controlled by the surgeon that can affect re-tear rates. Some surgeons prefer early mobilization after rotator cuff repair, whereas others prefer a period of immobilization to protect the repair site. The tendon-healing process incorporates biochemical and biomechanical responses to mechanical loading. Healing can be optimized with controlled loading. Complete load removal and chronic overload can be deleterious to the process. Several randomized clinical studies have also characterized the role of postoperative mobilization after rotator cuff repair.

Posterior shoulder instability in overhead athletes presents a unique and difficult challenge. Often, this group has an inherent capsular laxity and/or humeral retroversion to accommodate the range of motion necessary to throw. This adaptation makes the diagnosis of posterior capsulolabral pathology challenging, as the examiner must differentiate between adaptive capsular laxity and pathologic instability. Further complicating matters, the intraoperative surgeon must find the delicate balance of achieving stability while still allowing the necessary range of motion.

Distal biceps ruptures occur from eccentric loading of a flexed elbow. Patients treated nonoperatively have substantial loss of strength in elbow flexion and forearm supination. Surgical approaches include 1-incision and 2-incision techniques. Advances in surgical technology have facilitated the popularity of single-incision techniques through a small anterior incision. Recently, there is increased focus on the detailed anatomy of the distal biceps insertion and the important of anatomic repair in restoring forearm supination strength. Excellent outcomes are expected with early repair of the distal biceps, with restoration of strength and endurance to near-normal levels with minimal to no loss of motion.

Open fractures of the hand are a common and varied group of injuries. Although at increased risk for infection, open fractures of the hand are more resistant to infection than other open fractures. Numerous unique factors in the hand may play a role in the altered risk of postinjury infection. Current systems for the classification of open fractures fail to address the unique qualities of the hand. This article proposes a novel classification system for open fractures of the hand, taking into account the factors unique to the hand that affect its risk for developing infection after an open fracture.

Oncology

In the surgical management of solid tumors, adequacy of tumor resection has implications for local recurrence and survival. The standard method of intraoperative identification of tumor margin is frozen section pathologic analysis, which is time-consuming with potential for sampling error. Intraoperative tumor visualization has the potential to significantly improve surgical cancer care across disciplines, by guiding accuracy of biopsies, increasing adequacy of resections, directing adjuvant therapy, and even providing diagnostic information. We provide an outline of various methods of intraoperative tumor visualization developed to aid in the real-time assessment of tumor extent and adequacy of resection.

Limb preservation surgery has gained acceptance as a viable alternative to amputation for the treatment of extremity bone tumors in the growing child. There are several options for reconstructing the potential loss of a physis and the defect created by tumor excision. Metallic endoprosthesis, massive allograft, and allograft-prosthesis composites have been described in the skeletally immature population. With the development of expandable prostheses, even those far from skeletal maturity may be candidates for limb salvage. However, improvements in the literature are needed, including reporting surgical and functional outcomes in a rigorous manner, specific to age, anatomic location, and reconstruction.

Osteosarcoma is the most common primary bone malignancy in children. Treatment has evolved to include systemic chemotherapy and local control surgery. Although survival improved initially in a drastic fashion with this approach, recent decades have seen little to no further gains in this area. Limb salvage surgery evolved with effective chemotherapy and advances in imaging, and continues to improve in the recent era. This article serves as a review of survival in high-grade osteosarcoma: prognostic factors, advances in chemotherapy and surgery, late effects of chemotherapy and surgery in survivors, and future directions.

Dedication

Note from the Publisher: On behalf of Elsevier and *Orthopedic Clinics*, I would like to thank Asif M. Ilyas, MD, Shital N. Parikh, MD, Saqib Rehman, MD, Giles R. Scuderi, MD, and Felasfa M. Wodajo, MD for their years of service, dedication, and contributions to the publication. The January 2016 issue of *Orthopedic Clinics* will be the last one under this editorship. We wish them all well in their future endeavors.

Jennifer Flynn-Briggs
Senior Clinics Editor
Orthopedic Clinics

orthopedic.theclinics.com

Adult Reconstruction

Preface

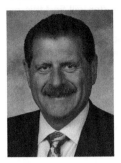

Giles R. Scuderi, MD
Editor

In this issue of *Orthopedic Clinics of North America*, there are several articles that review the complexity and complications associated with joint arthroplasty.

In the first article by Matsen and Parvizi, the authors review the new developments in the diagnosis of periprosthetic infections. The measurement of serum biomarkers, such as ESR and CRP, is routinely used to diagnosis an infection, but these biomarkers are elevated in several common inflammatory conditions. More specific synovial fluid biomarkers include synovial CRP, α-defensin, human β-defensin-2 (HBD-2) and HBD-3, leukocyte esterase, and cathelicidin LL-37. The era of serum and synovial biomarkers is upon us, and these biomarkers hold promise for the diagnosis of periprosthetic infections. The authors comment on the need for further research on developing diagnostic methods targeted to pathogen components and the products of their metabolic activity.

Once a periprosthetic infection is identified, two-stage exchange arthroplasty is the most preferred method of treating chronic periprosthetic infection following total hip arthroplasty; however, Zahar and Gehrke have advocated a protocol-based one-stage exchange arthroplasty. These authors report on their clinical experience and requirements for one-stage exchange arthroplasty. Their results appear promising with outcomes comparable to the two-stage exchange arthroplasty in a select group of patients.

Spinal deformity is commonly associated with arthritis of the hip and may influence the surgical technique and outcome of total hip arthroplasty. Blizzard and coauthors describe a comprehensive preoperative workup and component templating plan for implantation of components. The key to the management of these patients with interrelated pathologies is identification of potential changes in lumbar motion and pelvic alignment, and adjustment of the operative plan to reflect the increased pelvic tilt and increased propensity for impingement even if such adjustments violate the recommended "safe zone" for acetabular component positioning.

With the increasing interest in unicompartmental knee arthroplasty, it is well established that a high degree of accuracy of implant positioning and soft tissue balance is required to optimize durability and implant survivorship. Lonner reviews the latest generation robotic technology with an image-free hand-held robotic sculpting tool, which offers an alternative method for optimizing implant positioning and soft tissue balance without the need for advanced preoperative imaging.

Accuracy of component position is also important in total knee arthroplasty. Malrotation of femoral and tibial components is associated with poor functional outcomes. Nedopil and coauthors report on their experience with kinematic alignment versus mechanical alignment in posterior cruciate retaining total knee arthroplasty. Their kinematic aligned surgical technique demonstrated a wide range of tibial component rotational position, despite reportedly good functional results, which may be attributable to the relatively flat tibial

Orthop Clin N Am 47 (2016) xix–xx
http://dx.doi.org/10.1016/j.ocl.2015.10.004
0030-5898/16/$ – see front matter © 2016 Published by Elsevier Inc.

articular surface of the posterior cruciate retaining total knee design utilized by the authors.

In the final article in this section, Tripathi and co-authors report on their experience with con-strained total knee arthroplasty in obese patients. Total knee arthroplasty in the obese patient is associated with a greater number of preoperative comorbidities, more perioperative complications, and a shorter longevity than the patient with a normal body mass index. The authors report that the constrained total knee prosthesis in obese patients facilitates the operative procedure by improving the intramedullary alignment of the prosthesis and supporting the surrounding soft tissues. The clinical results were similar to a poste-rior stabilized prosthesis in the nonobese patient.

It is anticipated that the reader will find this ar-throplasty section of *Orthopedic Clinics of North America* to be insightful and to have an impact on the management of patients undergoing total knee and hip arthroplasty.

Giles R. Scuderi, MD
210 East 64th Street
New York, NY 10065, USA

E-mail address:
gscuderi@nshs.edu

Diagnosis of Periprosthetic Infection
Novel Developments

Laura Matsen Ko, MD[a],*, Javad Parvizi, MD, FRCS[b]

KEYWORDS

- Diagnosis • Periprosthetic joint infection • Serum markers • Synovial fluid markers
- Total joint arthroplasty

KEY POINTS

- Erythrocyte sedimentation rate and C-reactive protein (CRP) serum levels are elevated in multiple inflammatory conditions and, therefore, more specific biomarkers are required to diagnose periprosthetic joint infection (PJI).
- Serum biomarkers such as procalcitonin, interleukin (IL)-6, tumor necrosis factor (TNF)-α, short-chain exocellular lipoteichoic acid, soluble intercellular adhesion molecule-1, and monocyte chemoattractant protein–1 may be more specific to PJI.
- Synovial fluid biomarkers elevated in PJI include cytokines such as IL-1β, IL-6, IL-8, IL-17, TNF-α, interferon-δ, and vascular endothelial growth factor.
- More specific synovial fluid biomarkers include synovial CRP, α-defensin, human β-defensin (HBD)-2 and HBD-3, leukocyte esterase, and cathelicidin LL-37.

INTRODUCTION

Periprosthetic joint infection (PJI) is a devastating complication seen in total joint arthroplasty (TJA) patients. Traditionally, the serologic diagnosis of PJI was performed by measuring inflammatory factors of white blood cell (WBC) levels, erythrocyte sedimentation rate (ESR), and C-reactive protein (CRP). Microbiologic analysis of synovial fluid and periprosthetic tissue has also been performed using histology and synovial fluid culture, which may not be highly sensitive for detecting PJI. Modern use of novel molecular methods of diagnosis, along with the use of serum and synovial fluid biomarkers, may improve the diagnosis of PJI and provide markers that may be used to monitor the resolution of joint infection.

HISTORY AND PHYSICAL EXAMINATION

The first step for evaluating a patient with a possible PJI is to perform a thorough history and physical examination. The patient should be asked about a prior PJI because this has been shown to increase the risk of repeat PJI.[1,2] The postoperative course should be questioned for postoperative drainage, need for superficial washouts, or prolonged postoperative antibiotics. At

Disclosures: Nothing to disclose (L.M. Ko); Biomet; Covidien; National Institutes of Health (National Institute of Arthritis and Musculoskeletal and Skin Diseases [NIAMS] and National Institute of Child Health and Human Development [NICHD]); Salient Surgical; Smith & Nephew; Stryker; TissueGene; Zimmer; 3M; Musculoskeletal Transplant Foundation; Saunders/Mosby-Elsevier; SLACK Incorporated; Wolters Kluwer Health - Lippincott Williams & Wilkins; CD Diagnostics; SmartTech; United Healthcare (J. Parvizi).

[a] Rothman Institute, Thomas Jefferson University, 4703 33rd Avenue Northeast, Seattle, WA 98105, USA;
[b] Sidney Kimmel School of Medicine, Rothman Institute, Thomas Jefferson University, Sheridan Building, Suite 1000, 125 South 9th Street, Philadelphia, PA 19107, USA
* Corresponding author.
E-mail address: lauramatsenko@gmail.com

Orthop Clin N Am 47 (2016) 1–9
http://dx.doi.org/10.1016/j.ocl.2015.08.003
0030-5898/16/$ – see front matter © 2016 Elsevier Inc. All rights reserved.

orthopedic.theclinics.com

presentation, patients with PJI may report a history of fevers, chills, pain, and loss of function, including loss of range of motion and pain with ambulation.

On physical examination, the patient should be observed for signs of illness. The vital signs should be measured, including temperature, pulse, blood pressure, and respiration rate. Inspection of the joint is critical because erythema or drainage at the incision site, and swelling and warmth of the affected joint, may indicate a PJI. According to the Musculoskeletal Infection Society PJI criteria, the presence of a sinus tract from the surface of the skin to the implant is diagnostic of a PJI.[3] Thus, the diagnosis of PJI may be made on physical examination alone.

SEROLOGY: ERYTHROCYTE SEDIMENTATION RATE AND C-REACTIVE PROTEIN

The diagnosis of PJI still poses a significant challenge and there is no consensus on the most appropriate gold standard tests to diagnose PJI. Due to the ease and low-risk nature of blood draw, serum markers are an attractive diagnostic tool for PJI. However, serum markers are all subject to confounding comorbidities, such as systemic inflammation or other infections. When studies demonstrating the success of serum markers are carefully read,[4] it is almost invariably found that the study has excluded subjects with inflammatory comorbidities and subjects on antibiotics. When this confounded population is included,[5] the utility of serum biomarkers is found to decline. Inflammatory markers may be elevated in obesity.[6–8] The timing of infection must also be taken into account because ESR and CRP are routinely elevated in the postoperative period. ESR is elevated up to 6 weeks after surgery and CRP is elevated up to 2 weeks after surgery. If these laboratory test values are elevated postoperatively, they may not be reliable criteria for diagnosing infection. ESR and CRP levels should be measured in joint arthroplasty patients who present with pain; preoperative screening can point to the presence of infection.[9] The clinician must carefully consider whether the use of serum biomarkers will provide a reliable diagnosis in the patient being tested. To date, none of the serum biomarker tests have been developed and optimized specifically to detect PJI.

An ESR greater than 30 mm/hr or a CRP greater than 10 mg/L should raise the suspicion of PJI. Both the American Academy of Orthopaedic Surgeons (AAOS) and the recent International Consensus on Periprosthetic Joint Infection[10,11] recommend performing a joint aspirate for cell count, differential, and culture in the setting of elevated serology.

Of note, serum WBC may not be a reliable test for the diagnosis of infection because it has a low sensitivity (55%) and specificity (66%) for diagnosing PJI. Also, the test may not add to the synovial WBC test.[12,13]

If the ESR and CRP are not elevated, and the clinician has no suspicion of PJI, then a joint aspirate may be unnecessary. However, it must be kept in mind that PJI can exist in the setting of normal serology, especially with organisms such as *Propionibacterium acnes*, coagulase-negative *Staphylococcus*, *Candida*, *Corynebacterium*, *Mycobacterium*, and *Actinomyces* (**Box 1**).[14] **Fig. 1** provides an algorithm for diagnosing PJI using history, physical examination, serologic testing, and synovial fluid analysis.

Box 1
Seronegative infections

- Coagulase negative *Staphylococcus*
- *Candida*
- *Corynebacterium*
- *Mycobacterium*
- *Actinomyces*
- *Propionibacterium acnes*

Data from McArthur BA, Abdel MP, Taunton MJ, et al. Seronegative infections in hip and knee arthroplasty: periprosthetic infections with normal erythrocyte sedimentation rate and C-reactive protein level. Bone Joint J 2015;97-B(7):939–44.

SEROLOGY: BEYOND ERYTHROCYTE SEDIMENTATION RATE AND C-REACTIVE PROTEIN

There has been recent research evaluating other serum markers that can be used in the diagnosis of PJI. Procalcitonin (PCT) is a serum marker that is elevated in the presence of stimuli, such as bacteria, that are proinflammatory. Bottner and colleagues[5] measured serum levels of interleukin (IL)-6, PCT, tumor necrosis factor (TNF)-α, CRP, and ESR in 78 subjects undergoing revision total knee or hip replacement for PJI. CRP and IL-6 had the highest sensitivity (95%) for detecting PJI when the levels were higher than 3.2 mg/dL and 12 pg/mL, respectively, and the investigators recommended combining CRP and IL-6 as a screening test. PCT levels (>0.3 ng/mL) were very specific (98%) but had a low sensitivity (33%). On the other hand, Hügle and colleagues[15]

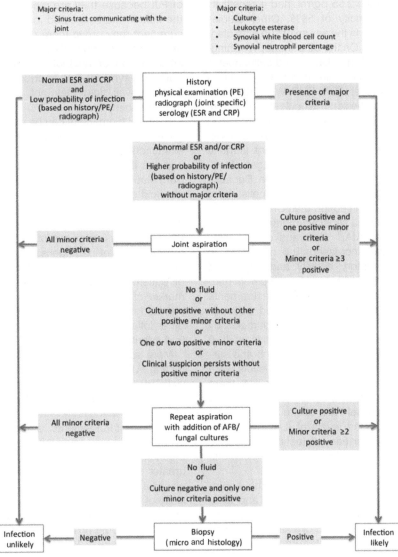

Major criteria:
- Sinus tract communicating with the joint

Major criteria:
- Culture
- Leukocyte esterase
- Synovial white blood cell count
- Synovial neutrophil percentage

Normal ESR and CRP and Low probability of infection (based on history/PE/radiograph)

History physical examination (PE) radiograph (joint specific) serology (ESR and CRP)

Presence of major criteria

Abnormal ESR and/or CRP or Higher probability of infection (based on history/PE/radiograph) without major criteria

Culture positive and one positive minor criteria or Minor criteria ≥3 positive

All minor criteria negative

Joint aspiration

No fluid or Culture positive without other positive minor criteria or One or two positive minor criteria or Clinical suspicion persists without positive minor criteria

Culture positive or Minor criteria ≥2 positive

All minor criteria negative

Repeat aspiration with addition of AFB/fungal cultures

No fluid or Culture negative and only one minor criteria positive

Infection unlikely   Negative   Biopsy (micro and histology)   Positive   Infection likely

Fig. 1. Algorithm for diagnosing PJI using history, physical examination, serologic testing of ESR and C-reactive protein, and synovial fluid analysis. AFB, acid-fast bacilli. (*From* Parvizi CJ, Gehrke T. Proceedings of the International Consensus Meeting on Periprosthetic Joint Infection. Brooklandville (MD): Data Trace Publishing Company; 2013. p. 160; with permission.)

reported that PCT had a higher sensitivity and specificity for diagnosing septic arthritis than CRP, with a sensitivity of 93% and specificity of 75% at a PCT cutoff of 0.25 ng/mL. Theoretically, this is possible because PCT is secreted by the mononuclear phagocyte system when stimulated by lipopolysaccharide. Based on these studies, PCT may be useful for distinguishing between bacterial infections of the joint and other causes of inflammation. Using this marker may also help determine whether an antimicrobial therapy might be effective that could reduce the duration of medication and minimize antimicrobial resistance.

Glehr and colleagues[16] compared PCT, IL-6, and interferon (IFN)-α as serum biomarkers to WBC and CRP levels for diagnosing PJI in revision arthroplasty patients. Blood samples were taken preoperatively and on the first, third, and seventh postoperative days. The results demonstrated that PCT, IL-6, CRP, and WBC correlated with the diagnosis of PJI, although IFN-α did not. IFN-α has an important role in antiviral immunity but not in antimicrobial immunity[17] and may not be detected in bacterial infections. In serum measurements, PCT greater than 0.35 ng/mL had a sensitivity of 80% and specificity of 37%, whereas the IL-6 greater than 2.55 pg/mL had a sensitivity of 92% and specificity of 59%. Other studies found similar results in the serum of subjects diagnosed with PJI.[18–21] On the other hand, Worthington and colleagues[22] and Drago and colleagues[23] found that PCT was not elevated in the serum of PJI subjects. However, ESR, CRP, WBC, IL-6, soluble intercellular adhesion molecule-1, and serum IgG to short-chain exocellular lipoteichoic acid were all elevated in subjects with septic loosening.[22,23] IL-6 is secreted by different immune cells, such as monocytes, macrophages, fibroblasts, and T2 lymphocytes after trauma. Because IL-6 triggers the release of CRP in liver cells, it can react much faster to infection than CRP[24] and has been reported to be a sensitive marker for bacterial infection after TJA.[5] Wirtz and colleagues[25] demonstrated that increased IL-6 correlates to increased inflammatory activity and suggested that IL-6 is a better indicator of postoperative inflammatory response than CRP measurements after TJA. This finding is confounded because monocytes respond to polyethylene particles by secreting IL-6, and high concentrations of IL-6 have been found in the interface membrane surrounding loose implants. Even if IL-6 levels were increased in the peripheral blood after TJA, there have been no clinical studies conducted that show a correlation between failure of an aseptic implant and increased levels of IL-6. Therefore, IL-6 maybe useful for early detection of a septic process and for monitoring success of antibiotic therapy.

Shah and colleagues[26] measured the serum levels of 25 different cytokines before and after TJA and identified cytokines associated with surgical trauma. Three of the 25 cytokines, including IL-6, monocyte chemoattractant protein (MCP)-1, and IL-2R, were associated with postsurgical trauma, which included 1 deep infection. The changes in IL-6 and MCP-1 seem to reflect increased inflammation in the subject with deep infection, and the levels of IL-2R in the same subject were lower than average but not markedly decreased. The investigators suggested that the combination of increased IL-6 at 6 hours and reduced levels of MCP-1 at 48 hours may be associated with infection.

SYNOVIAL FLUID MARKERS

In addition to serum biomarkers, synovial fluid biomarkers may aid in the diagnosis of PJI. To date, only the α-defensin test has been specifically optimized and made commercially available for the diagnosis of PJI.[27] Using these biomarkers may be beneficial for the diagnosis of PJI because they are measured directly from the fluid in the suspected joint. This direct measurement may prove more reliable in the setting of patients with comorbidities, such as systemic inflammation or antibiotic treatment. However, obtaining synovial fluid is an invasive procedure and synovial fluid may not always be drawn from the joint.

Synovial biomarkers can be divided into 2 categories: cytokines and biomarkers with antimicrobial functions.[28] At the site of infection, cytokines such as IL-1β, IL-6, IL-8, and IL-17 are released from macrophages and are increased in the synovial fluid of patients with diagnosed PJI.[29] Similar to serum biomarkers, TNF-α is elevated in synovial fluid.[30] IFN-δ is another cytokine that is elevated in PJI because it is a glycoprotein that is released in the presence of pathogens. Vascular endothelial growth factor is also increased in the synovial fluid of patients diagnosed with PJI because it is a marker of angiogenesis.[31] These markers are all elevated in synovial fluid but are also elevated in other inflammatory conditions, such as rheumatoid arthritis and vasculitis.

More specific synovial fluid biomarkers for detecting PJI have been evaluated, including synovial CRP, α-defensin, human β-defensin (HBD)-2, HBD-3, leukocyte esterase (LE), and cathelicidin LL-37. CRP, which is elevated in the serum and synovial fluid of PJI patients, is a liver protein that is synthesized during acute inflammation when there are increased macrophages.[32] Synovial fluid CRP greater than 9.5 mg/L in septic revision cases was found to have a sensitivity of 85% and a specificity of 95%, with an area under the curve (AUC) of 0.92.[33] Although this may be a valuable diagnostic test, some hospital laboratories are unwilling to measure CRP levels in synovial fluid because machines may only be calibrated for serum CRP.

α-Defensin is another synovial fluid biomarker for diagnosing PJI that has higher sensitivity and specificity than synovial fluid CRP. An α-defensin test has recently been developed and commercialized specifically for the purpose of diagnosing PJI. α-Defensins are released from neutrophils in the presence of bacteria. It has been shown that an α-defensin level greater than 5.2 μg/ml has been found to have a sensitivity of 97% and a specificity of 96%.[34] The diagnostic accuracy of α-defensin was demonstrated in a subject population that included those with systemic inflammatory diseases and antibiotic treatment. HBD-2 and HBD-3 are similar to α-defensin because they are secreted by neutrophils in inflammatory conditions and are active against gram-negative organisms and Candida. Synovial fluid HBD-3 was elevated in aspirates of PJI subjects with PJI with an AUC of 0.745.[30]

LE is another biomarker that is elevated in the urine of patients with urinary tract infections and has been diagnosed by the dipstick technique. Although the LE test was developed as a leukocyte count estimation for use in urinalysis, some investigators have reported its off-label use on synovial fluid. LE is specifically found in neutrophils and is measured in synovial fluid by lysis of neutrophils and measuring all intracellular and extracellular esterase activity, which could provide an estimation of the synovial fluid WBC count. This inexpensive and rapid test has 93.3% sensitivity and 77.0% specificity for diagnosing PJI when compared with microbiology culture.[35] This test must only be conducted on nonbloody synovial fluid because the presence of blood can interfere with the colorimetric change on the dipstick seen in this test.[36]

Human host defense peptide LL-37 is a member of the cathelicidin family and is an antimicrobial protein peptide that induces immune mediators such as IL-8, prevents the formation of biofilm, and regulates the inflammatory response.[37,38] Gollwitzer and colleagues[30] determined that LL-37 was elevated in the synovial fluid of PJI subjects and had a sensitivity of 80% and specificity of 85% for the diagnosis of PJI, with an AUC of 0.875.

SYNOVIAL CULTURE

If there is any clinical suspicion of PJI, a synovial fluid aspiration and culture should be considered. Although some clinicians may think that the culture result is diagnostic for PJI, many studies have demonstrated the failure of culture to provide for an accurate diagnosis.[39–41] There may be poor sensitivity of detection due to recent antibiotic use and less virulent organisms may not be detected by routine microbiology culture methods. When a low virulence microbial infection is suspected due to clinical symptoms, and preoperative culture demonstrate no bacterial growth, the incubation time of the culture sample should be extended to 14 days or more.[42] Sonication of explants can be performed in patients with suspected or confirmed PJI, with culture-negative results, or in patients treated with antibiotics before their operation. Sonication of hip, knee, and shoulder explants has been shown to not increase the contaminant rate and have increased the positive rate of pathogen detection.[43–49] If patients have suspected PJI, acid-fast bacilli and fungal cultures should be limited to patients who do not have pathogens detected by traditional culture methods. A single positive culture could be a false-positive result.[50–52] The diagnosis of PJI must be fully considered in conjunction with other diagnostic tests (see **Fig. 1**).

HISTOLOGY

Histologic analysis of tissue biopsies may be performed in parallel with culture analysis of tissue obtained during surgery for the diagnosis of PJI. Infections can be qualified as acute, chronic, or not present. The expression of infection in different tissue specimens of the same patient is sometimes very different, necessitating biopsies of a minimum of 3 different sites.[53] According to the AAOS clinical practice guidelines for diagnosing PJI,[9] frozen sections of peri-implant tissues have not been established or excluded in patients undergoing reoperation for the diagnosis of PJI. If using frozen section for the diagnosis of PJI, the number of neutrophils should be counted in a high-magnification microscopic field (400×), and the diagnosis PJI should be obtained by looking for 10 or more neutrophils in 5 high-power fields (HPFs). Intraoperative frozen sections may be beneficial for the diagnosis of inflammatory arthropathy and may also help distinguish aseptic loosening from PJI.

Although the AAOS published these guidelines for intraoperative frozen, there are still many investigators who question the standard of using intraoperative frozen section to diagnose PJI.[54,55] Tsaras and colleagues[56] conducted a meta-analysis evaluating the role of intraoperative frozen section histopathology in the diagnosis of PJI. They collected 26 studies involving 3269 subjects undergoing revision hip or knee arthroplasty. They demonstrated that the pooled diagnostic odds ratio (OR) was 54.7 (95% confidence interval [CI] 31.2–95.7), the likelihood ratio of a positive test was 12.0 (95% CI 8.4–17.2), and the likelihood ratio of a negative test was 0.23 (95% CI 0.15–0.35). They used the diagnostic criteria chosen by the investigating pathologist, including 5 or 10 polymorphonuclear leukocytes (PMNs) per HPF. Then, they analyzed 15 articles that adopted diagnostic criteria that used a threshold of 5 PMNs per HPF to define a positive frozen section in all 26 articles, whereas the other 6 studies used a diagnostic threshold of 10 PMNs per high-powered field. The results showed that 5 PMNs per HPF had a diagnostic OR of 52.6 (95% CI 23.7–116.2) and 10 PMN per HPF had a diagnostic OR of 69.8 (95% CI 33.6–145.0) for the diagnosis of PJI. They concluded that intraoperative frozen sections of periprosthetic tissues could perform well for diagnosing PJI; however, this only had moderate accuracy for ruling out the diagnosis. If a thorough preoperative evaluation is performed, frozen section histopathology at the time of surgery should be considered a valuable part of the diagnostic work-up for patients undergoing revision.

In most cases, a total of 23 PMNs per 10 HPF is thought to be a common criteria to diagnosis PJI.[57] Surface fibrin with neutrophils have no use in the diagnosis of PJI. The sample should not be removed by electrocautery but should be sharply dissected to avoid thermal damage to the sample.

MOLECULAR METHODS OF DIAGNOSIS

In recent years, molecular diagnostics have improved the process of clinical microbial identification. Now, advances in molecular diagnostic methodology are gradually improving protein and nucleic acid diagnostic accuracy. Highly sensitive molecular techniques may assist in identifying pathogens in the setting of culture negative infection. These techniques include the polymerase chain reaction (PCR) or matrix-assisted laser desorption/ionization time-of-flight mass spectrometry (MALDI-TOF MS) techniques.[45,58–67] The sensitivity of PCR ranges from 64% to 100%[61,62] and the specificity ranges between 0% and 100%.[58,61–64,68] The advantage of molecular techniques is that they do not require growth of the organism for detection.[45,65]

MALDI-TOF MS is a technique that performs soft laser ionization of intact bacteria and on the bacterial extract. It determines the molecular structure based on analyzing the mass differences between the fragmented ions of the parent molecule in the mass spectrum. Harris and colleagues[69] reported that they succeeded using MALDI-TOF MS to identify 158 characterized *Staphylococcal* isolates from the culture broth of PJIs using dedicated software.

Molecular techniques have also shown some promise in identifying genes associated with antibiotic resistance.[47,58,70] Although these genes have not reached clinical applicability for testing for antibiotic susceptibility, this is a potential future method of diagnosing PJI. For now, the cost and availability of this technology is limited. However, it may have broader applications in the future and may radically change the process of clinical microbial identification of PJI.

SUMMARY AND DISCUSSION

Serum and synovial biomarkers are more sensitive and specific methods for diagnosing PJI. Older methods, such as ESR and CRP serology, along with microbiology analysis using histology and culture, may become eclipsed by newer biomarker and molecular diagnostic methods. Future research should be focused on developing diagnostic methods targeted to pathogen components and the products of their metabolic activity, as well as to the human body's reaction to these microbiological agents.

REFERENCES

1. Jafari SM, Casper DS, Restrepo C, et al. Periprosthetic joint infection: are patients with multiple prosthetic joints at risk? J Arthroplasty 2012; 27(6):877–80.
2. Bedair H, Goyal N, Dietz MJ, et al. A history of treated periprosthetic joint infection increases the risk of subsequent different site infection. Clin Orthop Relat Res 2015;473(7):2300–4.
3. Parvizi J, Zmistowski B, Berbari EF, et al. New definition for periprosthetic joint infection: from the Workgroup of the Musculoskeletal Infection Society. Clin Orthop Relat Res 2011;469(11):2992–4.
4. Di Cesare PE, Chang E, Preston CF, et al. Serum interleukin-6 as a marker of periprosthetic infection following total hip and knee arthroplasty. J Bone Joint Surg Am 2005;87(9):1921–7.
5. Bottner F, Wegner A, Winkelmann W, et al. Interleukin-6, procalcitonin and TNF-alpha: markers of peri-prosthetic infection following total joint replacement. J Bone Joint Surg Br 2007;89(1):94–9.
6. Lee YH, Pratley RE. The evolving role of inflammation in obesity and the metabolic syndrome. Curr Diab Rep 2005;5(1):70–5.
7. Natali A, L'Abbate A, Ferrannini E. Erythrocyte sedimentation rate, coronary atherosclerosis, and cardiac mortality. Eur Heart J 2003;24(7):639–48.
8. Liu JZ, Saleh A, Klika AK, et al. Serum inflammatory markers for periprosthetic knee infection in obese versus non-obese patients. J Arthroplasty 2014; 29(10):1880–3.
9. Parvizi J, Della Valle CJ. AAOS clinical practice guideline: diagnosis and treatment of periprosthetic joint infections of the hip and knee. J Am Acad Orthop Surg 2010;18(12):771–2.
10. Cats-Baril W, Gehrke T, Huff K, et al. International consensus on periprosthetic joint infection: description of the consensus process. Clin Orthop Relat Res 2013;471(12):4065–75.
11. Parvizi J, Gehrke T, Chen AF. Proceedings of the International Consensus on Periprosthetic Joint Infection. Bone Joint J 2013;95-B(11):1450–2.
12. Toossi N, Adeli B, Rasouli MR, et al. Serum white blood cell count and differential do not have a role in the diagnosis of periprosthetic joint infection. J Arthroplasty 2012;27(8 Suppl):51–4.e1.
13. Zmistowski B, Restrepo C, Huang R, et al. Periprosthetic joint infection diagnosis: a complete

understanding of white blood cell count and differential. J Arthroplasty 2012;27(9):1589–93.

14. McArthur BA, Abdel MP, Taunton MJ, et al. Seronegative infections in hip and knee arthroplasty: periprosthetic infections with normal erythrocyte sedimentation rate and C-reactive protein level. Bone Joint J 2015;97-B(7):939–44.

15. Hügle T, Schuetz P, Mueller B, et al. Serum procalcitonin for discrimination between septic and nonseptic arthritis. Clin Exp Rheumatol 2008;26(3): 453–6.

16. Glehr M, Friesenbichler J, Hofmann G, et al. Novel biomarkers to detect infection in revision hip and knee arthroplasties. Clin Orthop Relat Res 2013; 471(8):2621–8.

17. Anders HJ, Lichtnekert J, Allam R. Interferon-alpha and -beta in kidney inflammation. Kidney Int 2010; 77(10):848–54.

18. Assicot M, Gendrel D, Carsin H, et al. High serum procalcitonin concentrations in patients with sepsis and infection. Lancet 1993;341(8844):515–8.

19. Carrol ED, Thomson AP, Hart CA. Procalcitonin as a marker of sepsis. Int J Antimicrob Agents 2002; 20(1):1–9.

20. Fottner A, Birkenmaier C, von Schulze Pellengahr C, et al. Can serum procalcitonin help to differentiate between septic and nonseptic arthritis? Arthroscopy 2008;24(2):229–33.

21. Gendrel D, Raymond J, Assicot M, et al. Measurement of procalcitonin levels in children with bacterial or viral meningitis. Clin Infect Dis 1997;24(6): 1240–2.

22. Worthington T, Dunlop D, Casey A, et al. Serum procalcitonin, interleukin-6, soluble intercellular adhesin molecule-1 and IgG to short-chain exocellular lipoteichoic acid as predictors of infection in total joint prosthesis revision. Br J Biomed Sci 2010;67(2): 71–6.

23. Drago L, Vassena C, Dozio E, et al. Procalcitonin, C-reactive protein, interleukin-6, and soluble intercellular adhesion molecule-1 as markers of postoperative orthopaedic joint prosthesis infections. Int J Immunopathol Pharmacol 2011;24(2):433–40.

24. Selberg O, Hecker H, Martin M, et al. Discrimination of sepsis and systemic inflammatory response syndrome by determination of circulating plasma concentrations of procalcitonin, protein complement 3a, and interleukin-6. Crit Care Med 2000;28(8): 2793–8.

25. Wirtz DC, Heller KD, Miltner O, et al. Interleukin-6: a potential inflammatory marker after total joint replacement. Int Orthop 2000;24(4):194–6.

26. Shah K, Mohammed A, Patil S, et al. Circulating cytokines after hip and knee arthroplasty: a preliminary study. Clin Orthop Relat Res 2009;467(4):946–51.

27. Deirmengian C, Kardos K, Kilmartin P, et al. The Alpha-defensin Test for Periprosthetic Joint Infection Responds to a Wide Spectrum of Organisms. Clin Orthop Relat Res 2015;473(7):2229–35.

28. Deirmengian C, Lonner JH, Booth RE Jr. The Mark Coventry Award: white blood cell gene expression: a new approach toward the study and diagnosis of infection. Clin Orthop Relat Res 2005;440:38–44.

29. Deirmengian C, Hallab N, Tarabishy A, et al. Synovial fluid biomarkers for periprosthetic infection. Clin Orthop Relat Res 2010;468(8):2017–23.

30. Gollwitzer H, Dombrowski Y, Prodinger PM, et al. Antimicrobial peptides and proinflammatory cytokines in periprosthetic joint infection. J Bone Joint Surg Am 2013;95(7):644–51.

31. Jacovides CL, Parvizi J, Adeli B, et al. Molecular markers for diagnosis of periprosthetic joint infection. J Arthroplasty 2011;26(6 Suppl):99–103.e1.

32. Parvizi J, Jacovides C, Adeli B, et al. Mark B. Coventry Award: synovial C-reactive protein: a prospective evaluation of a molecular marker for periprosthetic knee joint infection. Clin Orthop Relat Res 2012;470(1):54–60.

33. Parvizi J, McKenzie JC, Cashman JP. Diagnosis of periprosthetic joint infection using synovial C-reactive protein. J Arthroplasty 2012;27(8 Suppl):12–6.

34. Deirmengian C. Diagnosing PJI: the era of the biomarker has arrived. Philadelphia: Musculoskeletal Infection Society; 2013.

35. Koyonos L, Zmistowski B, Della Valle CJ, et al. Infection control rate of irrigation and debridement for periprosthetic joint infection. Clin Orthop Relat Res 2011;469(11):3043–8.

36. Wetters NG, Berend KR, Lombardi AV, et al. Leukocyte esterase reagent strips for the rapid diagnosis of periprosthetic joint infection. J Arthroplasty 2012;27(8 Suppl):8–11.

37. Overhage J, Campisano A, Bains M, et al. Human host defense peptide LL-37 prevents bacterial biofilm formation. Infect Immun 2008;76(9):4176–82.

38. Nijnik A, Hancock RE. The roles of cathelicidin LL-37 in immune defences and novel clinical applications. Curr Opin Hematol 2009;16(1):41–7.

39. Ali F, Wilkinson JM, Cooper JR, et al. Accuracy of joint aspiration for the preoperative diagnosis of infection in total hip arthroplasty. J Arthroplasty 2006;21(2):221–6.

40. Spangehl MJ, Masri BA, O'Connell JX, et al. Prospective analysis of preoperative and intraoperative investigations for the diagnosis of infection at the sites of two hundred and two revision total hip arthroplasties. J Bone Joint Surg Am 1999;81(5): 672–83.

41. Tigges S, Stiles RG, Meli RJ, et al. Hip aspiration: a cost-effective and accurate method of evaluating the potentially infected hip prosthesis. Radiology 1993;189(2):485–8.

42. Schafer P, Fink B, Sandow D, et al. Prolonged bacterial culture to identify late periprosthetic joint

infection: a promising strategy. Clin Infect Dis 2008; 47(11):1403–9.

43. Trampuz A, Fink B, Sandow D, et al. Sonication of explanted prosthetic components in bags for diagnosis of prosthetic joint infection is associated with risk of contamination. J Clin Microbiol 2006;44(2): 628–31.

44. Trampuz A, Piper KE, Jacobson MJ, et al. Sonication of removed hip and knee prostheses for diagnosis of infection. N Engl J Med 2007; 357(7):654–63.

45. Achermann Y, Vogt M, Leunig M, et al. Improved diagnosis of periprosthetic joint infection by multiplex PCR of sonication fluid from removed implants. J Clin Microbiol 2010;48(4):1208–14.

46. Bjerkan G, Witso E, Bergh K. Sonication is superior to scraping for retrieval of bacteria in biofilm on titanium and steel surfaces in vitro. Acta Orthop 2009; 80(2):245–50.

47. Kobayashi H, Oethinger M, Tuohy MJ, et al. Improving clinical significance of PCR: use of propidium monoazide to distinguish viable from dead Staphylococcus aureus and Staphylococcus epidermidis. J Orthop Res 2009;27(9):1243–7.

48. Monsen T, Lövgren E, Widerström M, et al. In vitro effect of ultrasound on bacteria and suggested protocol for sonication and diagnosis of prosthetic infections. J Clin Microbiol 2009;47(8):2496–501.

49. Piper KE, Jacobson MJ, Cofield RH, et al. Microbiologic diagnosis of prosthetic shoulder infection by use of implant sonication. J Clin Microbiol 2009; 47(6):1878–84.

50. Atkins BL, Athanasou N, Deeks JJ, et al. Prospective evaluation of criteria for microbiological diagnosis of prosthetic-joint infection at revision arthroplasty. The OSIRIS Collaborative Study Group. J Clin Microbiol 1998;36(10):2932–9.

51. Mikkelsen DB, Pedersen C, Højbjerg T, et al. Culture of multiple peroperative biopsies and diagnosis of infected knee arthroplasties. APMIS 2006;114(6): 449–52.

52. Muller M, Morawietz L, Hasart O, et al. Diagnosis of periprosthetic infection following total hip arthroplasty—evaluation of the diagnostic values of pre- and intraoperative parameters and the associated strategy to preoperatively select patients with a high probability of joint infection. J Orthop Surg Res 2008;3:31.

53. Pace TB, Jeray KJ, Latham JT Jr. Synovial tissue examination by frozen section as an indicator of infection in hip and knee arthroplasty in community hospitals. J Arthroplasty 1997;12(1):64–9.

54. Fehring TK, McAlister JA Jr. Frozen histologic section as a guide to sepsis in revision joint arthroplasty. Clin Orthop Relat Res 1994;(304):229–37.

55. Ko PS, Ip D, Chow KP, et al. The role of intraoperative frozen section in decision making in revision

hip and knee arthroplasties in a local community hospital. J Arthroplasty 2005;20(2):189–95.

56. Tsaras G, Maduka-Ezeh A, Inwards CY, et al. Utility of intraoperative frozen section histopathology in the diagnosis of periprosthetic joint infection: a systematic review and meta-analysis. J Bone Joint Surg Am 2012;94(18):1700–11.

57. Morawietz L, Tiddens O, Mueller M, et al. Twenty-three neutrophil granulocytes in 10 high-power fields is the best histopathological threshold to differentiate between aseptic and septic endoprosthesis loosening. Histopathology 2009;54(7):847–53.

58. Jacovides CL, Kreft R, Adeli B, et al. Successful identification of pathogens by polymerase chain reaction (PCR)-based electron spray ionization time-of-flight mass spectrometry (ESI-TOF-MS) in culture-negative periprosthetic joint infection. J Bone Joint Surg Am 2012;94(24):2247–54.

59. Clarke MT, Roberts CP, Lee PT, et al. Polymerase chain reaction can detect bacterial DNA in aseptically loose total hip arthroplasties. Clin Orthop Relat Res 2004;(427):132–7.

60. Esteban J, Alonso-Rodriguez N, del-Prado G, et al. PCR-hybridization after sonication improves diagnosis of implant-related infection. Acta Orthop 2012;83(3):299–304.

61. Gallo J, Kolar M, Dendis M, et al. Culture and PCR analysis of joint fluid in the diagnosis of prosthetic joint infection. New Microbiol 2008;31(1):97–104.

62. Gomez E, Cazanave C, Cunningham SA, et al. Prosthetic joint infection diagnosis using broad-range PCR of biofilms dislodged from knee and hip arthroplasty surfaces using sonication. J Clin Microbiol 2012;50(11):3501–8.

63. Mariani BD, Martin DS, Levine MJ, et al. The Coventry Award. Polymerase chain reaction detection of bacterial infection in total knee arthroplasty. Clin Orthop Relat Res 1996;(331):11–22.

64. Panousis K, Grigoris P, Butcher I, et al. Poor predictive value of broad-range PCR for the detection of arthroplasty infection in 92 cases. Acta Orthop 2005; 76(3):341–6.

65. Rak M, Barlič-Maganja D, Kavčič M, et al. Comparison of molecular and culture method in diagnosis of prosthetic joint infection. FEMS Microbiol Lett 2013;343(1):42–8.

66. Rasouli MR, Harandi AA, Adeli B, et al. Revision total knee arthroplasty: infection should be ruled out in all cases. J Arthroplasty 2012;27(6):1239–43.e1-2.

67. Tunney MM, Patrick S, Curran MD, et al. Detection of prosthetic hip infection at revision arthroplasty by immunofluorescence microscopy and PCR amplification of the bacterial 16S rRNA gene. J Clin Microbiol 1999;37(10):3281–90.

68. Portillo ME, Salvadó M, Sorli L, et al. Multiplex PCR of sonication fluid accurately differentiates between

prosthetic joint infection and aseptic failure. J Infect 2012;65(6):541–8.

69. Harris LG, El-Bouri K, Johnston S, et al. Rapid identification of staphylococci from prosthetic joint infections using MALDI-TOF mass-spectrometry. Int J Artif Organs 2010;33(9):568–74.

70. Kobayashi N, Inaba Y, Choe H, et al. Simultaneous intraoperative detection of methicillin-resistant Staphylococcus and pan-bacterial infection during revision surgery: use of simple DNA release by ultra-sonication and real-time polymerase chain reaction. J Bone Joint Surg Am 2009;91(12):2896–902.

One-Stage Revision for Infected Total Hip Arthroplasty

Akos Zahar, MD*, Thorsten A. Gehrke, MD

KEYWORDS

- Prosthetic joint infection (PJI) • One-stage septic exchange • Complication of total hip arthroplasty
- Cemented revision • Posterior approach

KEY POINTS

- The preoperative protocol of diagnostics includes joint aspiration and blood tests.
- The causative organisms and known susceptibility must be identified.
- All foreign material requires radical debridement and removal.
- Targeted antibiotic therapy is required both locally and systemically.
- Strict treatment protocol includes early mobilization with full weightbearing.

INTRODUCTION: NATURE OF THE PROBLEM

Prosthetic joint infection (PJI) is a most challenging complication following total hip arthroplasty (THA).[1] Despite all efforts to prevent this complication, infections occur in about 0.5% to 1.9% of primary hip arthroplasty; and in 8% to 10% after revisions.[2,3] Although the definitive diagnosis of PJI remains the key for success, a designated concept of preoperative planning and treatment is mandatory.[1,4,5] Treatment options can include irrigation and debridement[6] with retention of implants for acute infections and exchange arthroplasty either as a 1-stage or 2-stage procedure for deep, late infections.[7–11] In patients who fail all reconstructive options, consideration is given to salvage operations, including a Girdlestone-like resection arthroplasty or disarticulation.[7,12] Currently, the 2-stage exchange arthroplasty is the preferred method of treating chronic PJI of THA,[13,14] whereas a protocol-based, 1-stage exchange arthroplasty is advocated by a few specialized centers and has comparable outcomes.[15–18]

The therapeutic goal in 1-stage exchange arthroplasty is control of the infection in combination with the maintenance of joint function with a single surgery.[16] This technique is a viable option and, depending on the status of the patient,[19] the surgeon's expertise, and the hospital set-up should be used. The main objective is to reduce the bioburden by performing extensive and radical soft tissue debridement and removal of the biofilm-covered prosthesis.

Evaluating the current available literature and guidelines for the treatment of PJI,[20] there is no clear evidence that a 2-stage exchange arthroplasty has a higher success rate than a 1-stage approach.[9] Although the 2-stage technique is described in many articles as the gold standard for management of chronic PJI,[21] there are several unknowns regarding this procedure. Most important is the optimal timing of the reimplantation.[22]

The 1-stage exchange offers some advantages, including the need for only 1 operative procedure, reduced time on antibiotics, reduced hospitalization time, and reduced relative overall costs.[11] The reported outcome of this procedure is

HELIOS ENDO Klinik Hamburg, Holstenstrasse 2, Hamburg 22767, Germany
* Corresponding author.
E-mail address: akos.zahar@helios-kliniken.de

Orthop Clin N Am 47 (2016) 11–18
http://dx.doi.org/10.1016/j.ocl.2015.08.004
0030-5898/16/$ – see front matter © 2016 Elsevier Inc. All rights reserved.

orthopedic.theclinics.com

comparable to the 2-stage exchange arthroplasty.[18,23–25] Therefore, the 1-stage exchange at PJI of THA is getting more and more popular worldwide. There is, however, a need for randomized, prospective studies that can compare the outcome of these procedures.

This article provides a detailed description of current practice regarding the management of PJI of the hip, including diagnostics, preoperative planning, surgical treatment algorithm, possible complications, and postoperative care.

ONE-STAGE EXCHANGE ARTHROPLASTY

For obvious reasons, 1-stage exchange arthroplasty carries many advantages compared with the 2-stage exchange.[16] The 1-stage exchange arthroplasty, though commonly performed in specialized centers in Europe, has also been gaining popularity in North America.[26] One-stage exchange arthroplasty is a viable option for most patients with PJI.[27] At the Endo Klinik, approximately 85% of patients with PJI are treated with 1-stage exchange arthroplasty.[5] A main requirement for 1-stage exchange arthroplasty is that the infecting organism and its sensitivity must be determined before surgery.[28–30] This allows for delivery of local antibiotics, which are added to the cement.[31,32]

INDICATIONS FOR ONE-STAGE SEPTIC EXCHANGE OF THE HIP

One-stage septic exchange is in indicated by the following:

- PJI after THA in which infection is proven based on the International Consensus Group on Periprosthetic Infection of PJI (1 major or 3 minor criteria)[9]
- Late or chronic infection more than 30 days postoperatively or hematogenous infection more than 30 days after onset of the symptoms[33,34]
- Known germ with known susceptibility based on microbiological diagnostics
- Proper bone stock for cemented or, in some cases, uncemented reconstruction
- Possibility of primary wound closure.

CONTRAINDICATIONS OF ONE-STAGE PROCEDURE

One-stage procedure is contraindicated by the following:

- Culture-negative PJI
- Lack of appropriate antibiotics
- Systemic sepsis of the patient
- Failure of 2 or more previous 1-stage procedures[16]
- Infection involving the neurovascular bundles (femoral or sciatic nerve, iliac vessels)
- Extensive soft tissue involvement that would prevent closure of the wound
- Infection with a highly virulent organism, especially cases for which appropriate antibiotic impregnated cement is not available.

SURGICAL TECHNIQUE

The outcome of 1-stage exchange arthroplasty is technique-dependent. This procedure largely depends on the efficiency by which debridement and bioburden reduction is performed. The technique of 1-stage exchange arthroplasty is briefly outlined.

Preoperative Planning

In every case, preoperative plain radiographs (anteroposterior and lateral views) are performed (**Fig. 1**A). In some difficult cases with massive bone loss, computed tomography may be indicated. Preoperative templating using personal computer–based software (MediCAD, Hectec,

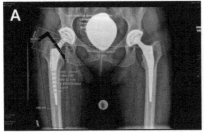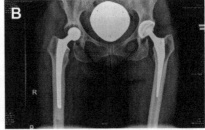

Fig. 1. (*A*) Preoperative anteroposterior (AP) pelvis radiograph and software-based templating of a 55-year-old female patient with PJI of right THA. Preoperative aspiration revealed *Staphylococcus capitis*. (*B*) Postoperative AP pelvis radiograph after 1-stage septic exchange of the right hip; both components were implanted with antibiotic-loaded bone cement.

Landshut, Germany) is done to reconstruct the proper leg-length, the lateral offset, and the center of rotation of the hip (see **Fig. 1**B). The proper implant sizes are templated, which can be intraoperatively double-checked.

Preparation and Patient Positioning

Patients are placed in the lateral decubitus position with a well-fixed pelvis and with a special cushion between the legs providing a stable positioning with the involved leg freely moved in all planes. The skin is prepped 4 times with an alcoholic (propanol) solution (Cutasept G, Bode Chemie, Hamburg, Germany); the acting time should be at least 2 minutes. If the skin is dry again after the disinfection, a standard hip draping is performed with single-use materials. The length of incision and possible extension of the surgical approach should be considered so there is enough space for extensive surgical preparation.

Surgical Approach

The authors recommend a posterolateral approach to the infected hip. Old scars and draining sinuses should be integrated into the approach, if possible. Detachment of the maximus sling (attachment of the gluteus maximus muscle) allows for better access to the posterior aspect of the joint and avoids the lesion of the sciatic nerve; rotational forces are also reduced and, therefore, periprosthetic femoral fracture can be avoided. With extra-articular preparation, the joint capsule is opened as late as possible to avoid contamination of the soft tissues. All capsule, synovia, and infective tissue are excised.

The advantage of the posterior approach is wide and unlimited access to all parts of the acetabulum and to the whole femur. Both endomedullary and periosteal preparation is easily performed. The approach can be extended to either direction; an access to the distal part of the femur can be achieved by preparation along the intermuscular septum. A neurolysis of the sciatic nerve can be performed, if necessary. Positioning of both the acetabular and femoral components is reported to be safer and more reliable when using the posterolateral approach. The disadvantage of the approach is a reportedly higher risk of dislocation, which can be avoided by proper positioning of the implants.

SURGICAL PROCEDURE
Step 1. Debridement and Explantation

The debridement begins by excising the previous scar. The sinus, if present, should be integrated into the skin incision and radically excised down to the joint capsule.[35] All nonbleeding tissues and related bone need to be radically excised. During the radical debridement, multiple tissue samples (4–6 for microbiology and 2 for pathohistology) are obtained and sent for further investigation.[36,37]

For removal of long and cemented stems, special instruments, such as curved chisels, long forceps, curetting instruments, long drills, high-speed burrs, and cement taps, are needed (**Fig. 2**). All implants and foreign material are removed (**Figs. 3** and **4**). Solid femoral implants may require a longitudinal osteotomy or, rarely, an extended trochanteric osteotomy. All cement and restrictors need to be removed. Generally, the debridement of bone and surrounding soft tissues must be as radical as possible. It must include all areas of bone loss and nonviable bone. Occasionally, resection of the greater trochanter or the proximal part of the femur becomes necessary, which necessitates the use of tumor-type, fully cemented, modular, long-stemmed revision implants and, sometimes, a higher level of constraint, such as a constrained liner or a dual-mobility cup.[11]

Step 2. Irrigation with Local Antiseptics

The authors recommend the general use of pulsatile lavage throughout the procedure; however, after complete implant removal and debridement, the intramedullary canals are packed with polymeric biguanide hydrochloride (polyhexanide)-soaked swabs (**Fig. 5**). After the completion of resection, if the surgical site is considered clean, during the acting time (10–15 minutes) of the local antiseptic solution, a new surgical setup is

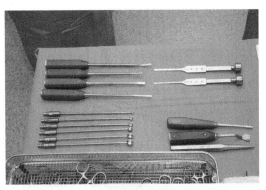

Fig. 2. Special chisels are needed to mobilize the solid implant to avoid femoral osteotomy. High-speed burrs facilitate the bone debridement and the interdigitation of the cement to achieve a good fixation for the cemented implant.

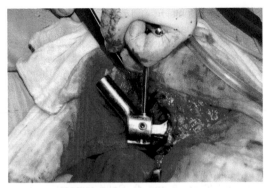

Fig. 3. A special explantation device is attached by drill holes and small screws to the taper of the solid implant, which is then removed by mallet taps.

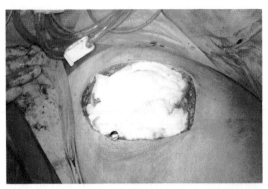

Fig. 5. The wound is packed with polyhexanide-soaked towels and swabs for 10 to 15 minutes to achieve a high concentration of the antiseptic solution. Meanwhile a new draping is performed.

performed. This consists of rescrub of the surgeons, redraping of the surgical field, changing of the suction tip, and the light handles. New surgical gowns and gloves are used. New instruments are brought into the operating theater for reimplantation. A complete new prepping of the patient is not possible because of the open wound. Intravenous antibiotics are given at this time according to the recommendation of the infectious disease specialist.[31]

Step 3. Reimplantation

The reimplantation proceeds, as do other types of revision, in an expeditious manner. To address bone loss, the authors prefer not to use allograft bone, although there have been favorable outcomes with the use of antibiotic-impregnated allografts.[24,38] Defects are filled with polymethyl methacrylate (PMMA) bone cement (Copal, Heraeus Medical, Hanau, Germany) or Tantalum Augments (Trabecular Metal, Zimmer Inc, Warsaw, IN, USA). Tantalum wedges, trabecular metal revision cups, or shim and buttress augments are used to

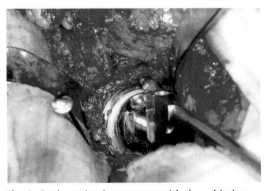

Fig. 4. Explantation instruments with sharp blades are used to mobilize the well-fixed uncemented cup.

reconstruct the bone stock of the acetabulum.[39] According to the defect situation, reconstruction rings and cages, such as Ganz-type or Burch-Schneider–type, are used in combination with antibiotic-loaded PMMA bone cement. Femoral reconstruction occurs with modular cemented revision stems (MP or MegaC modular systems, Waldemar Link, Hamburg, Germany) or standard cemented stems (SPII Lubinus, Waldemar Link, Hamburg, Germany). Consequently, a combined fixation of the cement with the prosthesis and tantalum cones offers an excellent addendum to the treatment portfolio. In addition, it has been suggested that tantalum may have protective effect against infection.[40]

In the meantime, antibiotic-loaded cement is prepared according to a strict protocol. Antibiotic-loaded bone cements may contain water-soluble, heat-resistant antibiotics in crystalline form. The powder should be mixed together with the powder of the PMMA bone cement before liquid is added. In general, manufactured antibiotic bone cements are used, such as Copal G+C or Copal G+V (Heraeus Medical, Wehrheim, Germany). However, according to the preoperative microbiological findings, an admixture of antibiotics may be indicated. When using the antibiotic-loaded cement for definitive fixation of a new implant during reimplantation, a maximum of 10% by weight antibiotic should be added to the cement to retain its biomechanical properties.[41] However, care should be taken with the total amount of local antibiotics used to prevent systemic toxicity. Although rarely described, topical antibiotics may be nephrotoxic and can lead to renal failure. It is essential that the antibiotic added to the cement have activity against the infecting organism; be in powder, not liquid, form; and be bactericidal.

Table 1
Complications and actions following surgical intervention

Complication	Severity	Action
Wound healing problem	Mild	Early revision
Dislocation	Mild	Closed reduction
Repeated dislocation	Moderate	Open reduction, revision of components
Persistent infection	Severe	Early revision, exchange of modular components, debridement, reloading with local antibiotics
Failed 1-stage exchange	Severe	2-stage exchange with antibiotic spacer

COMPLICATIONS AND MANAGEMENT

The persistence or recurrence of infection remains the most relevant complication following surgical intervention for PJI of the hip (**Table 1**). Failure rates with 2-stage exchange have been described to range from 9% to 20% with nonresistant bacteria. Recently published data regarding 1-stage septic exchange of the knee show comparable results for the 1-stage exchange arthroplasty at short and midterm follow-up.[18,25,42–48]

POSTOPERATIVE CARE
Postoperative Antibiotics

In the 1-stage approach, postoperative systemic antibiotic administration is usually continued for 10 to 14 days.[31] A central venous line is used during this period. In the case of PJI with *Streptococci*, a longer period of antibiotic therapy may be indicated. In the first 2 weeks, intravenous administration is recommended, after which oral therapy can be continued depending on the resistance profile of the infecting organism and the availability of an oral agent.[49] The antibiotic therapy is determined by the infectious disease specialist, who is a member of the multidisciplinary team that is involved in the whole diagnostic and therapy protocol of PJI patients.

Physiotherapy

A major advantage of the 1-stage technique is that patients can be ambulated early and allowed to start functional exercises. The physiotherapeutic approach at any stage cannot be generalized. Due to the variety of soft tissue and bone damage and the extent of infection, in most cases an individual plan is required. Postoperative rehabilitation in these patients aims to reduce associated muscular movement restrictions, stiffness, or fibrosis of the affected hip joint. The authors generally recommend early mobilization within the first postoperative days using walking aids such as crutches. Weightbearing should be adapted to the intraoperative findings and substance defects and might be increased to full weightbearing within the first 2 weeks after surgery, although most patients' immediate weightbearing is also allowed.

OUTCOMES

The 2-stage revision of PJI has become the gold standard for most members of orthopedic

Table 2
Summary of publications containing data about the infection control rate with one-stage septic exchange of total hip arthroplasty

Author, Year	Number of Patients	Follow-up (years)	Infection Control Rate (%)
Wroblewski,[25] 1986	102	3.2	91
Loty et al,[23] 1992	90	NA	91
Raut et al,[48] 1995	183	7.8	84
Winkler et al,[24] 2008	37	4.4	92
Klouche et al,[47] 2012	38	2.0	100
Hansen et al,[46] 2013	27	4.2	70
Choi et al,[44] 2013	17	5.2	82
Zeller et al,[18] 2014	157	5.0	95

Data from Refs.[18,23–25,44,46–48]

community,[50] with a reported failure rate in terms of incidence of reinfection between 9% and 20%. Despite the recommendations of mainstream publications, in our specialized hospital for bone and joint surgery, the authors established and have followed the 1-stage approach described in this article for almost 40 years.[5,15] There are good infection control rates for 1-stage septic exchange of infected TKA and success is seen in about 90% of all our total joint arthroplasty patients at 10-year follow-up.[42] The results of 1-stage septic exchange of THA are shown in **Table 2**.

When comparing the results published in the literature, far more studies have been published and emphasized the 2-stage approach. Only a few studies have evaluated the 1-stage exchange and its techniques in THA. However, these results show comparable success rates of 80% to 90%. Variations may result from different bacteria and follow-up times. As recent reports have shown, the overall results of 2-stage revisions might have even higher complication and lower success rates than reported previously, especially at multiresistant organisms such as methicillin-resistant *Staphylococcus aureus* (MRSA).[51,52]

SUMMARY

Although various surgical and nonsurgical options for the management of PJI of the knee exist, the outcome of all of these procedures is far from perfect. Most patients with PJI of the hip suffer a very protracted course of treatment. There is a desperate need for novel treatment modalities and improvement in care for these patients. In addition, effective strategies for prevention of PJI need to be implemented. Currently exciting research is in process that includes attempts to determine the genetic susceptibility of patients to host, design of numerous biofilm disruption technologies, and introduction of infection resistant implants. The future for the management of PJI of the knee needs to be different because the current status is unacceptable.

REFERENCES

1. Fink B, Makowiak C, Fuerst M, et al. The value of synovial biopsy, joint aspiration and C-reactive protein in the diagnosis of late peri-prosthetic infection of total knee replacements. J Bone Joint Surg Br 2008; 90(7):874–8.
2. Bozic KJ, Ries MD. The impact of infection after total hip arthroplasty on hospital and surgeon resource utilization. J Bone Joint Surg Am 2005; 87(8):1746–51.
3. Kurtz SM, Lau E, Schmier J, et al. Infection burden for hip and knee arthroplasty in the United States. J Arthroplasty 2008;23(7):984–91.
4. De Man FH, Sendi P, Zimmerli W, et al. Infectiological, functional, and radiographic outcome after revision for prosthetic hip infection according to a strict algorithm. Acta Orthop 2011;82(1):27–34.
5. Gehrke T, Zahar A, Kendoff D. One-stage exchange: it all began here. Bone Joint J 2013;95-B(11 Suppl A):77–83.
6. Romano CL, Manzi G, Logoluso N, et al. Value of debridement and irrigation for the treatment of peri-prosthetic infections. A systematic review. Hip Int 2012;22(Suppl 8):S19–24.
7. Cierny G 3rd, DiPasquale D. Periprosthetic total joint infections: staging, treatment, and outcomes. Clin Orthop Relat Res 2002;(403):23–8.
8. Hsieh PH, Shih CH, Chang YH, et al. Two-stage revision hip arthroplasty for infection: comparison between the interim use of antibiotic-loaded cement beads and a spacer prosthesis. J Bone Joint Surg Am 2004;86-A(9):1989–97.
9. ICG. International Consensus Group on Periprosthetic Infection. Consensus statements. Philadelphia: Thomas Jefferson University; 2013.
10. Parvizi J, Adeli B, Zmistowski B, et al. Management of periprosthetic joint infection: the current knowledge: AAOS exhibit selection. J Bone Joint Surg Am 2012;94(14):e104.
11. Zahar A, Webb J, Gehrke T, et al. One-stage exchange for prosthetic joint infection of the hip. Hip Int 2015;25(4):301–7.
12. Haddad FS, Masri BA, Garbuz DS, et al. The treatment of the infected hip replacement. The complex case. Clin Orthop Relat Res 1999;(369):144–56.
13. Cooper HJ, Della Valle CJ. The two-stage standard in revision total hip replacement. Bone Joint J 2013;95-B(11 Suppl A):84–7.
14. Engesaeter LB, Dale H, Schrama JC, et al. Surgical procedures in the treatment of 784 infected THAs reported to the Norwegian Arthroplasty Register. Acta Orthop 2011;82(5):530–7.
15. Buchholz HW, Elson RA, Engelbrecht E, et al. Management of deep infection of total hip replacement. J Bone Joint Surg Br 1981;63-B(3):342–53.
16. Gehrke T, Kendoff D. Peri-prosthetic hip infections: in favour of one-stage. Hip Int 2012;22(Suppl 8): S40–5.
17. Steinbrink K, Frommelt L. Treatment of periprosthetic infection of the hip using one-stage exchange surgery. Orthopade 1995;24(4):335–43 [in German].
18. Zeller V, Lhotellier L, Marmor S, et al. One-stage exchange arthroplasty for chronic periprosthetic hip infection: results of a large prospective cohort study. J Bone Joint Surg Am 2014;96(1):e1.
19. McPherson EJ, Woodson C, Holtom P, et al. Periprosthetic total hip infection: outcomes using a

staging system. Clin Orthop Relat Res 2002;(403): 8–15.

20. Parvizi J, Della Valle CJ. AAOS Clinical Practice Guideline: diagnosis and treatment of periprosthetic joint infections of the hip and knee. J Am Acad Orthop Surg 2010;18(12):771–2.

21. Romanò CL, Romanò D, Albisetti A, et al. Preformed antibiotic-loaded cement spacers for two-stage revision of infected total hip arthroplasty. Long-term results. Hip Int 2012;22(Suppl 8):S46–53.

22. Berend KR, Lombardi AV Jr, Morris MJ, et al. Two-stage treatment of hip periprosthetic joint infection is associated with a high rate of infection control but high mortality. Clin Orthop Relat Res 2013; 471(2):510–8.

23. Loty B, Postel M, Evrard J, et al. One stage revision of infected total hip replacements with replacement of bone loss by allografts. Study of 90 cases of which 46 used bone allografts. Int Orthop 1992; 16(4):330–8 [in French].

24. Winkler H, Stoiber A, Kaudela K, et al. One stage uncemented revision of infected total hip replacement using cancellous allograft bone impregnated with antibiotics. J Bone Joint Surg Br 2008;90(12):1580–4.

25. Wroblewski BM. One-stage revision of infected cemented total hip arthroplasty. Clin Orthop Relat Res 1986;211:103–7.

26. Jiranek WA, Waligora AC, Hess SR, et al. Surgical Treatment of Prosthetic Joint Infections of the Hip and Knee: Changing Paradigms? J Arthroplasty 2015;30(6):912–8.

27. Lichstein P, Gehrke T, Lombardi A, et al. One-stage vs two-stage exchange. J Arthroplasty 2014;29(2 Suppl):108–11.

28. Ince A, Rupp J, Frommelt L, et al. Is "aseptic" loosening of the prosthetic cup after total hip replacement due to nonculturable bacterial pathogens in patients with low-grade infection? Clin Infect Dis 2004;39(11):1599–603.

29. Parvizi J, Ghanem E, Menashe S, et al. Periprosthetic infection: what are the diagnostic challenges? J Bone Joint Surg Am 2006;88(Suppl 4):138–47.

30. Schinsky MF, Della Valle CJ, Sporer SM, et al. Perioperative testing for joint infection in patients undergoing revision total hip arthroplasty. J Bone Joint Surg Am 2008;90(9):1869–75.

31. Frommelt L. Principles of systemic antimicrobial therapy in foreign material associated infection in bone tissue, with special focus on periprosthetic infection. Injury 2006;37(Suppl 2):S87–94.

32. Hanssen AD, Spangehl MJ. Practical applications of antibiotic-loaded bone cement for treatment of infected joint replacements. Clin Orthop Relat Res 2004;(427):79–85.

33. Della Valle C, Parvizi J, Bauer TW, et al. Diagnosis of periprosthetic joint infections of the hip and knee. J Am Acad Orthop Surg 2010;18(12):760–70.

34. Osmon DR, Berbari EF, Berendt AR, et al. Executive summary: diagnosis and management of prosthetic joint infection: clinical practice guidelines by the Infectious Diseases Society of America. Clin Infect Dis 2013;56(1):1–10.

35. Raut VV, Siney PD, Wroblewski BM. One-stage revision of infected total hip replacements with discharging sinuses. J Bone Joint Surg Br 1994;76(5): 721–4.

36. Krenn V, Morawietz L, Perino G, et al. Revised histopathological consensus classification of joint implant related pathology. Pathol Res Pract 2014;210(12): 779–86.

37. Schafer P, Fink B, Sandow D, et al. Prolonged bacterial culture to identify late periprosthetic joint infection: a promising strategy. Clin Infect Dis 2008; 47(11):1403–9.

38. Winkler H, Kaudela K, Stoiber A, et al. Bone grafts impregnated with antibiotics as a tool for treating infected implants in orthopedic surgery - one stage revision results. Cell Tissue Bank 2006;7(4):319–23.

39. Schildhauer TA, Robie B, Muhr G, et al. Bacterial adherence to tantalum versus commonly used orthopedic metallic implant materials. J Orthop Trauma 2006;20(7):476–84.

40. Tokarski AT, Novack TA, Parvizi J. Is tantalum protective against infection in revision total hip arthroplasty? Bone Joint J 2015;97-B(1):45–9.

41. Fink B, Vogt S, Reinsch M, et al. Sufficient release of antibiotic by a spacer 6 weeks after implantation in two-stage revision of infected hip prostheses. Clin Orthop Relat Res 2011;469(11):3141–7.

42. Zahar A, Kendoff DO, Klatte TO, et al. Can good infection control be obtained in one-stage exchange of the infected TKA to a rotating hinge design? 10-year results. Clin Orthop Relat Res 2015. [Epub ahead of print].

43. Callaghan JJ, Katz RP, Johnston RC. One-stage revision surgery of the infected hip. A minimum 10-year followup study. Clin Orthop Relat Res 1999;(369):139–43.

44. Choi HR, Kwon YM, Freiberg AA, et al. Comparison of one-stage revision with antibiotic cement versus two-stage revision results for infected total hip arthroplasty. J Arthroplasty 2013;28(8 Suppl):66–70.

45. George DA, Konan S, Haddad FS, et al. Single-Stage Hip and Knee Exchange for Periprosthetic Joint Infection. J Arthroplasty 2015. http://dx.doi.org/10.1016/j.arth.2015.05.047.

46. Hansen E, Tetreault M, Zmistowski B, et al. Outcome of one-stage cementless exchange for acute postoperative periprosthetic hip infection. Clin Orthop Relat Res 2013;471(10):3214–22.

47. Klouche S, Leonard P, Zeller V, et al. Infected total hip arthroplasty revision: one- or two-stage procedure? Orthop Traumatol Surg Res 2012; 98(2):144–50.

48. Raut VV, Siney PD, Wroblewski BM. One-stage revision of total hip arthroplasty for deep infection. Long-term follow up. Clin Orthop Relat Res 1995;(321):202–7.

49. Kilgus DJ, Howe DJ, Strang A. Results of periprosthetic hip and knee infections caused by resistant bacteria. Clin Orthop Relat Res 2002;(404):116–24.

50. Wongworawat MD. Clinical faceoff: One- versus two-stage exchange arthroplasty for prosthetic joint infections. Clin Orthop Relat Res 2013; 471(6):1750–3.

51. Mortazavi SM, O'Neil JT, Zmistowski B, et al. Repeat 2-stage exchange for infected total hip arthroplasty: a viable option? J Arthroplasty 2012;27(6):923–6.e1.

52. Mortazavi SM, Vegari D, Ho A, et al. Two stage exchange arthroplasty for infected total knee arthroplasty: predictors of failure. Clin Orthop Relat Res 2011;469(11):3049–54.

The Impact of Lumbar Spine Disease and Deformity on Total Hip Arthroplasty Outcomes

Daniel J. Blizzard, MD, MS*, Brian T. Nickel, MD,
Thorsten M. Seyler, MD, PhD, Michael P. Bolognesi, MD

KEYWORDS

- Spinal deformity • Scoliosis • Kyphosis • Lumbar • THA • Total hip arthroplasty • Pelvic tilt
- Sagittal balance

KEY POINTS

- Spinal deformities can significantly restrict lumbar range of motion and lumbar lordosis, leading to pelvic obliquity and increased pelvic tilt.
- A comprehensive preoperative workup and component templating are essential to ensure appropriate compensation for altered pelvic parameters for implantation of components according to functional positioning.
- Pelvic obliquity from scoliosis must be measured to calculate appropriate leg length.
- Cup positioning should be templated on standing radiograph to limit potential impingement from cup malposition.
- In cases of spinal deformity, the optimal position of the cup that accommodates pelvic parameters and limits impingement may lie outside the classic parameters of the safe zone.

INTRODUCTION

Osteoarthritis (OA) is a systemic and inevitable disease of aging that can affect the hip and spine concurrently, producing substantial pain and disability.[1–11] The degenerative changes of end-stage arthritis in the hip and spine can significantly alter body kinematics and spinopelvic alignment.[5,12–18] Accordingly, the diagnosis and treatment of patients with simultaneous hip and spine disease require consideration of the relative contributions of each region to clinical symptoms, postural balance, and locomotion.

LUMBAR RANGE OF MOTION

Lumbar disease, low back pain (LBP), and guarding from fear of LBP cause a significant reduction in lumbar range of motion (ROM).[12–16] In addition, McGregor and colleagues[19] showed that patients with disk prolapse, degenerative disk disease, and stenosis have a predictable reduction in lumbar ROM in flexion/extension, lateral bending, and rotation compared with age-matched controls. In more obvious cases, patients with ankylosing spondylitis and those undergoing multilevel spinal fusion procedures

Study funding: none.
Department of Orthopaedic Surgery, Duke University Medical Center, Durham, NC, USA
* Corresponding author. DUMC Box 3000, Durham, NC 27710.
E-mail address: daniel.blizzard@duke.edu

can have profound, fixed reductions in lumbar ROM.

To complete activities of daily living (ADLs) that demand spinopelvic motion, patients with lumbar disease compensate for decreased lumbar motion from stiffness or fusion by increasing motion through the hip joints.

SPINOPELVIC MOTION AND PELVIC PARAMETERS

Spinopelvic flexion and extension are the sum of intrinsic motion from the hip joints and extrinsic motion from the lumbosacral joints.[18] Duval-Beaupere and colleagues[20,21] introduced the concept of pelvic incidence (PI) to describe the anatomic relationship between the alignment and motion of the spine and pelvis.[22] PI, defined by the angle between a line drawn from the center of the femoral head to the midpoint of the S1 end plate on a lateral radiograph (**Fig. 1**), can vary significantly from person to person but remains an anatomic constant for each individual after puberty throughout all pelvic ROM. Sacral slope (SS), defined by the angle between a line parallel to the S1 end plate and a horizontal line, is a measure of the inclination of the pelvis base and is variable throughout spinopelvic motion, increasing from the sitting position to standing and from standing to lying supine.[5,18,23] Pelvic tilt (PT), defined by the angle between a line drawn from the midpoint of the S1 end plate and a vertical line, is a measure of the position of the pelvis relative to the acetabulum and varies reciprocally with SS, decreasing, or becoming less posterior, from the sitting position to standing and further decreasing from standing to lying supine. The relationship between the geometric measures is PI = SS + PT.

Pelvic parameters and spine measures are connected by a linear relationship between SS and lumbar lordosis. This relationship was initially described by Stagnara and colleagues[24] in 1982 and subsequently confirmed by other investigators showing a correlation of $r = 0.84$ to 0.86 between the measures.[22,25] The implication of this

relationship is that as lumbar lordosis decreases, SS concurrently decreases and PT increases, retroverting the pelvis.

INFLUENCE OF BODY POSITION ON PELVIC PARAMETERS

Although PI remains constant throughout spinopelvic motion, SS and PT significantly vary with body position.[5,18,23,26] While lying supine, lumbar lordosis and SS (often exceeding 45°) are accentuated, the pelvis is tilted forward, and acetabular version and abduction are low to permit maximal hip extension. Moving from lying supine to standing, the pelvis tilts slightly backward and SS decreases slightly (between 35° and 45°), and acetabular version and abduction increase. Moving from standing to sitting, the pelvis is further tilted backward and the SS decreases to 25° or less, and acetabular version and abduction further increase to permit further hip flexion.[18,27]

In multiple studies, Lazennec and colleagues[5,18,23,27] documented the variable radiographic position of total hip arthroplasty (THA) cups on anteroposterior (AP) and lateral films in the sitting and standing positions. These investigators reported changes in the AP inclination of the cup from 49° to 52° in the standing position to 57° to 64° in the seated position and changes in the sagittal inclination of the cup from 36° to 47° standing to 51° to 58° in the seated position. Patients with limited lumbar ROM from lumbar disease or resultant fusion show little variation in pelvic orientation based on position.[5,18,23] That is, there is little change in SS, PT, or acetabular version or abduction with body positioning, inherently limiting the ability to accommodate additional hip flexion when seated or extension when standing or lying supine.

CORONAL AND SAGITTAL ALIGNMENT AND SPINOPELVIC MECHANICS

Coronal imbalance is governed by scoliosis and pelvic obliquity. Although idiopathic adolescent scoliosis and degenerative scoliosis arise de novo,

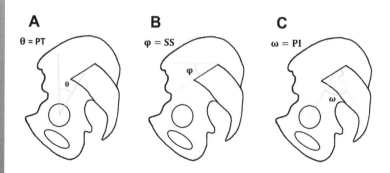

A $\theta = PT$

B $\varphi = SS$

C $\omega = PI$

Fig. 1. (A) PT. Defined by the angle (θ) between a line drawn from the center of the femoral head to the midpoint of the S1 end plate on a lateral radiograph. (B) SS. Defined by the angle (φ) between a line parallel to the S1 end plate and a horizontal line. (C) PI. Defined by the angle (ω) between a line drawn from the midpoint of the S1 end plate and a vertical line.

compensatory lumbar and thoracic scoliosis can also arise from limb length deformity secondary to multiple causes, including end-stage degenerative changes in the hip.[28,29] Uncorrected pelvic obliquity accelerates degenerative changes in the lumbosacral spine and can significantly affect normal gait.[29]

Sagittal alignment is a measure of an individual's adaptation to variations in anatomy and disease to produce a functional and balanced posture.[5,18,26] Sagittal balance is the net effect of thoracic kyphosis and lumbar lordosis and can be influenced by axial musculature, spinal disease, and surgical interventions.

Degenerative changes in the spine are manifested through hypertrophy and cystic changes of the facets, degeneration of intervertebral disks, osteophytosis of the vertebra, and atrophy of spinal extensor muscles, which lead to a net effect of hypolordosis.[30–34] Compared with age-matched control individuals, patients with degenerative spine disease and LBP have a significant reduction in lumbar lordosis and SS and significant increase in PT (or posterior tilt).[33,35,36]

Lumbar spine fusion can provide reliable and durable stabilization and symptom relief for degenerative spinal conditions, including spondylolisthesis and scoliosis. The advent of interbody fusion techniques from the anterior, lateral, transforaminal, and posterior approaches has increased the frequency of the procedures and provided new strategies to treat complex deformities.

The goals of spinal deformity surgery are stabilization of unstable segments and restoration of lumbar lordosis and coronal and sagittal balance.[37,38] The restoration of lumbar lordosis is influenced by multiple factors, including operative table and positioning, osteotomies, and single or combined anterior and posterior approaches. Failure to restore appropriate lordosis can result in positive sagittal balance, chronic LBP, and accelerated adjacent segment disease.[17]

The term flatback syndrome was coined by Moe and Denis in 1977[39] to describe a fixed, iatrogenic positive sagittal imbalance resulting from spinal fusion. Although initially resulting nearly exclusively from Harrington rod constructs,[40–43] the increase in interbody fusion surgery over the last 2 decades has led to an increase in reports of flatback syndrome.[44,45] Poor sagittal alignment can result from inadequate restoration of lordosis in patients with significant preoperative positive sagittal balance or from iatrogenic causes, including hypolordotic positioning on the operative table and undercontouring of rods.

The compensatory mechanisms to restore postural balance in patients with lumbar hypolordosis include thoracic hyperextension (or loss of kyphosis), forward tilt of the trunk, knee flexion, hip extension, and increased or posterior PT.[17,30,46] The net compensatory effect is positive sagittal balance and relative retroversion of the pelvis, resulting in excessive acetabular anteversion.[26]

IMPINGEMENT AND INSTABILITY

The combined effect of hypolordosis and posterior PT and limited lumbar ROM in patients with degenerative spine disease and deformity decrease the functional ROM of the hip before impingement occurs.[5,18,23] In the standing position, the compensation of increased posterior PT for hypolordosis increases anteversion and abduction of the acetabulum and forces the hips into a hyperextended position and can cause posterior hip impingement and create anterior instability. Conversely, in the seated position, a rigid lumbar spine is unable to contribute to combined spinopelvic flexion and the hip joints are hyperflexed, leading to potential posterior instability.

INDICATIONS/CONTRAINDICATIONS

The well-recognized poor correlation between radiographic severity of hip arthritis and clinical signs and symptoms poses a significant diagnostic challenge when patients present with concurrent LBP, hip pain, or leg pain and have radiographic polyarticular disease. The absolute indications for THA do not differ in this population; however, the overlap of symptoms between lumbar and hip disease makes it difficult to assess the respective effects that each anatomic location has on morbidity and disability.

Hip-spine syndrome, first coined by Offierski and MacNab in 1983, is defined as the concurrent existence of OA and degenerative lumbar spinal stenosis.[7] Spine disease can present with pain and symptoms that mimic many common disorders, including hip arthritis, trochanteric bursitis, iliopsoas impingement, sacroiliac arthritis, and piriformis syndrome. Similarly, studies have shown that THA can result in significant improvement in lumbar spine pain.[1] Although multiple studies have shown high sensitivity and specificity using diagnostic anesthetic hip injections to distinguish between lumbar disease and hip disease when the anatomic source of pain is ambiguous,[47,48] more often, the existence of concurrent hip and lumbar spine disease is only realized after pain persists after operative treatment of the spine or the hip.

Currently, there exist no evidence-based guidelines regarding the order or operative treatment of concurrent hip and spine disease. Most surgeons recommend treating the most symptomatic disease first; however, the acetabular cup positioning and stability are dependent on lumbar lordosis, SS, and PT, which can all be altered by spine procedures. In a recent study, it was shown that patients with lumbar spine disease undergoing THA had significantly less improvement in pain and functionality and greater medical charges and longer episodes of care after THA than did patients without lumbar spine disease.[49]

SURGICAL PROCEDURE
Preoperative Planning

Understanding the effect of PT on acetabular cup positioning is the crux of THA preoperative planning in patients with concomitant lumbar spine disease (**Fig. 2**). The traditional radiographic AP pelvis plane was described by Murray[50] and is based on coronal plane projection of the pelvis. Conversely, computer navigation is based on the anterior pelvic plane (APP) defined by the plane between the anterior superior iliac spines and the pubic symphysis.[51] When the APP and coronal plane of the standing body are equal, the pelvis has no tilt and any navigation based on the APP is reflective of a patient's functional anatomy.

This alignment occurs in only a few patients. Specifically, only 6.1% of 477 patients were found to have zero PT.[52] Most patients fell in a narrow range close to neutral PT, with 83.9% of patients having less than 10° of tilt. However, the outlier patients would have a cup implanted correctly according to anterior reference points, but functionally, the acetabular cup would be malpositioned, leading to possible dislocation and impingement in extreme positions.

A similar study of 138 THA primary patients reported that 17% of patients had greater than 10° of PT.[53] Because of the significant percentage of outliers, computed tomography (CT) navigation measurements based on the APP are not directly comparable with AP radiographs. Also, the approximate 16.5% of patients with a significant PT may be the outliers who have component malposition on CT despite excellent cup position on AP pelvic radiographs as a result of the lack of sagittal alignment influence on AP radiographs.

In simplistic terms, an increase in PT changes the normal AP pelvis view to modified outlet view. This finding is not parallax, but a true dynamic change in orientation of the acetabulum. Studies have quantified the impact of PT on acetabular inclination as approximately each degree of posterior tilt leads to a 0.7° increase in

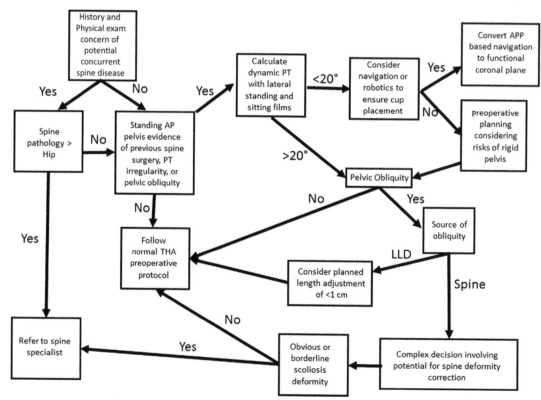

Fig. 2. Clinical decision-making flow chart for preoperative evaluation for THA.

acetabular inclination.[51,53,54] Similarly, anatomic version progressively increases from supine to standing to sitting, from 24.2° to 31.7° to 38.8°, respectively, with a mean of 7.1° increase in version from standing to sitting in relation to a 14.5° increase in posterior tilt.[55] This linear relationship also holds with the lateral radiographic parameter of anteinclination, defined as the sagittal cup position based on change in standing to sitting on lateral radiographs.[56] The importance of analyzing and considering acetabular version and abduction in the standing position for THA templating was highlighted by Tiberi and colleagues,[57] who showed that 43% of patients had greater than a 5° change in acetabular inclination and 53% patients had great than a 5° change in version between supine and standing films.

Understanding the normal effect of PT on cup position is crucial to understanding the implications of stiff or hypermobile spinopelvic motion. Pelvic stiffness is defined as the difference in PT between standing and sitting on lateral radiographs. Normal pelvises have a 20° to 35° increase in PT, stiff pelvises have less than 20°, and hypermobile greater than 35°. The variation between stiff and hypermobile pelvises results in a minimum of 15° difference in functional cup positioning. This variation may lead to malpositioning of the cup at certain positions during ADLs, leading to potential impingement, subluxation, dislocations, or accelerated wear.

Functional consequences of pelvic tilt on acetabular cup position

Acetabular cup position is dynamic to accommodate hip extension while standing or lying supine and hip flexion while sitting. Limited lumbar spine motion forces the body to compensate with increased hip extensions or flexion to achieve a functional position. Extreme flexion/extension can then lead to impingement, subluxation, and dislocation despite excellent cup position on an AP radiograph. Classically, the safe zone described by Lewinnek and colleagues[58] in 1978 has been used to define ideal cup position of 40° ± 10° and 15° ± 10°. Major limitations to this definition include the lack of consideration for lumbar spine dynamics, implant design and wear, and relatively small sample size of 300 patients. Most importantly, these parameters are based on two-dimensional coronal imaging and do not account for three-dimensional position of the cup.

Patients with spinal deformity are vulnerable to dislocation both anteriorly and posteriorly, regardless of the direction of the surgical approach. Patients undergoing anterior approach surgery have a near equal incidence of anterior and posterior dislocation,[59,60] whereas patients undergoing posterior approach surgery are more predisposed to posterior dislocation.[59,61] Patients with lumbar spine rigidity and compensatory PT are at risk for instability anteriorly with requisite hip hyperextension while standing or lying supine and posteriorly with the requisite hyperflexion while sitting.[18] In addition, increased PT leading to verticalization of the cup is a risk factor for increased surface wear and liner fracture.[62,63]

The compensatory position of the pelvis and acetabulum for lumbar rigidity and deformity may explain why most (58%) dislocated THAs have cups placed in the safe zone, leading investigators to recommend advanced analysis of dynamic factors.[64–66]

Pelvic Obliquity

Coronal imbalance must be addressed during THA planning to determine proper leg length. Pelvic obliquity resulting from severe degenerative changes of the hip joint can be corrected by templating the prosthesis to match the ipsilateral hip. However, pelvic obliquity caused primarily by scoliosis can be more challenging. In their 2015 study, Abe and colleagues[29] showed improvement in pelvic obliquity in 79% of patients with preoperative scoliosis obliquity through intentional leg lengthening with THA, although their algorithm to determine amount of lengthening was not given. The amount of leg lengthening is inherently limited by soft tissue compliance and potential neural stretch injury, but any plan to intentionally lengthen the leg to address pelvic obliquity resulting from scoliosis should also factor the potential for subsequent spine surgery to directly correct the spinal deformity. That is, a THA with intentional lengthening of the leg to compensate for pelvic obliquity could result in iatrogenic pelvic obliquity in the opposite direction from leg length discrepancy if the spinal deformity is corrected.

In their 2013 series, Meftah and colleagues[67] described their method to address pelvic obliquity from fixed spinal deformity during THA templating for the goal of orienting the cup in a position of function. These investigators described drawing a horizontal line that crosses the teardrop and planning their cup abduction according to that line, noting the relative position of the lateral edge of the cup to the most lateral margin of the acetabulum to use for comparison intraoperatively. Although this technique does not alter pelvic obliquity, it ensures cup orientation according to functional positioning.

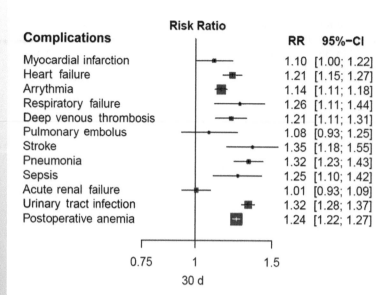

Fig. 3. Forest plot of medical complications at 30 days postoperative listing RR (and 95% confidence intervals [95%-CI]).

Clinical assessment

- Thorough history and physical to identify potential concurrent spine disease, including overlapping symptoms
- Obtain a standing AP radiograph of the pelvis
- Obtain standing and sitting lateral radiographs in all patients with lumbar spine symptoms, previous spine surgery, pelvic obliquity, or PT irregularity on AP pelvis radiograph
- Calculate dynamic PT between sitting and standing to determine lumbar rigidity
- Calculate pelvic obliquity according to method of Meftah and colleagues[67]
- Template arthroplasty components, accounting for pelvic obliquity and PT and balancing the risk of anterior impingement in hip flexion with a flattened cup and posterior impingement in hip extension with a vertical cup[53,56,68]
  - If using CT navigation, consider converting the CT-based APP cup positioning to a functional positioning based on preoperative sitting and standing radiographs
- Counsel patients regarding increased risk of THA given concurrent spine disease

Operative considerations

Intraoperative imaging has been shown to be a quick, reliable, readily available option to evaluate cup position with limited cost, and almost half of all cases required an adjustment to either the acetabular or femoral component.[69,70] However, it is important to interpret the intraoperative radiograph in relation to the preoperative standing and sitting radiographs, to account for potential variances in the plane of the AP images.

Although there are no published data, it may be reasonable to consider a constrained liner, larger heads, or even bipolar or tripolar heads for primary THA in cases of extreme PT and lumbar rigidity.

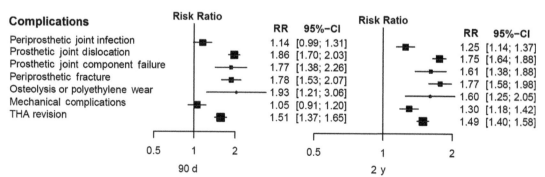

Fig. 4. Forest plot of surgical complications at 30 days and 2 years postoperative listing RR (and 95% confidence intervals [95%-CI]).

Complications and management

The principal surgical complications after THA include periprosthetic joint infection, dislocation, periprosthetic fracture, component failure or loosening, osteolysis or polyethylene wear, and revision THA. Analysis of a large cohort of patients from the Medicare database from 2005 to 2012 showed that patients undergoing THA with coexisting spinal deformities including kyphosis and thoracic and lumbar scoliosis have a significantly increased relative risk (RR) of several postoperative medical (**Fig. 3**) and surgical (**Fig. 4**) complications compared with patients without spinal deformities. At 90 days after THA, patients with spinal deformity have a significantly increased risk of prosthetic hip dislocation (RR = 1.86), prosthetic component failure (RR = 1.77), periprosthetic fracture (RR = 1.78), and early revision THA (RR = 1.51) compared with control patients without spine deformity (see **Fig. 4**). At 2 years after THA, patients with spine deformity have a significantly higher RR of all surgical complications measured (see **Fig. 4**).

Again, the explanation for the marked increase in operative complications for patients with spinal deformity after THA is not entirely understood; however, the increased rates of dislocation, component failure or loosening, osteolysis and polyethylene wear, and revision THA likely result, at least in part, from the aforementioned anterior and posterior impingement from a spinal deformity.

Postoperative Care

Although no formal adjusted algorithms have been published for patients with concurrent spine disease undergoing THA, it may be beneficial to adjust perioperative ROM protocols according to preoperative spinopelvic motion. A person with limited lumbar flexion and extension requires increased flexion and extension through the hip

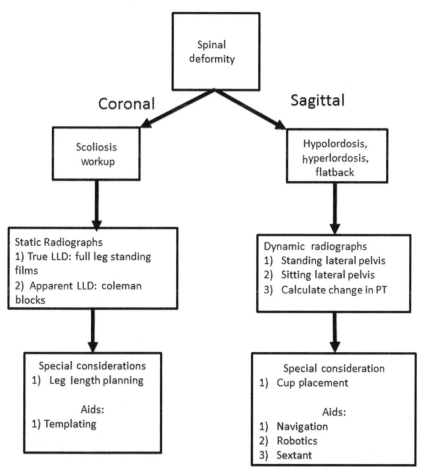

Fig. 5. Proposed workup algorithm based on deformity plane and special considerations for treatment. LLD, leg length discrepancy.

joints to accomplish ADLs, including sitting on a toilet and dressing. Even a radiographically ideally placed hip prosthesis faces increased stresses if lumbar motion is limited. Accordingly, patients identified preoperatively with limited lumbar ROM could benefit from therapy recommendations or instructions that further restrict ROM limits to prevent positions of instability (ie, deep hip flexion for a posterior approach).

SUMMARY

Patients with spinal disease and deformity present a unique challenge to the arthroplasty surgeon. The key to management of these patients with interrelated diseases is identification of potential changes in lumbar motion and pelvic alignment and adjustment of the operative plan or template to reflect the increased PT and increased propensity for impingement even if such adjustments violate the safe zone described by Lewinnek and colleagues **(Fig. 5)**.

REFERENCES

1. Ben-Galim P, Ben-Galim T, Rand N, et al. Hip-spine syndrome: the effect of total hip replacement surgery on low back pain in severe osteoarthritis of the hip. Spine (Phila Pa 1976) 2007;32(19):2099–102.
2. Bohl WR, Steffee AD. Lumbar spinal stenosis. A cause of continued pain and disability in patients after total hip arthroplasty. Spine (Phila Pa 1976) 1979; 4(2):168–73.
3. Devin CJ, McCullough KA, Morris BJ, et al. Hip-spine syndrome. J Am Acad Orthop Surg 2012; 20(7):434–42.
4. Fogel GR, Esses SI. Hip spine syndrome: management of coexisting radiculopathy and arthritis of the lower extremity. Spine J 2003;3(3):238–41.
5. Lazennec JY, Riwan A, Gravez F, et al. Hip spine relationships: application to total hip arthroplasty. Hip Int 2007;17(Suppl 5):S91–104.
6. McNamara MJ, Barrett KG, Christie MJ, et al. Lumbar spinal stenosis and lower extremity arthroplasty. J Arthroplasty 1993;8(3):273–7.
7. Offierski CM, MacNab I. Hip-spine syndrome. Spine (Phila Pa 1976) 1983;8(3):316–21.
8. Parvizi J, Pour AE, Hillibrand A, et al. Back pain and total hip arthroplasty: a prospective natural history study. Clin Orthop Relat Res 2010;468(5):1325–30.
9. Saito J, Ohtori S, Kishida S, et al. Difficulty of diagnosing the origin of lower leg pain in patients with both lumbar spinal stenosis and hip joint osteoarthritis. Spine (Phila Pa 1976) 2012;37(25):2089–93.
10. Saunders WA, Gleeson JA, Timlin DM, et al. Degenerative joint disease in the hip and spine. Rheumatol Rehabil 1979;18(3):137–41.
11. Sembrano JN, Polly DW Jr. How often is low back pain not coming from the back? Spine (Phila Pa 1976) 2009;34(1):E27–32.
12. Esola MA, McClure PW, Fitzgerald GK, et al. Analysis of lumbar spine and hip motion during forward bending in subjects with and without a history of low back pain. Spine (Phila Pa 1976) 1996;21(1):71–8.
13. Porter JL, Wilkinson A. Lumbar-hip flexion motion. A comparative study between asymptomatic and chronic low back pain in 18- to 36-year-old men. Spine (Phila Pa 1976) 1997;22(13):1508–13 [discussion: 1513–4].
14. Thomas E, Silman AJ, Papageorgiou AC, et al. Association between measures of spinal mobility and low back pain. An analysis of new attenders in primary care. Spine (Phila Pa 1976) 1998;23(3):343–7.
15. Thomas JS, France CR. The relationship between pain-related fear and lumbar flexion during natural recovery from low back pain. Eur Spine J 2008; 17(1):97–103.
16. Wong TK, Lee RY. Effects of low back pain on the relationship between the movements of the lumbar spine and hip. Hum Mov Sci 2004;23(1):21–34.
17. Barrey C, Darnis A. Current strategies for the restoration of adequate lordosis during lumbar fusion. World J Orthop 2015;6(1):117–26.
18. Lazennec JY, Brusson A, Rousseau MA. Hip-spine relations and sagittal balance clinical consequences. Eur Spine J 2011;20(Suppl 5):686–98.
19. McGregor AH, McCarthy ID, Doré CJ, et al. Quantitative assessment of the motion of the lumbar spine in the low back pain population and the effect of different spinal pathologies of this motion. Eur Spine J 1997;6(5):308–15.
20. Duval-Beaupere G, Robain G. Visualization on full spine radiographs of the anatomical connections of the centres of the segmental body mass supported by each vertebra and measured in vivo. Int Orthop 1987;11(3):261–9.
21. Duval-Beaupere G, Schmidt C, Cosson P. A barycentremetric study of the sagittal shape of spine and pelvis: the conditions required for an economic standing position. Ann Biomed Eng 1992; 20(4):451–62.
22. Legaye J, Duval-Beaupère G, Hecquet J, et al. Pelvic incidence: a fundamental pelvic parameter for three-dimensional regulation of spinal sagittal curves. Eur Spine J 1998;7(2):99–103.
23. Lazennec JY, Brusson A, Rousseau MA. Lumbar-pelvic-femoral balance on sitting and standing lateral radiographs. Orthop Traumatol Surg Res 2013;99(1 Suppl):S87–103.
24. Stagnara P, De Mauroy JC, Dran G, et al. Reciprocal angulation of vertebral bodies in a sagittal plane: approach to references for the evaluation of kyphosis and lordosis. Spine (Phila Pa 1976) 1982; 7(4):335–42.

25. Vaz G, Roussouly P, Berthonnaud E, et al. Sagittal morphology and equilibrium of pelvis and spine. Eur Spine J 2002;11(1):80–7.
26. Sariali E, Lazennec JY, Khiami F, et al. Modification of pelvic orientation after total hip replacement in primary osteoarthritis. Hip Int 2009;19(3):257–63.
27. Lazennec JY, Rousseau MA, Rangel A, et al. Pelvis and total hip arthroplasty acetabular component orientations in sitting and standing positions: measurements reproductibility with EOS imaging system versus conventional radiographies. Orthop Traumatol Surg Res 2011;97(4):373–80.
28. Papaioannou T, Stokes I, Kenwright J. Scoliosis associated with limb-length inequality. J Bone Joint Surg Am 1982;64(1):59–62.
29. Abe Y, Sato S, Abe S, et al. The impact of the leg-lengthening total hip arthroplasty on the coronal alignment of the spine. Scoliosis 2015;10(Suppl 2):S4.
30. Barrey C, Roussouly P, Le Huec JC, et al. Compensatory mechanisms contributing to keep the sagittal balance of the spine. Eur Spine J 2013;22(Suppl 6): S834–41.
31. Gelb DE, Lenke LG, Bridwell KH, et al. An analysis of sagittal spinal alignment in 100 asymptomatic middle and older aged volunteers. Spine (Phila Pa 1976) 1995;20(12):1351–8.
32. Jackson RP, Kanemura T, Kawakami N, et al. Lumbopelvic lordosis and pelvic balance on repeated standing lateral radiographs of adult volunteers and untreated patients with constant low back pain. Spine (Phila Pa 1976) 2000;25(5):575–86.
33. Jackson RP, McManus AC. Radiographic analysis of sagittal plane alignment and balance in standing volunteers and patients with low back pain matched for age, sex, and size. A prospective controlled clinical study. Spine (Phila Pa 1976) 1994;19(14): 1611–8.
34. Le Huec JC, Faundez A, Dominguez D, et al. Evidence showing the relationship between sagittal balance and clinical outcomes in surgical treatment of degenerative spinal diseases: a literature review. Int Orthop 2015;39(1):87–95.
35. Charosky S, Guigui P, Blamoutier A, et al. Complications and risk factors of primary adult scoliosis surgery: a multicenter study of 306 patients. Spine (Phila Pa 1976) 2012;37(8):693–700.
36. Lafage V, Schwab F, Patel A, et al. Pelvic tilt and truncal inclination: two key radiographic parameters in the setting of adults with spinal deformity. Spine (Phila Pa 1976) 2009;34(17):E599–606.
37. Baghdadi YM, Larson AN, Dekutoski MB, et al. Sagittal balance and spinopelvic parameters after lateral lumbar interbody fusion for degenerative scoliosis: a case-control study. Spine (Phila Pa 1976) 2014;39(3):E166–73.
38. Glassman SD, Berven S, Bridwell K, et al. Correlation of radiographic parameters and clinical

39. Moe JH, Denis F. The iatrogenic loss of lumbar lordosis. Orthop Trans 1977;1:131.
40. Swank SM, Mauri TM, Brown JC. The lumbar lordosis below Harrington instrumentation for scoliosis. Spine (Phila Pa 1976) 1990;15(3):181–6.
41. La Grone MO. Loss of lumbar lordosis. A complication of spinal fusion for scoliosis. Orthop Clin North Am 1988;19(2):383–93.
42. van Dam BE, Bradford DS, Lonstein JE, et al. Adult idiopathic scoliosis treated by posterior spinal fusion and Harrington instrumentation. Spine (Phila Pa 1976) 1987;12(1):32–6.
43. Aaro S, Ohlen G. The effect of Harrington instrumentation on the sagittal configuration and mobility of the spine in scoliosis. Spine (Phila Pa 1976) 1983; 8(6):570–5.
44. Stephens GC, Yoo JU, Wilbur G. Comparison of lumbar sagittal alignment produced by different operative positions. Spine (Phila Pa 1976) 1996;21(15): 1802–6 [discussion: 1807].
45. Godde S, Fritsch E, Dienst M, et al. Influence of cage geometry on sagittal alignment in instrumented posterior lumbar interbody fusion. Spine (Phila Pa 1976) 2003;28(15):1693–9.
46. Lafage V, Schwab F, Skalli W, et al. Standing balance and sagittal plane spinal deformity: analysis of spinopelvic and gravity line parameters. Spine (Phila Pa 1976) 2008;33(14):1572–8.
47. Byrd JW, Jones KS. Diagnostic accuracy of clinical assessment, magnetic resonance imaging, magnetic resonance arthrography, and intra-articular injection in hip arthroscopy patients. Am J Sports Med 2004;32(7):1668–74.
48. Pateder DB, Hungerford MW. Use of fluoroscopically guided intra-articular hip injection in differentiating the pain source in concomitant hip and lumbar spine arthritis. Am J Orthop (Belle Mead NJ) 2007;36(11): 591–3.
49. Prather H, Van Dillen LR, Kymes SM, et al. Impact of coexistent lumbar spine disorders on clinical outcomes and physician charges associated with total hip arthroplasty. Spine J 2012;12(5):363–9.
50. Murray DW. The definition and measurement of acetabular orientation. J Bone Joint Surg Br 1993; 75(2):228–32.
51. Wan Z, Malik A, Jaramaz B, et al. Imaging and navigation measurement of acetabular component position in THA. Clin Orthop Relat Res 2009;467(1):32–42.
52. Zhu J, Wan Z, Dorr LD. Quantification of pelvic tilt in total hip arthroplasty. Clin Orthop Relat Res 2010; 468(2):571–5.
53. Maratt JD, Esposito CI, McLawhorn AS, et al. Pelvic tilt in patients undergoing total hip arthroplasty: when does it matter? J Arthroplasty 2015;30(3): 387–91.

symptoms in adult scoliosis. Spine (Phila Pa 1976) 2005;30(6):682–8.

54. Lembeck B, Mueller O, Reize P, et al. Pelvic tilt makes acetabular cup navigation inaccurate. Acta Orthop 2005;76(4):517–23.

55. Lazennec JY, Boyer P, Gorin M, et al. Acetabular anteversion with CT in supine, simulated standing, and sitting positions in a THA patient population. Clin Orthop Relat Res 2011;469(4):1103–9.

56. Kanawade V, Dorr LD, Wan Z. Predictability of acetabular component angular change with postural shift from standing to sitting position. J Bone Joint Surg Am 2014;96(12):978–86.

57. Tiberi JV 3rd, Antoci V, Malchau H, et al. What is the fate of THA acetabular component orientation when evaluated in the standing position? J Arthroplasty 2015;30:1555–60.

58. Lewinnek GE, Lewis JL, Tarr R, et al. Dislocations after total hip-replacement arthroplasties. J Bone Joint Surg Am 1978;60(2):217–20.

59. Woo RY, Morrey BF. Dislocations after total hip arthroplasty. J Bone Joint Surg Am 1982;64(9): 1295–306.

60. Biedermann R, Tonin A, Krismer M, et al. Reducing the risk of dislocation after total hip arthroplasty: the effect of orientation of the acetabular component. J Bone Joint Surg Br 2005;87(6):762–9.

61. Pierchon F, Pasquier G, Cotten A, et al. Causes of dislocation of total hip arthroplasty. CT study of component alignment. J Bone Joint Surg Br 1994; 76(1):45–8.

62. Gallo J, Havranek V, Zapletalova J. Risk factors for accelerated polyethylene wear and osteolysis in ABG I total hip arthroplasty. Int Orthop 2010;34(1): 19–26.

63. Leslie IJ, Williams S, Isaac G, et al. High cup angle and microseparation increase the wear of hip surface replacements. Clin Orthop Relat Res 2009; 467(9):2259–65.

64. Esposito CI, Gladnick BP, Lee YY, et al. Cup position alone does not predict risk of dislocation after hip arthroplasty. J Arthroplasty 2015;30(1):109–13.

65. Reize P, Geiger EV, Suckel A, et al. Influence of surgical experience on accuracy of acetabular cup positioning in total hip arthroplasty. Am J Orthop (Belle Mead NJ) 2008;37(7):360–3.

66. Abdel MP, von Roth P, Jennings MT, et al. What safe zone? The vast majority of dislocated THAs are within the Lewinnek safe zone for acetabular component position. Clin Orthop Relat Res 2015. [Epub ahead of print].

67. Meftah M, Yadav A, Wong AC, et al. A novel method for accurate and reproducible functional cup positioning in total hip arthroplasty. J Arthroplasty 2013;28(7):1200–5.

68. McCollum DE, Gray WJ. Dislocation after total hip arthroplasty. Causes and prevention. Clin Orthop Relat Res 1990;(261):159–70.

69. Ezzet KA, McCauley JC. Use of intraoperative X-rays to optimize component position and leg length during total hip arthroplasty. J Arthroplasty 2014;29(3):580–5.

70. Hofmann AA, Bolognesi M, Lahav A, et al. Minimizing leg-length inequality in total hip arthroplasty: use of preoperative templating and an intraoperative x-ray. Am J Orthop (Belle Mead NJ) 2008; 37(1):18–23.

Robotically Assisted Unicompartmental Knee Arthroplasty with a Handheld Image-Free Sculpting Tool

Jess H. Lonner, MD

KEYWORDS

- Robotic • Unicompartmental knee arthroplasty • Treatment • Implant positioning
- Soft tissue balance

KEY POINTS

- Unicompartmental arthroplasty is a successful procedure for the treatment of focal arthritis or osteonecrosis of the medial or lateral compartments of the knee.
- This article reviews the next-generation robotic technology (an image-free handheld robotic sculpting tool), which offers an alternative method for optimizing implant positioning and soft tissue balance without the need for preoperative computed tomography (CT) scans and with price points that make it suitable for use in an outpatient surgery center.
- The Navio robotic sculpting system does not compromise precision or safety; it represents a considerable savings on multiple levels, including savings of time, inconvenience, and radiation exposure related to the elimination of the preoperative CT scan; savings on space requirements; and savings on capital and per-case costs.

INTRODUCTION

The popularity of unicompartmental knee arthroplasty (UKA) continues to grow, currently accounting for roughly 10% of all knee arthroplasty procedures; the percentage is anticipated to increase to more than 20% in the future.[1-3] The use of UKA increased between 1998 and 2005 at an average rate of 32.5% compared with the growth of 9.4% in the rate of total knee arthroplasty in the United States.[1] Interest in UKA continues to expand as an early intervention strategy and is viewed as a more conservative procedure than total knee arthroplasty, with better kinematics and functionability.[4,5] UKA is also a particularly relevant option when considering that our knee

replacement patients today tend to be more active, younger, and often present with an earlier stage of arthritis than in years past.[6] Even without expanding the appropriate surgical indications, a growing interest in outpatient knee arthroplasty procedures and the emerging use of surgery centers for UKA will likely increase training and endorsement of these procedures by a growing volume of surgeons.

Successful results and durability of UKA are affected by a variety of factors, including appropriate surgical indications, implant design, component alignment and fixation, and soft tissue balance. Early mechanical failure has been shown to occur in the setting of excessive posterior tibial slope or varus of the tibial component or both.[7-9]

This article is modified from: Lonner JH. Robotically assisted unicompartmental knee arthroplasty with a handheld image-free sculpting tool. Oper Tech Orthop 2015;25:104–13. Copyright © 2015 JH Lonner. Published by Elsevier Inc.

Rothman Institute, Department of Orthopedic Surgery, Thomas Jefferson University, 925 Chestnut Street, Philadelphia, PA 19107, USA

E-mail address: Jesslonner@comcast.net

Orthop Clin N Am 47 (2016) 29–40
http://dx.doi.org/10.1016/j.ocl.2015.08.024
0030-5898/16/$ – see front matter © 2016 Elsevier Inc. All rights reserved.

Achieving consistently accurate alignment of the tibial component in UKA using conventional approaches is difficult.[7,10–12] Outliers beyond 2° of the desired alignment may occur in as many as 40% to 60% of cases using conventional methods[12,13]; the range of component alignment varies considerably, even in the hands of skilled knee surgeons.[7] The problem is compounded when using minimally invasive surgical approaches.[10,11,14] In a study analyzing the results of 221 consecutive UKAs performed through a minimally invasive approach, tibial component alignment had a mean of 6° (standard deviation ±4) of varus and a range from 18° varus to 6° valgus.[11]

Computer navigation was introduced in an effort to reduce the number of outliers and improve the accuracy of UKA. Even with computer navigation, the incidence of outliers (beyond 2° of the preoperatively planned implant position) may approach 15% resulting from imprecision with the use of standard cutting guides and conventional methods of bone preparation.[12] Semiautonomous robotic guidance was, therefore, introduced to not only capitalize on the improvements seen with computer navigation but also to further refine and enhance the accuracy of bone preparation, even with minimally invasive techniques, by better interfacing and integrating the planning and performance of bone preparation.[13,15–24] Although the emergence of robotics in knee and hip arthroplasty has been gradual, semiautonomous robotic technology is currently being used in more than 15% of the UKA cases performed in the United States.[25] Enhanced precision and optimized outcomes have raised substantially the interest in semiautonomous robotics for UKA (and increasingly other procedures), but the challenge facing the robotics sector is to produce technologies that are also efficient and economically feasible. Although first-generation semiautonomous robotic technology was found to significantly improve precision and reduce error of bone preparation and component positioning in UKA, broader adoption of robotic technology was impeded by several factors: the high capital and maintenance costs of the first-generation systems; soft tissue complications observed with an autonomous (active) robotic system used for a brief time by several centers for total hip and knee arthroplasty primarily in Asia and Europe; skepticism regarding the importance of optimizing precision in UKA; expense, inconvenience, and delays associated with having to obtain preoperative computed tomography (CT) scans for planning and mapping; and concern regarding the potential carcinogenic risk associated with radiation exposure with CT-based planning.[18,20,26,27]

The story of the evolution of robotics in knee arthroplasty is a study in the characteristic pattern that defines technological progress and innovation, in general, whereby exponential developments occur along with declining capital and maintenance costs, smaller space requirements, broadening access, and increased use.[28] A newer image-free semiautonomous robotic technology (Navio PFS [Precision Free-Hand Sculptor], Blue Belt Technologies, Plymouth, MN) is an alternative to the first-generation autonomous and semiautonomous CT-based systems, with data in the first 1000 cases showing optimization of accuracy and no compromise of safety. This technology is reviewed herein.

NAVIO PRECISION FREE-HAND SCULPTOR SYSTEM OVERVIEW

The Navio PFS robotic system is a handheld image-free open-platform sculpting device available worldwide for assistance in UKA and patellofemoral arthroplasty (PFA), having received initial CE Mark and US Food and Drug Administration (FDA) clearances in February and December 2012, respectively (**Fig. 1**). This lightweight robotic tool combines image-free intraoperative registration, planning, and navigation with precise bone preparation and dynamic soft tissue balancing. As a semiautonomous system, it augments the surgeon's movements, with safeguards in place to optimize both accuracy and safety. The system continuously tracks the position of the patients' lower limb as well as the handheld burr, so that the limb position and degree of knee flexion can be changed constantly during the surgical procedure to gain exposure to different parts of the knee during registration and bone preparation through a minimally invasive approach.[29]

After percutaneous insertion of bicortical partially threaded pins into the proximal tibia and distal femur and attachment of optical tracking arrays, mechanical and rotational axes of the limb are determined intraoperatively by establishing the hip and knee centers and the center of the ankle. The kinematic, anteroposterior (Whiteside), or transepicondylar axes of the knee are identified and selected to determine the rotational position of the femoral component (**Fig. 2**). Osteophytes are excised, and the condylar anatomy is mapped out by painting the surfaces with the optical probes (**Fig. 3**). A virtual model of the knee is created (see **Fig. 3**). In this way, intraoperative mapping supplants the predicate system that required a preoperative CT scan.

A dynamic soft tissue balancing algorithm is initiated. With an applied valgus stress to tension

A

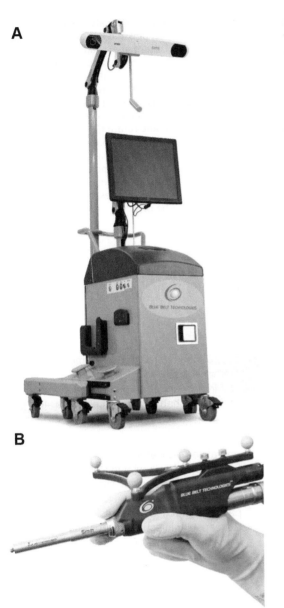

B

Fig. 1. (*A, B*) Navio PFS. (*Courtesy of* Blue Belt Technologies, Plymouth, MN).

balance (see **Fig. 5**). By adjusting the implant positions, including tibial slope, depth of resection, and anteriorization or distalization of the femoral component, virtual dynamic soft tissue balance can be achieved.

Either a 5- or 6-mm handheld sculpting burr is used to prepare the bone on the condylar surfaces (**Figs. 6** and **7**). Unlike its predecessors, Navio PFS does not rely on haptic feedback. Rather, it provides protective control against inadvertent bone removal by modulating the exposure and speed of the motorized burr. In exposure-control mode, the Navio PFS system modulates the exposure of the burr tip beyond the protective sheath. These position data are continuously updated in real time, resulting in fluid adjustments in position of the burr tip. In speed-control mode, the passive exposure guard is removed from the Navio PFS hand piece and the system modulates the rotational speed of the burr based on proximity to the target surface. This allows the burr to spin and remove the intended bone but slows and stops the burr when the tip has reached the final preparation position. Speed-control mode is ideal for preparing the lug holes, as the algorithms inherently allow the user to find the correct plunge trajectory, prevent cutting bone beyond the walls of a lug hole, and stop the burr from cutting bone at the bottom of the lug hole.

After bone preparation, the surfaces are assessed and trial components impacted into place for assessment of range of motion and stability. Limb alignment, range of motion, implant position, and gap balance can be quantified and compared with the preoperative plan (**Fig. 8**). If necessary, additional bone can be removed by making adjustments to slope or depth of resection in the surgical plan on the computer and then resculpting the bone surfaces. Once the knee is considered adequately aligned and balanced, the final components are cemented into place (**Figs. 9** and **10**).

PERIOPERATIVE MANAGEMENT

For most patients, UKA and PFA are performed on an outpatient basis, at either a surgery center or a hospital. Successful implementation of outpatient partial knee arthroplasties requires a good deal of preoperative preparation, medical risk stratification, patient education and expectation management, scheduling of postoperative physical therapy, commitment from the patient's family or friends to provide assistance after surgery, and prescription provision for venous thromboembolism prophylaxis, antibiotics, and pain management.

Intraoperative fluid management, minimization of intraoperative sedation, low-dose spinal

the medial collateral ligament (for medial UKA) or a varus stress to tension the lateral structures (for lateral UKA), the 3-dimensional positions of the femur and the tibia are captured throughout a passive range of knee motion and implant sizes, position, and orientation are virtually established (**Figs. 4** and **5**). A graphic representation of gap spacing through an entire range of flexion is created, and determination is made regarding whether the planned position of the femoral and tibial components is adequate or adjustments can be made to achieve the desired soft tissue

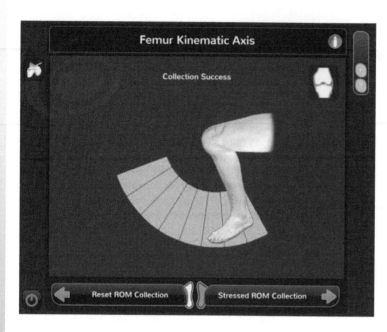

Fig. 2. After attachment of bicortical pins and optical trackers to the distal femoral and proximal tibial metaphyses, and establishment of the hip center and mechanical axes of the femur and tibia, the knee is flexed through a full range of motion to determine the kinematic rotational axis of the knee. This is the basis for establishing the rotational position of the femoral component. Alternatively, the anteroposterior or transepicondylar axes of the femur can be used.

anesthesia with bupivacaine, and perioperative nausea control are critical to secure early discharge. Standard-risk patients are typically discharged within 2 to 6 hours after surgery, and higher-risk patients can stay for 23 hours; occasionally patients are admitted overnight depending on circumstances. Patients are encouraged to ambulate immediately with a cane, crutches, or walker with immediate range-of-motion exercises initiated via an interactive Web-based program or simple preprinted handout. Formal outpatient physical therapy should be commenced within 2 to 5 days of surgery. Use of a cane can be terminated once patients recover adequate balance and strength. Many patients may be able to ambulate without a cane as soon as 2 to 3 weeks after surgery.

Effective postoperative pain management is one of the most important factors contributing to a successful UKA outcome. Patients whose pain is well controlled are more likely to participate in physical therapy, facilitate early hospital/surgery center discharge, and resume independent unassisted ambulation. Although perioperative protocols are reevaluated periodically and may evolve over time, the author's current protocol, which he has been using for the past few years, includes the following, unless contraindicated owing to allergy, medical comorbidity, age-related issues, or drug interactions:

Preoperative medications
- Celecoxib 200 mg daily is started 2 days before surgery.
- Oxycodone hydrochloride 10 mg is given the morning of surgery.
- Within 2 hours of surgery, patients are given acetaminophen 975 mg, celecoxib 400 mg, and pregabalin 75 mg (orally).

Intraoperative medications
- Spinal anesthesia with low-dose bupivacaine (7.5–10.0 mg) is used. Indwelling catheters, epidural anesthesia, and postoperative patient-controlled anesthesia are avoided.
- Pericapsular injections are given currently using either 40 mL of 0.5% ropivacaine or a combination of 30 mL of 0.5% plain bupivacaine and 266 mg of liposomal-based bupivacaine diluted in 40 mL of 0.9% saline (comparative study is ongoing).
- Tranexamic acid is administered intravenously (IV), using weight-adjusted dosing.
- Patients are well hydrated during surgery.

Postoperative medications
- Postoperatively, the goal is to avoid overuse of IV medications and narcotics. Although most patients are discharged within a few hours after surgery and do not require these additional medications, the author's preferred medications while in the surgical center or hospital include the following: standing orders of orally administered acetaminophen 650 mg, every 6 hours (starting 12 hours after first dose); pregabalin 75 mg every 12 hours (avoid in patients older than 80 years); and

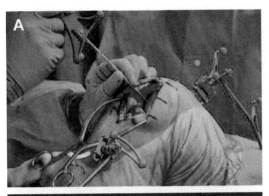

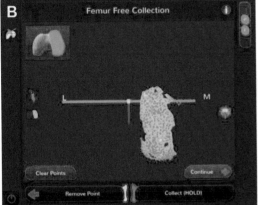

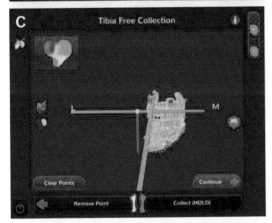

Fig. 3. Condylar anatomy is mapped out by painting the surfaces of the femoral condyle and tibial hemi-plateau with an optical probe: (*A*) intraoperative photograph, (*B*) mapping of the femoral surface, and (*C*) mapping of the tibial surface.

ketorolac tromethamine 30 mg IV every 6 hours (modify dose to 15 mg IV for elderly patients). For breakthrough pain, oxycodone immediate release 10 mg every 4 hours and tramadol 50 mg every 6 hours can be given orally as needed.

- Patients are discharged on oxycodone hydrochloride and acetaminophen 5/325 mg every 4 to 6 hours as needed.

- A compressive cold wrap with freezable gel packs is encouraged as an effective adjuvant to postoperative pain management.
- Ondansetron hydrochloride 4 mg 1 to 2 pills every 6 to 8 hours is given as needed for nausea.
- Some form of venous thromboembolism prophylaxis is recommended for 4 to 6 weeks. Most standard-risk patients are adequately protected with enteric-coated aspirin, 325 mg twice daily (with pantoprazole sodium 40 mg daily), although surgeons should use their preferred method of thromboprophylaxis. Higher-risk patients inject low-molecular-weight heparin 30 mg twice daily starting in the morning after surgery (12–24 hours postoperatively).
- For patients discharged home on the day of surgery, oral antibiotics are given for postoperative use, either cephalexin 500 mg or ciprofloxacin 500 mg, 1 pill taken at 8-hour intervals for 3 doses.

RESULTS

Several key preclinical and clinical studies have been completed and others are currently being conducted to evaluate robotically assisted UKA with the Navio sculptor.

In an initial feasibility study of Navio PFS, Smith and colleagues[30,31] assessed the accuracy of bone preparation in 20 synthetic lower extremities (10 right and 10 left) and found root-mean-square (RMS) errors across all angular orientations (flexion-extension, varus-valgus, and rotation) ranging from 1.05° to 1.52° for the femoral implant and 0.66° to 1.32° for the tibial implant. RMS translational errors averaged 0.61 mm, with a maximum of 1.18 mm. Mean surface overcut or undercut was 0.14 mm and 0.21 mm for the femoral and tibial surfaces, respectively.

A follow-up study by Lonner and colleagues[17] evaluated the precision of bone preparation using Navio PFS in 25 cadaveric specimens. The planned and actual angular, translational, and rotational positions of the components were compared. The RMS angular errors were 1.42° to 2.34° for the 3 directions for the femoral implant and 1.95° to 2.60° for the 3 directions of the tibial implant. The RMS translational errors were 0.92 to 1.61 mm for the femoral implant and 0.97 to 1.67 mm for the tibial implant. The results are further summarized in **Table 1**, with comparison made with other series reviewing the implant position with robotic and conventional technologies.

A clinical study by Picard and colleagues[32] reported on 65 patients undergoing medial UKA

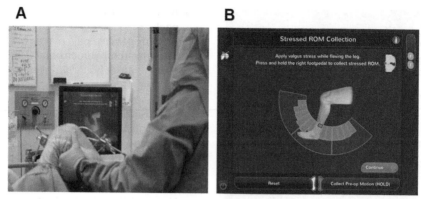

Fig. 4. After osteophyte excision, a dynamic soft tissue balancing algorithm is initiated. In the case of a medial UKA, a valgus stress is applied to tension the medial collateral ligament and other medially based soft tissues (*A*, *B*).

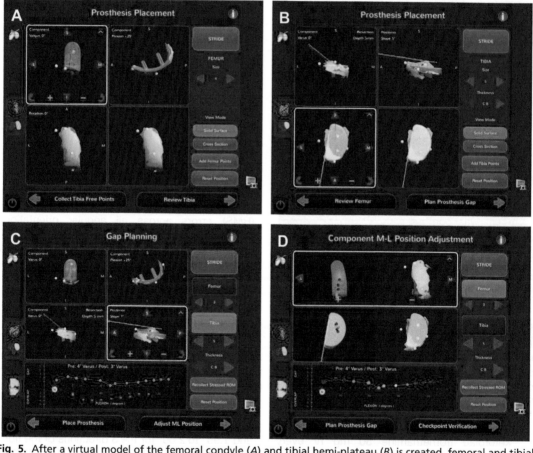

Fig. 5. After a virtual model of the femoral condyle (*A*) and tibial hemi-plateau (*B*) is created, femoral and tibial component sizes, alignment, and position are determined. Note in (*A*), the anterior-most edge of the femoral component would overhang slightly anteromedial to the tide mark of the medial femoral condyle. The plan was adjusted and the surface prepared for an implant one size smaller. A virtual graphic representation of gap spacing (relative laxity or tightness) is provided through a full range of motion, and an assessment can be made regarding the planned positions of the femoral and tibial components and anticipated correction of limb alignment (*C*). In this case, the plan determined that limb alignment would be corrected from 4° to 3° of mechanical varus. Contact points showing virtually where the femur is anticipated to be tracking on the tibia based on implant position and soft tissue balance are also shown (*D*). Adjustments in position can be made accordingly. M-L, medio-lateral.

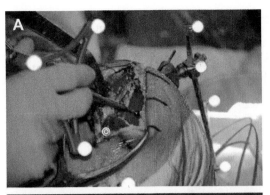

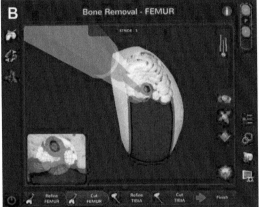

Fig. 6. Real-time (*A*) and virtual views (*B*) of femoral preparation with the 6-mm burr attached to the handheld robotic sculpting tool.

using Navio. The planned mechanical axis alignment was compared with the postsurgical alignment using full-length, double-stance, weight-bearing radiographs. The average preoperative alignment was 4.5° mechanical varus (standard deviation = 2.9°, range: 0–12° varus). The average postoperative mechanical axis was corrected to 2.1° (range: 0°–7° varus). The

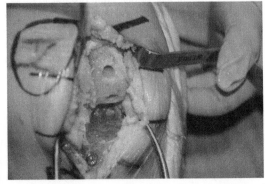

Fig. 7. Intraoperative view of the precisely prepared femoral and tibial surfaces.

postoperative mechanical axis alignment in the coronal plane was within 1° of the intraoperative plan in 91% of the cases. Of 6 cases with postoperative alignment greater than 1° from the plan, 3 resulted from an increase in the thickness of the tibial polyethylene insert implanted. The average difference between the planned intraoperative mechanical axis alignment and the postoperative long leg, weight-bearing mechanical axis alignment was 1.8°.

Surgeon endorsement and technology use in the case of joint arthroplasty requires proof of precision and safety; however, advances observed with innovative technologies must not substantially prolong surgical times or come at the expense of a lengthy learning curve to achieve the desired surgical outcome. A study by Gregori and colleagues[33] examined the number of surgeries required to reach the steady-state surgical time among 5 surgeons in consecutive UKA cases performed using the Navio robotic system. The surgeons had each performed at least 15 surgeries. *Steady state* was defined as the point in which 2 consecutive cases were completed within the 95% confidence interval of the surgeon's steady-state time. The average surgical time (tracker placement to trial acceptance) from all surgeons across their first 15 cases was 56.8 minutes (range: 27–102 minutes). The average improvement was 46 minutes from slowest to quickest surgical times, with the cutting phase decreasing on average by 31 minutes during the initial 15 cases. On average, it took 8 procedures (range: 5–11) to reach a steady-state surgical time. The average steady-state surgical time was 50 minutes (range: 37–55 minutes).

Schwarzkopf and colleagues[34] found that complexity of revision from UKA to total knee arthroplasty is substantially more challenging and the need for augments greater when a thicker polyethylene insert is used at the time of UKA. In an unpublished series, this author retrospectively compared the distribution of polyethylene insert sizes implanted using conventional and robotic-assisted techniques for UKA. Several manufacturers provided a listing of consecutive polyethylene insert sizes used in UKA. The analysis included 7902 robotic-assisted UKA cases and 27,989 conventional UKA cases. In the robotic and conventional groups, 8- and 9-mm polyethylene inserts were used in 94% and 85% of knees, respectively. Polyethylene inserts larger than 10 mm were used in 0.1% and 5.6% of robotic and conventional cases, respectively. Robotic-assisted UKA produced a maximum tibial resection of 11 mm; conventional UKA yielded a maximum polyethylene thickness of 14 mm. The

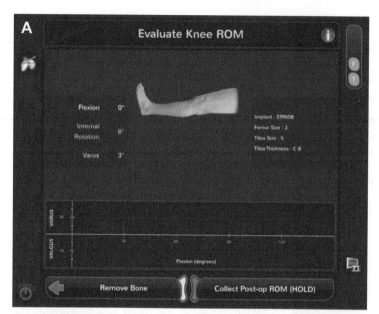

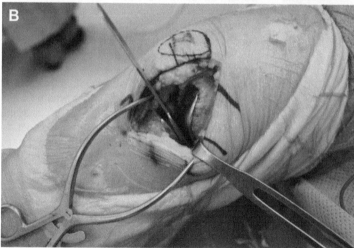

Fig. 8. (*A*, *B*) With trials in place, limb alignment and soft tissue balance are reconfirmed. In this case, final limb alignment in full extension is 3° varus, consistent with the preoperative plan (*A*). A 1- to 2-mm shim can be inserted to confirm reasonable balance through a range of motion (*B*).

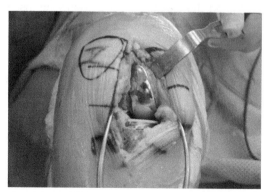

Fig. 9. Intraoperative appearance of medial UKA cemented into place.

percentage of polyethylene inserts of 10 mm or less was statistically significantly greater in cases performed with robotic assistance ($P<.0001$). No significant differences were noted in the percentages of polyethylene sizes between Navio and Mako (Mako, Stryker Mako, Fort Lauderdale, FL) cases.

CT technology has experienced expanded diagnostic and clinical applications in health care. However, emerging data are raising concerns regarding the potential carcinogenic risks from radiation exposure from CT scans and prompting discussion about whether the risks of radiation exposure are offset by their potential substantial medical benefits or whether alternative diagnostic studies and surgical procedures that do not require

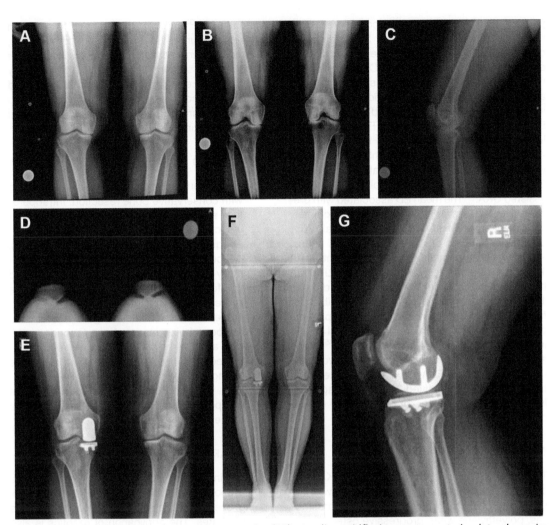

Fig. 10. (*A–G*) Standing preoperative anteroposterior (AP), standing midflexion posteroanterior, lateral, sunrise radiographs showing isolated anteromedial osteoarthritis of the right knee in a 58-year-old woman. (*E–G*) Standing postoperative AP, full-length AP, and lateral radiographs after medial UKA using Navio PFS.

Table 1
Summary of positioning: robotic techniques versus conventional

RMS Error	Mako Rio[19] (Stryker Mako, Fort Lauderdale, FL)	Acrobot[13] (Stanmore Implants, Elstree, UK)	Navio PFS[17]	Conventional[19]
Flex-ext (deg)	2.1	2.1	1.8	6.0
Varus-valgus (deg)	2.1	1.7	2.5	4.1
Int-ext (deg)	3.0	3.1	1.7	6.3
Prox-dist (mm)	1.0	1.0	1.3	2.8
Ant-post (mm)	1.6	1.8	1.3	2.4
Med-lat (mm)	1.0	0.6	1.0	1.6

Abbreviations: Ant-post, Anterior-posterior; deg, degrees; Flex-ext, Flexion-extension; Int-ext, Internal-external; Med-lat, Medial-lateral; mm, millimeter; Prox-dist, Proximal-distal.
Data from Refs.[13,17,19]

preoperative CT scans should be considered. In the realm of robot-assisted UKA, 2 systems are currently available for use in the United States: one that requires a preoperative CT scan for planning and one that does not. A study by Ponzio and Lonner[26] analyzed the radiation avoidance by switching from a CT scan–based system (Mako, Stryker Mako, Fort Lauderdale, FL) to the Navio image-free system discussed in this article. The effective dose (ED, millisievert [mSv]) of radiation was calculated from the preoperative CT scans of 211 patients (236 knees) undergoing Mako robot-assisted UKA.[26] The mean ED associated with preoperative CT was 4.8 ±3.0 mSv (approximately equivalent to 48 chest radiographs). Overall, 25% of patients had one or more additional CT scans, amounting to a cumulative ED per patient up to 103 mSv. Taken in the context that the US FDA has stated that an effective CT radiation dose of 10 mSv may be associated with the possibility of fatal cancer in approximately 1 in 2000 patients compared with the natural incidence of fatal cancer in the United States (≈1 chance in 5),[35] steps should be taken to mitigate exposure to avoidable radiation, as the US FDA has warned.[36] The radiation avoidance associated with the image-free Navio system is, thus, of substantial clinical consequence.

COMPLICATIONS

Typical complications observed after UKA with conventional techniques may also occur with robotic control, including loosening of the prostheses, polyethylene wear, progressive osteoarthritis of the unresurfaced compartments of the knee, infection, stiffness, instability, thromboembolic complications, and others.

Specific complications related to robot-assisted UKA include issues with pin placement, longer initial operative times, and case conversion owing to mechanical or hardware issues. The pin tracts for the optical tracking arrays create a stress riser in the cortical bone, which poses a risk for fracture; therefore, it is highly advised that the tracking pins be inserted in the metaphyseal regions of the femur and tibia rather than the diaphyses, to minimize the fracture risk.[37] Inadvertent pin placement could also theoretically cause neurovascular laceration. Most concerning, however, is the risk of inadvertent soft tissue complications during bone preparation with the robotic tool. A study by Chun and colleagues[38] reported the need to abandon 22% of cases using an autonomous robot-assisted technology. Overall, 5% were due to patellar tendon disruption; the remainder was a result of technical or mechanical glitches of

various sorts.[39] In contrast, the need to abandon the procedure with the semiautonomous, surgeon-driven technology used by this author has been less than 0.5%. Unlike the relatively high incidence of soft tissue injuries reported with autonomous systems, there have been no soft tissue injuries with the Navio semiautonomous robotic sculpting tool in the initial 1000 cases.

PEARLS AND PITFALLS

- Follow sound principles of implant positioning with conservative bone resection. Intraoperative adjustments can be made, but over-resection cannot be corrected.
- Adequate surgical exposure is critical. Although the procedure is amenable to minimally invasive techniques, the surgeon should comfortably visualize all aspects of the surgery.
- Trace the field before starting the burr. Ensure the bone being resected corresponds to the plan and makes sense before proceeding.
- Protect soft tissue structures with retractors during all aspects of the case.
- With the trial components in place, assess component position and kinematic balance of the knee. Make adjustments if necessary.

SUMMARY

Robotic innovation is a growing method of bone preparation and soft tissue balance for UKA, now being used in more than 15% of cases in the United States. The application of robotics is also expanding into other procedures, such as PFA, total hip arthroplasty, femoral acetabular impingement, spine surgery, and beyond, with anticipation that there will be continued growth of robotic use over the next few years. The Navio robotic sculpting system described in this review is a second-generation semiautonomous robot that, unlike its predecessors, does not require a preoperative CT scan. Without compromising precision or safety, Navio represents considerable savings on multiple levels, including savings of time, inconvenience, and radiation exposure related to the elimination of the preoperative CT scan; savings on space requirements; and savings on capital and per-case costs. These benefits are clear for the key stakeholders: payers, hospitals, surgeons, and patients. Navio dovetails nicely into the transition we are seeing nationwide whereby partial knee arthroplasties are increasingly being performed on an outpatient basis, with greater use in surgery centers rather than hospitals. Its reduced costs, small foot print, and diminished storage needs are perfectly suited for use in these outpatient centers.

Although it is anticipated that improved component alignment and quantified soft tissue balance achieved with this technology will translate to improved midterm and long-term outcomes and survivorship, we currently can only use these measures as surrogates for improved clinical outcomes. Prospectively tracking our patients will be necessary to determine whether the added precision of Navio will correlate with better durability. Proponents of semiautonomous robotics anticipate that functional outcomes, implant durability, and preservation of the adjacent tibiofemoral compartment will indeed be optimized with these technologies.

REFERENCES

1. Riddle DL, Jiranek WA, McGlynn FJ. Yearly incidence of unicompartmental knee arthroplasty in the United States. J Arthroplasty 2008;23:408–12.

2. Lonner JH. Modular bicompartmental knee arthroplasty with robotic arm assistance. Am J Orthop (Belle Mead NJ) 2009;38(Suppl 2):28–31.

3. Arno S, Maffei D, Walker PS, et al. Retrospective analysis of total knee arthroplasty cases for visual, histological, and clinical eligibility of unicompartmental knee arthroplasties. J Arthroplasty 2011;26: 1396–403.

4. Noticewala M, Geller J, Lee J, et al. Unicompartmental knee arthroplasty relieves pain and improves function more than total knee arthroplasty. J Arthroplasty 2012;27(Suppl 8):99–105.

5. Felts E, Parratte S, Pauly V, et al. Function and quality of life following medial unicompartmental knee arthroplasty in patients 60 years of age or younger. Orthop Traumatol Surg Res 2010;96:861–7.

6. Kurtz SM, Lau E, Ong K, et al. Future young patient demand for primary and revision joint replacement: national projections from 2010 to 2030. Clin Orthop Relat Res 2009;467:2606–12.

7. Collier MB, Eickmann TH, Sukezaki F, et al. Patient, implant, and alignment factors associated with revision of medial compartment unicondylar arthroplasty. J Arthroplasty 2006;21(6 Suppl 2):108–15.

8. Hernigou P, Deschamps G. Alignment influences wear in the knee after medial unicompartmental arthroplasty. Clin Orthop Relat Res 2004;(423):161–5.

9. Hernigou P, Deschamps G. Posterior slope of the tibial implant and the outcome of unicompartmental knee arthroplasty. J Bone Joint Surg Am 2004;86-A: 506–11.

10. Fisher DA, Watts M, Davis KE. Implant position in knee surgery: a comparison of minimally invasive, open unicompartmental, and total knee arthroplasty. J Arthroplasty 2003;18(7 Suppl 1):2–8.

11. Hamilton WG, Collier MB, Tarabee E, et al. Incidence and reasons for reoperation after minimally invasive unicompartmental knee arthroplasty. J Arthroplasty 2006;21(6 Suppl 2):98–107.

12. Keene G, Simpson D, Kalairajah Y. Limb alignment in computer-assisted minimally-invasive unicompartmental knee replacement. J Bone Joint Surg Br 2006;88:44–8.

13. Cobb J, Henckel J, Gomes P, et al. Hands-on robotic unicompartmental knee replacement: a prospective, randomised controlled study of the acrobot system. J Bone Joint Surg Br 2006;88:188–97.

14. Romanowski MR, Repicci JA. Minimally invasive unicondylar arthroplasty: eight-year follow-up. J Knee Surg 2002;15:17–22.

15. Lonner JH. Indications for unicompartmental knee arthroplasty and rationale for robotic arm-assisted technology. Am J Orthop (Belle Mead NJ) 2009; 38(Suppl 2):3–6.

16. Sinha RK. Outcomes of robotic arm-assisted unicompartmental knee arthroplasty. Am J Orthop (Belle Mead NJ) 2009;38(Suppl 2):20–2.

17. Lonner JH, Smith JR, Picard F, et al. High degree of accuracy of a novel image-free handheld robot for unicondylar knee arthroplasty in a cadaveric study. Clin Orthop Relat Res 2015;(473):206–12.

18. Conditt MA, Bargar WL, Cobb JP, et al. Current concepts in robotics for the treatment of joint disease. Adv Orthop 2013;2013:948360.

19. Dunbar NJ, Roche MW, Park BH, et al. Accuracy of dynamic tactile-guided unicompartmental knee arthroplasty. J Arthroplasty 2012;27:803–8.e1.

20. Lang JE, Mannava S, Floyd AJ. Specialty update: general orthopaedics: robotic systems in orthopaedic surgery. J Bone Joint Surg Br 2011;93:1296–9.

21. Lonner JH, John TK, Conditt MA. Robotic arm-assisted UKA improves tibial component alignment: a pilot study. Clin Orthop Relat Res 2010;(468):141–6.

22. Conditt MA, Roche MW. Minimally invasive robotic-arm-guided uni-compartmental knee arthroplasty. J Bone Joint Surg Am 2009;91(Suppl 1):63–8.

23. Roche M, O'Loughlin PF, Kendoff D, et al. Robotic arm-assisted unicompartmental knee arthroplasty: preoperative planning and surgical technique. Am J Orthop (Belle Mead NJ) 2009;38(Suppl 2):10–5.

24. Swank ML, Alkire M, Conditt M, et al. Technology and cost effectiveness in knee arthroplasty: computer navigation and robotics. Am J Orthop (Belle Mead NJ) 2009;38(Suppl 2):32–6.

25. Orthopedic Network News. Hip and knee implant review. 2013. Available at: www.OrthopedicNetwork News.com. 24, 2013.

26. Ponzio DY, Lonner JH. Preoperative mapping in unicompartmental knee arthroplasty using computed tomography scans is associated with radiation exposure and carries high cost. J Arthroplasty 2015;30(6):964–7.

27. Lonner JH. Robotically assisted unicompartmental knee arthroplasty. In: Austin MS, Klein GR, editors. World clinics: orthopedics: current controversies in joint replacement. Philadelphia: Jaypee Brothers Medical Publishers LTD; 2014. p. 120–34.

28. Brynjolfsson E, McAfee A. The second machine age: work, progress, and prosperity in a time of brilliant technologies. New York: W.W. Norton & Company; 2014.

29. Lonner JH. Robotically-assisted unicompartmental knee arthroplasty with a hand-held image-free sculpting tool. In: Ranawat AS, Satalich J, editors. Operative techniques in orthopaedics, vol. 25. New York: Elsevier; 2015. p. 104–13.

30. Smith JR, Picard F, Rowe PJ. The accuracy of a robotically-controlled freehand sculpting tool for unicondylar knee arthroplasty. J Bone Joint Surg Br 2013;95(Suppl):68.

31. Smith JR, Riches PE, Rowe PJ. Accuracy of a free-hand sculpting tool for unicondylar knee replacement. Int J Med Robot 2014;10:162–9.

32. Picard F, Gregori A, Bellemans J, et al. Handheld robot-assisted unicondylar knee arthroplasty: a clinical review. 14th annual meeting of the International Society for Computer Assisted Orthopaedic Surgery. Milan, Italy, June 18-21, 2014.

33. Gregori A, Picard F, Bellemans J et al. The learning curve of a novel handheld robotic system for unicondylar knee arthroplasty. 14th annual meeting of the International Society for Computer Assisted Orthopaedic Surgery. Milan, Italy, June 18-21, 2014.

34. Schwarzkopf R, Mikhael B, Li L. Effect of initial tibial resection thickness on outcomes of revision UKA. Orthopedics 2013;36:e409–14.

35. Radiation-emitting products. Available at: http://www.fda.gov/Radiatio n-EmittingProducts/Radiation EmittingProductsandProcedures/default. htm. Accessed February 25, 2014.

36. Initiative to reduce unnecessary radiation exposure from medical imaging, 2010. Available at: http://www.fda.gov/Radiation-Emitting Products/Radiation Safety/RadiationDoseReduction/ucm199904.htm. Accessed February 20, 2014.

37. Wysocki RW, Sheinkop MB, Virkus WW, et al. Femoral fracture through a previous pin site after computer-assisted total knee arthroplasty. J Arthroplasty 2008;23:462–5.

38. Chun YS, Kim KI, Cho YJ, et al. Causes and patterns of aborting a robot-assisted arthroplasty. J Arthroplasty 2011;26:621–5.

39. Honl M, Dierk O, Gauck C, et al. Comparison of robotic-assisted and manual implantation of a primary total hip replacement. A prospective study. J Bone Joint Surg Am 2003;85-A:1470–8.

Does Malrotation of the Tibial and Femoral Components Compromise Function in Kinematically Aligned Total Knee Arthroplasty?

Alexander J. Nedopil, MD[a],*, Stephen M. Howell, MD[b],
Maury L. Hull, PhD[c]

KEYWORDS

- Knee arthroplasty • Internal and external rotation • Malrotation of components
- Kinematic alignment • Oxford knee and WOMAC scores • Function

KEY POINTS

- Association between femoral component rotation and function.
- Association between tibial component rotation and function.
- WOMAC and Oxford Knee Score determined function.
- High function after kinematic aligned total knee arthroplasty.
- Weak association between component rotation bounded by the ranges reported in the present study and function.

INTRODUCTION

Internal and external (I-E) malrotation of the femoral and tibial components is associated with poor function after total knee arthroplasty (TKA).[1,2] In mechanically aligned TKA, there are several reference lines in use to minimize I-E malrotation of the femoral and tibial components. Three reference lines used to set I-E rotation of the femoral component are

1. The line parallel to the anterior-posterior (A-P) axis of the trochlear groove,
2. The line parallel to the transepicondylar axis, or
3. The line 3° externally rotated to the posterior condylar line of the femur.[3]

Four reference lines used to set I-E rotation of the tibial component are

1. The line between the most medial and most lateral points of the plateau,
2. The line between the medial one-third of the tubercle and the center of the PCL attachment,
3. The line between the medial border of the tubercle and the PCL, and
4. The line between the projection of the anterior crest and the PCL.[4]

Disclosures: The authors have not received grant support or research funding and do not have any proprietary interests in the materials described in the article.
[a] Department of Orthopaedics, University of California, Davis, 4860 Y Street, Suite 3800, Sacramento, CA 95817, USA; [b] Department of Biomedical Engineering, University of California, Davis, Sacramento, CA 95817, USA; [c] Department of Mechanical Engineering, University of California, Davis, Sacramento, CA 95817, USA
* Corresponding author.
E-mail address: nedopil@ucdavis.edu

orthopedic.theclinics.com

However, the range of I-E malrotation of the femoral component ($-13°$ internal to $16°$ external; SD $\pm 7°$) and of the tibial component ($-44°$ internal to $46°$ external; SD $\pm 28°$) reported for these reference lines is high, which indicates the placement of these lines is not reproducible.[3,4]

Kinematic alignment is a new method that has gained interest because 2 studies showed that patients with a kinematically aligned TKA reported better pain relief, better function, better flexion, and a more normal-feeling knee than patients with a mechanically aligned TKA.[5,6] The goal of kinematic alignment is to correct the arthritic deformity of the limb to the constitutional alignment of the patient with the intent of positioning the femoral and tibial components so that the natural tibial-femoral articular surface, alignment, and laxities of the knee are restored. This is accomplished in part by setting the A-P axes of the femoral and tibial components parallel to the flexion-extension (F-E) plane of the extended knee (**Fig. 1**). The F-E plane of the extended knee is aligned perpendicular to the F-E axis of the tibia that connects the 2 centers of the circular portion of the posterior femoral condyles from about $20°$ to $120°$ and parallel to the F-E axis of the patella and the natural distal and posterior femoral joint lines.[7–13]

Surgically, the A-P axis of the femoral component is set parallel to the F-E plane of the extended knee by placing a $0°$ rotation posterior referencing guide in contact with the posterior femoral condyles at $90°$ and removing posterior femoral resections within ± 0.5 mm of the thickness of the condyles of the femoral component after compensating for cartilage wear and kerf.[14] Surgically, the A-P axis of the tibial component is set parallel to the F-E plane of the extended knee by aligning the A-P axis of the tibial component parallel to the major axis of the elliptical-shaped boundary of the lateral tibial condyle (**Fig. 2**).[15] However, there are no data reporting the range of I-E malrotation of the femoral and tibial components when these methods of rotational alignment are used to perform a kinematically aligned TKA.

The objectives of the present study were to determine the range of I-E malrotation for both components in a case series of patients treated with a kinematically aligned TKA and then determine whether the degree of I-E malrotation of the femoral and tibial components compromised function as measured by the Oxford Knee Score (OKS) and the Western Ontario and McMaster Universities Osteoarthritis Index (WOMAC) score.

METHODS

An institutional review board approved the analyses of 101 consecutive patients (101 knees) treated with a primary kinematically aligned TKA from June to September, 2012, by an inventor surgeon (S.M.H.) who were prospectively followed for 6 months. When feasible, patients were scheduled for a preoperative MRI scan to evaluate cartilage wear and plan the thickness of the posterior resections from the femur. Thirty patients were excluded because they were unable to have our protocol preoperative MRI because of a pacemaker, hardware about the knee, insurance refused to authorize, or an MRI had been performed with a different protocol. The indications for performing kinematically aligned TKA were

1. Disabling knee pain and functional loss unresolved with standard of care, nonoperative, treatment modalities;
2. Radiographic evidence of advanced arthritis indicated by a Kellgren-Lawrence grade of 3 or 4; and
3. Any severity of varus and valgus deformity and flexion contracture.

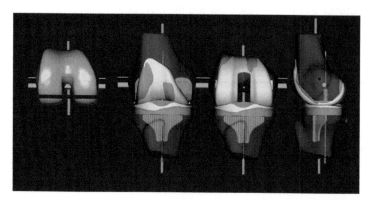

Fig. 1. A right femur with posterior femoral resections equal in thickness to the condyle of the femoral component and 3 views of a kinematically aligned TKA. The green line in the femur is the F-E axis of the tibia. The magenta line in the femur is the F-E axis of the patella. The orange line is parallel to the F-E plane of the extended knee, which is perpendicular to the F-E axis of the tibia, the F-E axis of the patella, and a line tangent to the distal and posterior femoral condyles.

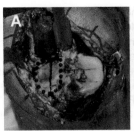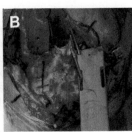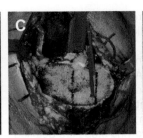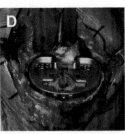

Fig. 2. Intraoperative proximal view of a right tibia and the surgical steps for kinematically aligning the I-E rotation of the A-P axis of the tibial component parallel to the F-E plane of the extended knee. The black dots outline the boundary of the articular surface of the lateral tibial condyle, and the blue line is the approximate long axis connecting the most anterior and distal points on the boundary (*A*). Two pins are drilled parallel to the blue line through the articular surface of the medial tibial condyle with a guide (*B*). On the cut surface of the tibia, 2 lines are drawn parallel to the 2 drill holes (*C*). The rotation of the A-P axis of the tibial component is set parallel to these 2 lines (*D*).

Seventy-one patients (71 knees) with an average (SD) age of 68 ± 8.6 years, of whom 30 were men, met our inclusion criterion and were included in the analysis (**Table 1**). The number (percent) of patients with a 5° to 10° varus deformity was 22 (31%), 11° to 15° varus deformity was 18 (26%), greater than 16° varus deformity was 9 (12%), 10° to 15° valgus deformity was 12 (17%), 16° to 20° valgus deformity was 7 (10%), and greater than 20° valgus deformity was 3 (4%). Patient-reported OKS and WOMAC score at 6 months determined function. Function was measured at 6 months because the New Zealand Joint Registry 2014 showed that 6-month OKSs predict the revision rate at 2 years and the function at 5 years.[16]

The preoperative MRI scan was obtained in an oblique sagittal plane oriented parallel to the F-E plane of the extended knee with a 1.5-T scanner and a dedicated knee coil (General Electric Medical Systems, Milwaukee, WI, USA). The F-E plane of the extended knee is perpendicular to F-E axes of the tibia and patella, and the distal and posterior joint lines of the femur.[17] The following parameters were used: fast-relaxation fast-spin-echo proton density, echo time, 30 to 35 milliseconds, repetition time, 2800 to 3400 milliseconds; bandwidth, 31.25 Hz; a minimum of 2 excitations with a

Table 1
Preoperative demographics and clinical characteristics for the patients treated in the present study

Preoperative Demographics and Clinical Characteristics	Number of Patients or Knees	Mean (SD) or Number (%)	Range
Demographics			
Age (years)	N = 71	68 (8.6)	45–86
Sex (male)	N = 30	42%	—
Body mass index (kg/m²)	N = 71	31 (5.1)	19–42
Anesthesia Society of Anesthesiologists Score (ASA) (1 is best, 4 is worst)	N = 71	1 (0%), 2 (69%), 3 (23%), 4 (8%)	—
Preoperative motion and deformity			
Extension (degrees)	N = 69	11 (8.2)	0–40
Flexion (degrees)	N = 69	112 (9.5)	80–150
Varus (+)/valgus (−) deformity (degrees)	N = 71	1 (13.5)	−30–20
Preoperative function and mental scores			
Oxford Score (48 is best, 0 is worst)	N = 69	23 (7.7)	3–36
Knee Society Score (100 is best, 0 is worst)	N = 69	34 (11.7)	8–74
Knee Function Score (100 is best, 0 is worst)	N = 69	52 (17.8)	0–100
SF-12 Physical Score (50 average)	N = 68	29 (6.1)	14–47
SF-12 Mental Score (50 average)	N = 68	53 (10.4)	24–68

16-cm field of view centered at the joint line of the knee, 256 × 224 matrix; slice thickness, 2 mm; and no spacing/gap.

Each kinematically aligned TKA was performed with US Food and Drug Administration-approved generic instruments and cruciate-retaining, fixed-bearing components (Triathlon; Stryker, Inc, Mahwah, NJ, USA), and with a technique previously described.[14,15,18] The following steps are detailed because they set the varus-valgus (V-V), proximal-distal (P-D), I-E, A-P, and F-E locations of the femoral and tibial components when performing kinematically aligned TKA.

For the placement of the femoral component, the V-V and P-D locations of the distal femoral resection were set using an offset distal femoral referencing guide that contacted the distal medial and lateral femoral condyles. The offset was selected to compensate for 2 mm of cartilage wear on the worn condyle(s), which corrected the V-V deformity caused by wear. The P-D level of the distal femoral resection was set so that the thickness of the resections of the distal medial and lateral femoral condyles equaled the condylar thickness of the femoral component after compensating for cartilage wear and kerf.[14,19] The A-P and I-E locations of the posterior femoral resection were set parallel to the F-E plane of the extended knee by placing a 0° rotation posterior referencing guide in contact with the posterior femoral condyles at 90° and removing posterior femoral resections within ± 0.5 mm of the thickness of the condyles of the femoral component after compensating for cartilage wear and kerf.[14] The thickness of each posterior resection was measured with a caliper. Over or under resection of 1 or 2 mm was corrected by adjustment of the position of the chamfer block and then performing the anterior and chamfer cuts to hold the new position of the femoral component. Compensation for cartilage and bone wear at 90° on the posterior femoral condyles was rarely needed when treating grade 3 and 4 Kellgren-Lawrence osteoarthritic knees.[19]

For the placement of the tibial component, the V-V, P-D, and F-E locations of the tibial resection were set using an extramedullary tibial guide and an angel wing inserted in the saw slot alongside the medial border of the tibia. The V-V position of the tibial component was set by medial translation of the slider at the ankle section of the guide until the saw slot was parallel to the tibial articular surface after a visual compensation for cartilage and bone wear. When the extension gap was asymmetric or trapezoidal, the V-V angle of the tibial resection was fine-tuned in increments of 1° to 2° until the gap was symmetric and V-V laxity was eliminated. Elimination of the V-V laxity with the knee in extension minimized any confounding effect that the V-V angles of the resection might have had on I-E rotation of the components. The F-E position of the tibial component was set by adjustment of the slope of the tibial guide until the angel wing was parallel to the slope of the medial joint line. The P-D position of the tibial component was set by adjustment of the level of the saw slot to remove enough tibia to accommodate a 10-mm-thick tibial component.[14] The I-E rotation of the A-P axis of the tibial component was set parallel to the F-E plane of the extended knee by alignment of the A-P axis parallel to the long axis of the boundary of the lateral tibial condyle (see Fig. 2).[15] The long axis was defined as the line connecting the most anterior and posterior points on the boundary. In all cases, the patella was resurfaced and all components were cemented. A 1.25-mm thick axial computed tomography (CT) scan of the hip, knee, and ankle was performed on each patient before discharge using a previously described technique.[15,20]

The following technique computed the I-E malrotation of the A-P axis of the femoral and tibial components from the F-E plane of the extended knee using free image-analysis software (OsiriX Imaging Software, http://www.osirix-viewer.com) by 1 author (A.J.N.) blinded to the function scores (Fig. 3). The CT scan was opened with the 3D MPR tool. The axial view was optimized by orienting the image plane tangential to the distal surface of the tibial baseplate, which required adjustment of the P-D and V-V plane in the coronal window and adjustment of the F-E plane in the sagittal window. The DICOM export tool was used to export the optimized axial plane of the knee at a 1.25-mm slice thickness. The axial images of the preoperative MRI and postoperative CT scans were opened side by side. The P-D level of each scan was adjusted until the projection of the femoral epicondyles on the MRI and CT scans matched. The matched images were linked with the sync tool. The femoral reference line connecting the medial and lateral epicondyles was drawn on the MRI and CT scan. The P-D level was adjusted until the posterior condylar axis of the tibia was viewed on the MRI and CT scans. The tibial reference line was drawn tangent to the posterior tibia on the MRI and CT scans. The P-D level was adjusted until the largest dimension of the intercondylar notch was viewed on the MRI scan. A line parallel to the F-E axis of the extended knee was drawn perpendicular to the posterior condylar axis of the femur. The P-D level was adjusted until the lugs on the femoral component were viewed on the CT scan. The A-P axis of the femoral component was drawn perpendicular to a line connecting the lugs. The P-D

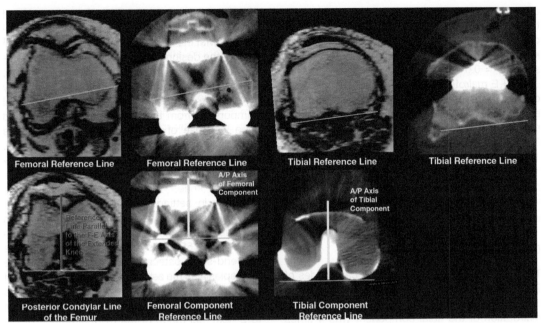

Fig. 3. Matched axial views of the femur and tibia on the preoperative MRI and postoperative CT scans. The femoral reference line connects the femoral epicondyles. The tibial reference line connects the posterior tibial condyles. The reference line perpendicular to the posterior condylar line of the femur on the MRI is parallel to the F-E plane of the extended knee. The A-P axis of the femoral component is perpendicular to the femoral component reference line. The A-P axis of the tibial component is perpendicular to the tibial component reference line.

level was adjusted until the posterior border of the tibial component or liner was viewed on the CT scan. The A-P axis of the tibial component was drawn perpendicular to a line tangent to the posterior condylar axis of the tibial component or liner. On the MRI scan, the angle between the femoral and the tibial reference lines and the line parallel to the F-E plane of the extended knee was computed. On the CT scan, the angle between the femoral reference line and the A-P axis of the femoral component was computed. On the CT scan, the angle between the tibial reference line and the A-P axis of the tibial component was computed. These angles enabled the determination of the I-E malrotation of the A-P axis of the femoral and tibial components on the CT scan from the line parallel to the F-E axis of the extended knee on the MRI scan (+ indicated external and − indicated internal malrotation of the components from the F-E plane of the extended knee).

Statistical Analysis

The reproducibility of the measurement of the I-E malrotation of the femoral and tibial components from the F-E plane of the extended knee was determined by computing the intraclass correlation coefficient (ICC) with use of measurements

made on 10 randomly selected knees by 2 observers. The arithmetic mean, SD, and 95% confidence interval (CI) of the mean and SD were computed for each measured quantity when appropriate (JMP, 10.02, http://www.jmp.com). A simple regression determined the strength of the association between the I-E malrotation of the femoral and tibial component from the F-E plane of the extended knee and patient-reported function (OKS and WOMAC score). Significance was $P < .05$.

RESULTS

The ICC of 0.91 for the measurement of I-E malrotation of the femoral component and the ICC of 0.97 for the measurement of I-E malrotation of the tibial component indicated high (first class) measurement reproducibility.

The best achievable OKS is 48 (range 0–48), and the mean patient-reported OKS was 42 ± 4.5 (95% CI, 41.2 to 43.4). The best achievable WOMAC score is 100 (range 0–100), and the mean WOMAC score was 89 ± 9.7 (95% CI, 86.7–91.3).

The I-E malrotation of the A-P axis of the femoral component ranged from −3° internal to 2° external (mean 0.3° ± 1.1°; 95% CI of the mean, 0°–0.6°; 95% CI of the SD, 0.9°–1.3°) from the F-E plane of the extended knee. There was a weak association between the I-E malrotation of the femoral component from the F-E plane of the extended knee and the OKS (r^2 = 0.0284) and the WOMAC score (r^2 = 0.011) (**Fig. 4**).

The I-E malrotation of the A-P axis of the tibial component ranged from −11° internal to 12° external (mean −1.0° ± 5.4°; 95% CI of the mean, −2.3° to 0.30°; 95% CI of the SD, 4.7°–6.5°) from the F-E plane of the extended knee. There was a weak association between the I-E malrotation of the tibial component from the F-E plane of the extended knee and the OKS (r^2 = 0.0265) and the WOMAC score (r^2 = 0.0256) (**Fig. 5**).

DISCUSSION

The most important findings in this case series of 71 patients treated with a kinematically aligned, cruciate-retaining TKA were that the range of I-E malrotation of the tibial component was 4 times greater than the range of I-E malrotation of the femoral component, and that the range of I-E malrotation of the femoral component from −3° internal to 2° external and the range of I-E malrotation of the tibial component from −11° internal to 12° external were not associated with compromised function as measured by the OKS and WOMAC score.

Six limitations should be discussed as they could affect the generalization of the findings. First, the range of I-E malrotation of the femoral and tibial components is specific for both kinematically aligned TKA performed with generic instruments and the specific design of the tibial liner used in the present study that had a fairly flat articular surface that might accommodate tibial malrotation better than more constrained designs. Accordingly, these results might not apply to mechanically aligned TKA and tibial liners with a more constrained tibial articular surface. Second, the present study used an MR imaging plane that was rotationally aligned parallel to the F-E plane of the extended knee.[17] The use of an MR imaging plane not rotationally aligned parallel to the F-E plane of the extended knee might yield different results from the present study. Third, although the New Zealand Joint Registry has shown that a high self-reported OKS at 6 months prognosticates a low revision rate at 2 years and high function at 5 years, the present study's functional analysis at 6 months is only predictive and does not determine long-term patient function and survival of the implant.[16] However, the reported mid-term outcomes of the kinematic alignment TKA surgical technique at a mean of 6.3 years

(range, 5.8–7.2 years) had a survivorship of 97.5% and an average OKS of 43, which is comparable with the score of 42 in the present study.[21] Fourth, the design features of the femoral component and tibial insert may affect the results. Fifth, the unique method described in the present study to compute I-E rotation of the femoral and tibial components from the F-E plane of the extended knee with use of MRI and CT images requires additional clinical evaluation and validation. Finally, dysplasia of a femoral condyle, in particular the lateral femoral condyle in the valgus osteoarthritic knee, could adversely affect the accuracy in setting the I-E rotation of the A-P axis of the femoral component when a 0° rotation posterior referencing guide is used. However, an analysis of 155 varus and 44 valgus deformities with end-stage osteoarthritis showed no evidence of dysplasia as the asymmetry between the radii of the medial and lateral femoral condyles was ≤0.2 mm.[17] In the present study, the −3° internal to 2° external range of the I-E malrotation of the 59 varus and 22 valgus deformities confirms that dysplasia, if present, had a negligible clinical effect on setting the I-E rotation of the A-P axis of the femoral component parallel to the F-E plane of the extended knee.

The present study strived to align the I-E rotation of the femoral component parallel to the F-E plane of the extended knee, which is a less variable and a different alignment target than the 3 femoral reference lines used in mechanical alignment. Eleven arthroplasty surgeons each working with 10 cadaveric specimens reported that identifying the mechanical alignment femoral reference lines resulted in high variability as shown by the range of −11° internal to 16° external rotation for the transepicondylar axis, −12° internal to 15° external rotation for the A-P axis of the trochlear groove, and −10° internal to 12° external rotation for the line 3° externally rotated from the posterior condylar line.[4] These mechanical alignment femoral reference lines are neither parallel nor perpendicular to the F-E plane of the extended knee, and when used may cause a ≥2 mm instability in a compartment between 0° and 90° of flexion that is uncorrectable by a collateral ligament release in 42% to 80% of knees.[7,22,23] In contrast, the −3° internal to 2° external range of malrotation of the femoral component for a single arthroplasty surgeon in the present study was 4 to 5 times narrower. Because the limits of agreement of −1.9° to 2.2°, defined as the mean ± 2 SDs, are small enough to be clinically unimportant in terms of function, because the use of a posterior referencing guide is straightforward, and because the use of caliper is a simple check that the

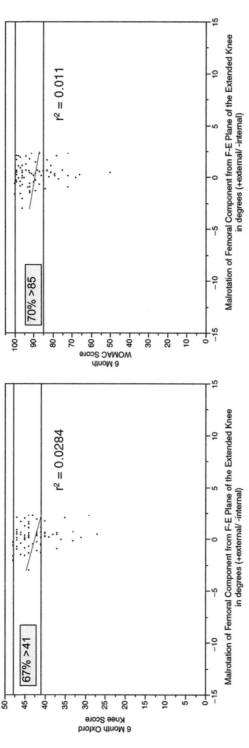

Fig. 4. Scatterplots show the weak association of the malrotation of the femoral component, which ranges from −3° internal to 2° external from the F-E plane of the extended knee, and the OKS (r^2 = 0.0284) and the WOMAC score (r^2 = 0.011) at 6 months. Percentages indicate the proportion of patients with a function score greater than the indicated value.

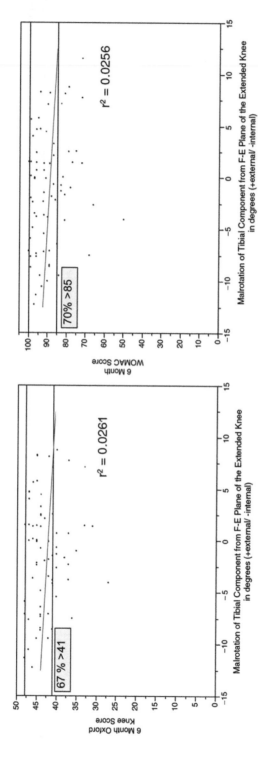

Fig. 5. Scatterplots show the weak association of the malrotation of the tibial component, which ranges from −11° internal to 12° external from the F-E plane of the extended knee, and the OKS ($r^2 = 0.0265$) and the WOMAC score ($r^2 = 0.0256$) at 6 months. Percentages indicate the proportion of patients with a function score greater than the indicated value.

intraoperative thickness of each posterior resection is correct, the ranges of agreement might not inflate to a clinically important level when this alignment method is used by other surgeons.

The present study strived to align the I-E rotation of the A-P axis of the tibial component parallel to the F-E plane of the extended knee with use of the long axis of the boundary of the articular surface of the lateral tibial condyle, which is a less variable and different target than the tibial reference lines commonly used in mechanical alignment. Eleven arthroplasty surgeons each working with 10 cadaveric specimens reported that identifying the mechanical alignment tibial reference lines resulted in high variability as shown by the range from −43° internal to 42° external rotation for the line connecting the center of the posterior cruciate ligament fossa to the medial border of the tibial tubercle, range from −40° internal to 46° external rotation for the line connecting the center of the posterior cruciate ligament fossa to the medial one-third of the tibial tubercle, and range from −20° internal to 32° external rotation for the line connecting the center of the posterior cruciate ligament fossa to the most anterior point of the tibial tubercle.[3] The mechanical alignment tibial reference lines that reference the tibial tubercle are not useful landmarks when the goal is to set the I-E rotation of the A-P axis of the tibial component parallel to F-E plane of the extended knee because there is 15 mm of mediolateral variability of the location of the tibial tubercle on the tibia.[18] In contrast, the method used in the present study to set I-E rotation of the tibial component, which yielded a −11° internal to 12° external range, was 2 to 3 times narrower. Although the limits of agreement of −7.4° to 10.4° are small enough to be clinically unimportant in terms of function, the use the long axis of the boundary of the articular surface of the lateral tibial condyle to set the I-E rotation of the tibial component requires intraoperative judgment and the ranges of agreement might inflate to a clinically important level when this alignment method is used by other surgeons.

In summary, even though the range of I-E malrotation of the tibial component can be 4 times greater than the range of I-E malrotation of the femoral component, this degree of I-E malrotation does not compromise function in kinematically aligned TKA with use of a fairly flat tibial articular surface. Hence, surgeons analyzing CT scans of kinematically aligned TKA should understand that I-E malrotation of the femoral and tibial components that are bounded by the ranges reported in the present study are compatible with a well-functioning TKA.

REFERENCES

1. Barrack RL, Schrader T, Bertot AJ, et al. Component rotation and anterior knee pain after total knee arthroplasty. Clin Orthop Relat Res 2001;(392):46–55.
2. Windsor RE, Scuderi GR, Moran MC, et al. Mechanisms of failure of the femoral and tibial components in total knee arthroplasty. Clin Orthop Relat Res 1989;(248):15–9 [discussion: 19–20].
3. Siston RA, Goodman SB, Patel JJ, et al. The high variability of tibial rotational alignment in total knee arthroplasty. Clin Orthop Relat Res 2006;452:65–9.
4. Siston RA, Patel JJ, Goodman SB, et al. The variability of femoral rotational alignment in total knee arthroplasty. J Bone Joint Surg Am 2005;87(10): 2276–80.
5. Dossett HG, Estrada NA, Swartz GJ, et al. A randomised controlled trial of kinematically and mechanically aligned total knee replacements: two-year clinical results. Bone Joint J 2014;96-B(7): 907–13.
6. Nam D, Nunley RM, Barrack RL. Patient dissatisfaction following total knee replacement: a growing concern? Bone Joint J 2014;96-B(11 Suppl A):96–100.
7. Eckhoff DG, Bach JM, Spitzer VM, et al. Three-dimensional mechanics, kinematics, and morphology of the knee viewed in virtual reality. J Bone Joint Surg Am 2005;87(Suppl 2):71–80.
8. Hollister AM, Jatana S, Singh AK, et al. The axes of rotation of the knee. Clin Orthop Relat Res 1993;(290):259–68.
9. Iwaki H, Pinskerova V, Freeman MA. Tibiofemoral movement 1: the shapes and relative movements of the femur and tibia in the unloaded cadaver knee. J Bone Joint Surg Br 2000;82(8):1189–95.
10. Pinskerova V, Iwaki H, Freeman MA. The shapes and relative movements of the femur and tibia at the knee. Orthopade 2000;29(Suppl 1):S3–5.
11. Weber WE, Weber EFM. Mechanik der menschlichen Gehwerkzeuge. Göttingen (Germany): Verlag der Dietrichschen Buchhandlung; 1836.
12. Coughlin KM, Incavo SJ, Churchill DL, et al. Tibial axis and patellar position relative to the femoral epicondylar axis during squatting. J Arthroplasty 2003; 18(8):1048–55.
13. Iranpour F, Merican AM, Dandachli W, et al. The geometry of the trochlear groove. Clin Orthop Relat Res 2010;468(3):782–8.
14. Howell SM, Papadopoulos S, Kuznik KT, et al. Accurate alignment and high function after kinematically aligned TKA performed with generic instruments. Knee Surg Sports Traumatol Arthrosc 2013;21(10): 2271–80.
15. Nedopil AJ, Howell SM, Rudert M, et al. How frequent is rotational mismatch within 0±10 in kinematically aligned total knee arthroplasty? Orthopedics 2013;36(12):e1515–20.

16. Listed NA. The New Zealand joint registry fourteen year report. Available at: http://www.nzoa.org.nz/nz-joint-registry. Accessed December 20, 2014.

17. Howell SM, Howell SJ, Hull ML. Assessment of the radii of the medial and lateral femoral condyles in varus and valgus knees with osteoarthritis. J Bone Joint Surg Am 2010;92(1):98–104.

18. Howell SM, Chen J, Hull ML. Variability of the location of the tibial tubercle affects the rotational alignment of the tibial component in kinematically aligned total knee arthroplasty. Knee Surg Sports Traumatol Arthrosc 2013;21(10):2288–95.

19. Nam D, Lin KM, Howell SM, et al. Femoral bone and cartilage wear is predictable at 0 degrees and 90 degrees in the osteoarthritic knee treated with total knee arthroplasty. Knee Surg Sports Traumatol Arthrosc 2014;22(12):2975–81.

20. Bedard M, Vince KG, Redfern J, et al. Internal rotation of the tibial component is frequent in stiff total knee arthroplasty. Clin Orthop Relat Res 2011;469(8):2346–55.

21. Howell SM, Papadopoulos S, Kuznick K, et al. Does varus alignment adversely affect implant survival and function six-years after kinematically aligned total knee arthroplasty? Int Orthop 2015. [Epub ahead of print].

22. Eckhoff D, Hogan C, DiMatteo L, et al. Difference between the epicondylar and cylindrical axis of the knee. Clin Orthop Relat Res 2007;461:238–44.

23. Gu Y, Roth JD, Howell SM, et al. How frequently do four methods for mechanically aligning a total knee arthroplasty cause collateral ligament imbalance and change alignment from normal in white patients? J Bone Joint Surg Am 2014;96(12):e101.

The Utility of Increased Constraint in Primary Total Knee Arthroplasty for Obese Patients

Mohan S. Tripathi, MD[a], Colin C. Heinle, MD[a],
Moiz I. Manaqibwala, MD[a], Alfred J. Tria Jr, MD[b],*

KEYWORDS

- Primary TKA • Obese patients • Constrained condylar knee • Complications • Longevity

KEY POINTS

- Total knee arthroplasty for the obese patient is associated with a greater number of preoperative comorbidities, more perioperative complications, and a shorter longevity than the patient with a normal body mass index.
- The purpose of this retrospective study is to determine if the clinical result and longevity of the constrained implant in the obese patient is the same as that of the normal weight patient with a standard prosthesis.
- The constrained condylar knee for obese patients facilitates the operative procedure by improving the intramedullary alignment of the prosthesis and supporting the surrounding soft tissues. The clinical results are similar to standard implants in the nonobese with similar longevity at midterm follow-up.

INTRODUCTION

According to the World Health Organization (WHO), obesity is a global epidemic and incidence is expected to surpass undernutrition.[1] In the United States, 1 in 3 adults are obese.[2] Furthermore, obesity is an independently recognized modifiable risk factor for the development and progression of osteoarthritis (OA).[3,4] Compared with normal weight patients, obese patients have a 3-fold to 5-fold increased risk of developing knee OA.[5,6] It is thought that increased body mass results in increased forces across a joint, thus progressing[7] OA. Other studies demonstrate that arthritis has earlier onset in the obese than that shown by radiographic progression.[8]

Total knee arthroplasty (TKA) in the obese patient presents a challenge for both the patient and the surgeon. Obesity is associated with several systemic medical comorbidities, including type II diabetes, obstructive sleep apnea, cardiovascular disease, cancer, and other musculoskeletal pathologic conditions.[1,9–11] Compared with nonobese patients, obese patients have longer operative times, longer hospital stays, and higher morbidity and mortality.[6,10,12]

The surgery, itself, can be fraught with difficulty. Intraoperatively, the increased adiposity makes dissection and retraction of soft tissues more difficult and obscures bony landmarks typically needed for extramedullary alignment techniques.

Disclosure: The senior author receives consulting and royalty fees from Smith and Nephew Orthopedics unrelated to the topic of this paper.
[a] Department of Orthopaedic Surgery, Rutgers-Robert Wood Johnson Medical School, 1 Robert Wood Johnson Place, MEB 401, New Brunswick, NJ 08901, USA; [b] Department of Orthopaedic Surgery, The Orthopaedic Center of New Jersey, St. Peter's University Hospital, 1527 State Highway 27, Suite 1300, Somerset, NJ 08873, USA
* Corresponding author.
E-mail address: Atriajrmd@aol.com

Orthop Clin N Am 47 (2016) 51–55
http://dx.doi.org/10.1016/j.ocl.2015.08.007
0030-5898/16/$ – see front matter © 2016 Elsevier Inc. All rights reserved.

Together, these factors can contribute to component malalignment and may portend a worse outcome. Additionally, postoperative periprosthetic joint infection (PJI) is of great concern to both the patient and surgeon. Obese patients have 3.3 to 9.0 times higher prevalence of PJI than the normal weight patient.[13–15]

Component alignment is critical to a successful TKA. A study by Werner and colleagues[16] suggests that as little as 3° of malalignment of the mechanical axis can result in altered load distribution between the medial and lateral compartments of the implant. In obese patients, increased forces borne by the implant coupled with improper component alignment may ultimately predispose a prosthetic joint to premature failure. Given the difficulty with extramedullary alignment techniques in the obese, a combination of intramedullary cutting guides as well as intramedullary prosthetic stems for both the tibial and femoral components can support correct alignment in the coronal plane (**Fig. 1**).

Furthermore, the obese knee can have a decreased arc of motion compared with a nonobese knee secondary to the excess adipose tissue on the posterior aspect of the lower extremity. This excess adipose may cause the thigh to contact the calf at 100° (or less) of flexion (**Fig. 2**). This decrease in the thigh-to-calf angle leads to abnormal forward pressure on the posterior tibia as the knee flexes (**Fig. 3**). When a posterior stabilized knee design is used, the tibia will shift forward with forced flexion and the polyethylene post can dislocate beneath the femoral cam. The posterior stabilized constrained condylar knee (CCK) designs include increased constraint in the coronal plane as well as a higher post with increased jump distance for dislocation. Given the increase in thigh girth, this additional constraint may prevent dislocation.

In the present study, a CCK implant was used in all of the obese patients (body mass index [BMI] >30), both for the added stability in the sagittal plane and for coronal alignment in the operating room. The intramedullary stems also decrease the total surgical time by facilitating the positioning of the components with respect to the intramedullary canals.

The authors sought to answer 2 questions with our study: Would the obese patients have similar clinical results (as defined by the Knee Society Scores and designated complications) and would the CCK allow similar longevity compared with a matched group of normal weight patients with a standard primary posterior stabilized knee implant?

MATERIALS AND METHODS

Ninety consecutive records were reviewed of patients who had a BMI greater than 30, resulting in a total of 100 knees. There were 10 bilateral surgeries. The operations were performed from 1996 to 2000. All of the obese knees were replaced with CCK-type prostheses. The prosthesis was chosen if the patient BMI was greater than 30 and if the range of motion of the knee was limited at its end by the thigh touching the calf (ie, a mechanical block secondary to the soft tissues impinging on themselves in flexion; see **Fig. 2**). Ninety-two consecutive patient records were reviewed for patients undergoing primary TKA with a BMI of 30 or less during the same time period. There were 8 bilateral surgeries in this group. All of the normal weight TKAs were performed with a posterior stabilized primary TKA. The charts were reviewed for standard patient-identifying data. Preoperative comorbidities were recorded, including obesity, cardiac disease (myocardial infarction, hypertension, arrhythmia, pacemaker), diabetes, respiratory disease (asthma, chronic obstructive pulmonary disease, sleep apnea), gastrointestinal disease, renal disease, and cancer. The postoperative physical examination findings, Knee Society Scores, and radiograph summaries were reviewed and all revisions were recorded.

Statistical Methods

Data analysis was performed using SPSS software (version 16.0; Chicago, Illinois). The data were checked for normality using the Shapiro-Wilk W-test. The comparison between groups

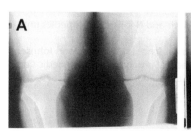
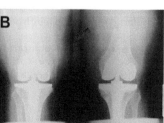

Fig. 1. (*A, B*) The preoperative and postoperative anteroposterior radiographs of a bilateral TKA in an obese patient.

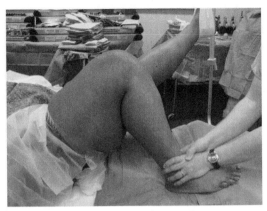

Fig. 2. The thigh-to-calf limitation in the obese patient.

used the Student's t-test. The comparison between the preoperative and postoperative data of each group used the paired t-test for the normal distribution and the Wilcoxon test for skewed data. A P value of less than 0.05 was considered to be significant. The confidence interval at certain points was calculated with the Greenwood formula.

RESULTS

The obese group included 100 knees, 57 right and 43 left. There were 85 female and 15 male knees. Ten patients underwent bilateral surgery. The comparison group included 100 knees, 51 right and 49 left. There were 73 female and 27 male knees, with 8 bilateral surgeries.

Table 1 summarizes the results. There were 3 reoperations in the obese group: 1 prosthetic loosening, 1 incision and drainage for a superficial infection, and 1 proximal realignment for a

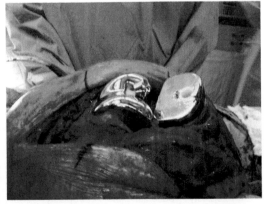

Fig. 3. The tibial component is shifted anteriorly as the obese leg is flexed on the operating room table.

dislocating patella without component malalignment. There was 1 revision for loosening in the control group and 1 manipulation for decreased range of motion.

DISCUSSION

The obese patients were younger, perhaps because of the stress on the knee joints or due to a greater degree of perceived pain (lower Knee Society preoperative pain score). The higher preoperative comorbidities were expected. The decreased range of motion was primarily due to the thigh-to-calf angle limitation. Although the obese function score was not equal to that of the control group, the postoperative pain scores were the same. The complications and the revisions were the same.

The literature has expressed a strong concern for the use of constrained implants in a primary setting because of decreased motion in all 3 planes of the knee and possible resultant loosening of the device. The obese patients in this study did not experience increased failures or complications related to the use of the constrained knee. The obese are often less active than their normal weight counterparts and this decreased activity may partially account for the similar longevity.

We asked 2 questions for this study. First, would the postoperative clinical results be the same? The pain relief was equal but the function level did not improve to that of the controls. In the obese patients the knee disease is probably not the only factor leading to functional limitation. The complications were not different and there were no deep infections or tibiofemoral dislocations. Second, would the CCK implant, itself, lead to a shorter longevity with the additional constraint? There was only 1 revision for loosening and that was the same for the control group. There were no other impending failures noted. The follow-up is only midterm (2–12.5 years) but certainly supports use of the device.

Most papers report compromised results in the obese patients with increased complications, infections, and early revision. The CCK device in the obese makes the alignment and balancing of the knee easier with the intramedullary stems and the constrained post. The timely operative procedure combined with the increased stability decreases the complications around the time of surgery with no compromise in the longevity at midterm. The authors conclude that the CCK represents a viable choice for TKA in the obese.

Table 1
Comparison of 100 obese patients who underwent primary TKA with a constrained condylar prosthesis with 100 nonobese patients who underwent primary TKA with a standard knee prosthesis

	Obese	Nonobese	P Value<.05 Significant
BMI	40.7 (Range 31–55)	26.4 (Range 22–30)	<0.001
Average Age	59 y (Range 45–70)	65 y (Range 45–75)	<0.001
Comorbidities	2.3	0.9	<0.001
Preoperative ROM	113°	117°	<0.001
Change in ROM	+6.1°	+2.4°	0.013
Surgical Time	96.min	79.min	0.015
Knee Society Preoperative Pain	39	43	0.004
Knee Society Postoperative Pain	96	96	—
Change in Knee Society Pain	57	53	0.005
Knee Society Preoperative Function	33	39	<0.001
Knee Society Postoperative Function	79	83	0.03
Change in Knee Society Function	46	44	0.49
Average Length of Follow-up	6.9 y	6.1 y	0.02
Complications	8	8	—
Reoperations	3	2	—
Average Preoperative Radiograph Varus	6.3°	5.6°	0.15
Average Preoperative Radiograph Valgus	11.2°	8.3°	<0.001
Average Postoperative Valgus Alignment	All 3°–7°	All 3°–7°	—

Abbreviation: ROM, range of motion.

REFERENCES

1. [Internet]Obesity: preventing and managing the global epidemic. World Health Organization; 2004. Available at: www.who.int/nutrition/publications/obesity/WHO_TRS_ 894/en/index.html. Accessed July 10, 2015.
2. Ogden CL, Carroll MD, Flegal KM. Prevalence of obesity in the United States. JAMA 2014;312(2):189–90.
3. Salih S, Sutton P. Obesity, knee osteoarthritis and knee arthroplasty: a review. BMC Sports Sci Med Rehabil 2013;5(1):25.
4. Bijlsma JW, Berenbaum F, Lafeber FP. Osteoarthritis: an update with relevance for clinical practice. Lancet 2011;377(9783):2115–26.
5. Blagojevic M, Jinks C, Jeffery A, et al. Risk factors for onset of osteoarthritis of the knee in older adults: a systematic review and meta-analysis. Osteoarthritis Cartilage 2010;18(1):24–33.
6. Odum SM, Springer BD, Dennos AC, et al. National obesity trends in total knee arthroplasty. J Arthroplasty 2013;28(8 Suppl):148–51.
7. Wang Y, Simpson JA, Wluka AE, et al. Relationship between body adiposity measures and risk of primary knee and hip replacement for osteoarthritis: a prospective cohort study. Arthritis Res Ther 2009; 11(2):R31.
8. Sridhar MS, Jarrett CD, Xerogeanes JW, et al. Obesity and symptomatic osteoarthritis of the knee. J Bone Joint Surg Br 2012;94(4):433–40.
9. Chesney D, Sales J, Elton R, et al. Infection after knee arthroplasty a prospective study of 1509 cases. J Arthroplasty 2008;23(3):355–9.
10. Bray GA. Overweight is risking fate. Definition, classification, prevalence, and risks. Ann N Y Acad Sci 1987;499:14–28.
11. Flegal KM, Graubard BI, Williamson DF, et al. Excess deaths associated with underweight, overweight, and obesity. JAMA 2005;293(15):1861–7.
12. Turgeon TR, Santore RF, Coutts RD, editors. Influence of obesity on outcome following primary hip replacement surgery. Presented at the Annual Meeting of the Hip Society. Iowa City (IA), September 2006.
13. Namba RS, Paxton L, Fithian DC, et al. Obesity and perioperative morbidity in total hip and total knee arthroplasty patients. J Arthroplasty 2005; 20(7 Suppl 3):46–50.

14. Dowsey MM, Choong PF. Obese diabetic patients are at substantial risk for deep infection after primary TKA. Clin Orthop Relat Res 2009;467(6): 1577–81.

15. Malinzak RA, Ritter MA, Berend ME, et al. Morbidly obese, diabetic, younger, and unilateral joint arthroplasty patients have elevated total joint arthroplasty infection rates. J Arthroplasty 2009; 24(6 Suppl):84–8.

16. Werner FW, Ayers DC, Maletsky LP, et al. The effect of valgus/varus malalignment on load distribution in total knee replacements. J Biomech 2005;38(2):349–55.

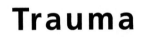

Trauma

Preface
Going Out with a Bang

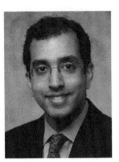

Saqib Rehman, MD
Editor

You may have noticed the unusually large size of this issue of the *Orthopedic Clinics of North America*, and the trauma section has eight articles on an assortment of contemporary issues facing surgeons who care for injured patients.

Whereas most surgeons in developed countries have the luxury of fluoroscopic-assisted intramedullary nailing, this technology is simply not available in much of the developing world. The SIGN program has allowed surgeons in developing nations, where trauma is a growing health care burden, to provide interlocked medullary nailing. Dr Zirkle and coauthors share their extensive experience with their techniques in this issue of the *Orthopedic Clinics of North America*.

Nonunions are challenging problems to treat even without infection and bone loss. Drs Brinker and O'Connor share their insights and management tips in their review article entitled "Management of Aseptic Tibial and Femoral Diaphyseal Nonunions Without Bony Defects."

Fractures about the knee and elbow, such as patellar, distal femur, and elbow fractures, require a thorough appreciation of the local biomechanics and fixation options. Patellar fractures, often considered relatively straightforward problems, do not do as well as we seem to think. Drs Kakazu and Archdeacon give their tips and techniques to try and help you achieve good results. Similarly, Drs Gangavalli and Nwachuku review the surgical management options to optimize results when treating distal femur fractures. Dr Jennings and coauthors review the complexities of adult elbow fracture dislocations and their management strategies.

The Morel Lavallée lesion is frequently diagnosed late, or when not missed, is simply difficult to manage. Dr Greenhill and colleagues review this important condition that should be recognized early by surgeons who treat orthopedic trauma patients.

Upper extremity amputations leave patients extremely disabled and can present to surgeons who are not accustomed to managing these injuries acutely. Preservation of limb length is arguably even more critical than in the lower extremity, and Dr Solarz and coauthors review this topic in their review article.

Minimizing intraoperative blood loss continues to be an important issue in orthopedic practice and research. Tranexamic acid has emerged as a therapeutic option in other disciplines of surgery, but its use in orthopedics has been relatively limited. Dr Jennings and colleagues review this therapy and its applications and potential in orthopedic surgery and trauma.

This is my last issue editing the trauma section, and I hope you enjoy it as much as I have enjoyed working with the surgeon-author community and the editors at the *Orthopedic Clinics of North America*.

Saqib Rehman, MD
Department of Orthopaedic Surgery
Temple University Hospital
3401 North Broad Street
Philadelphia, PA 19140, USA

E-mail address:
Saqib.rehman@tuhs.temple.edu

Orthop Clin N Am 47 (2016) xxi
http://dx.doi.org/10.1016/j.ocl.2015.10.005
0030-5898/16/$ – see front matter © 2016 Published by Elsevier Inc.

Interlocked Intramedullary Nail Without Fluoroscopy

Lewis G. Zirkle, MD[a],*, Faseeh Shahab, MBBS[b],
Shahabuddin, MBBS, FCPS (Ortho)[c]

KEYWORDS

- Education • Appropriate implants • Visual versus tactile sense • SIGN family of surgeons
- Interlocked intramedullary nail • Fluoroscopy

KEY POINTS

- Education and implants that can be used without power equipment are key to enable interlocked intramedullary nailing without fluoroscopy in developing countries.
- The same implants and instruments are used to treat all long bone fractures.
- Open reduction is usually necessary.
- Results of Surgical Implant Generation Network surgery are equivalent to series of other implants in developed countries.

ORTHOPEDIC CLINICS: INTERLOCKED INTRAMEDULLARY NAIL WITHOUT FLUOROSCOPY

Five key points must interconnect to enable interlocked intramedullary nailing without fluoroscopy in developing countries:

- Patients who need this technology
- Skilled surgeons who understand the need for intramedullary nail interlocking screw system to treat their patients
- Appropriate implants designed to be used in austere environments
- Appropriate instruments designed for these implants and other conditions in austere environments
- Education for the surgeons using these implants and instruments
- Validation of surgical results using these implants and instruments.

Increasing Numbers of Patients with High-Energy Fractures

The numbers of patients in developing countries who need stabilization of high-energy fractures due to road traffic accidents are predicted to increase 67% by the year 2020. Every year, 20 to 50 million people are injured or disabled by road traffic accidents.[1] Global conflicts are causing increasing numbers of fractures. Blast injuries are an extreme example of high-energy open

Disclosure Statement: L.G. Zirkle (president and founder of SIGN Fracture Care International) does not receive any payment or financial benefits. He is on the International Humanitarian Committee of OTA and is a reviewer for Journal of Bone and Joint Surgery. F. Shahab does not receive any financial benefits and has no disclosures. Shahabuddin does not receive any financial benefits and has no disclosures. Hospitals receive free-of-cost implants from SIGN Fracture Care International.

[a] SIGN Fracture Care International, 451 Hills Street, Suite B, Richland, WA 99354, USA; [b] Rehman Medical Institute, House 146, Street 7, Sector P-1, Phase 4, Hayatabad, Peshawar, Pakistan; [c] Department of Orthopaedics and Traumatology, Lady Reading Hospital, House 146, Street 7, Sector P-1, Phase 4, Hayatabad, Peshawar, Pakistan
* Corresponding author.
E-mail address: lewis.zirkle@signfracturecare.org

Orthop Clin N Am 47 (2016) 57–66
http://dx.doi.org/10.1016/j.ocl.2015.08.008
0030-5898/16/$ – see front matter © 2016 Elsevier Inc. All rights reserved.

fractures. The SIGN system is being used to treat civilians in Iraq, Afghanistan, Syria, South Sudan, and Pakistan, and is used in hospitals in 48 other developing countries.

Collaboration with Surgeons in Developing Countries

The development of the SIGN system has been facilitated by the combined efforts of many surgeons throughout the world. These surgeons work hard to treat the increasing number of severe fractures. They work hard because there are not enough orthopedic surgeons in developing countries.

Not only do these surgeons have an increasing number of patients with high-energy fractures to treat but treatment of these fractures is more difficult because the patients often have surgeries 2 to 6 weeks after injury. Surgical reduction of these fractures takes longer as the number of patients awaiting surgery increases (**Fig. 1**).

SIGN was originally designed for stabilization of tibia fractures because a delay in treating an open tibia fracture has serious consequences for the patient. In developing countries, the patient and the family must purchase their implant before surgery can be done. This delays surgery while the funds for the implant are gathered by the family. SIGN was founded when we observed the need to combine education with the appropriate implants to implement the education. In 2011, 2.8 billion people in the world were living on less than 2 dollars per day and, therefore, could not afford the proper implant to stabilize the fracture.[2]

Often, no fluoroscopy is available. Surgeons must use tactile sense to substitute for the visual images seen on C-arm screens. They feel vibrations coming from the far end of the instrument

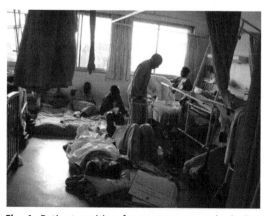

Fig. 1. Patients waiting for surgery occupy beds that could be used for other patients. (*Courtesy of* SIGN Fracture Care International; with permission.)

and internally visualize the location of the far end of the instrument instead of concentrating on the near end of the instrument while looking at a fluoroscopy image. For example, during reaming, they recognize the tactile difference as the increasing size of the reamers become tighter in the canal and produce chatter. They place the interlocking screws accurately and efficiently using instruments designed to be guided by tactile sense.

Surgical Implant Generation Network Technique for Tibial Nailing

The SIGN technique can be used in treatment of a high-energy tibia fracture or fractures of the femur and humerus.

A fractured tibia can be treated by closed reduction within 1 week of injury (**Fig. 2**). Tactile sense facilitates this reduction. The hand reamers and nail are passed across the fracture site using vibratory sense. Development of tactile sense is procedural memory similar to riding a bicycle. The vibrations from the seat and handlebars keep us from falling off. This ability to feel vibrations and discern their meaning is not easily forgotten. Procedural memory allows a person to return to riding a bicycle years later without falling.

Reduction is accomplished by closed methods if possible. It is very difficult to reduce a fractured tibia closed 10 days after surgery. The fracture is stressed in all directions before attempting reduction; these maneuvers are repeated during reaming and placement of the nail. The surgeon has a baseline of instability before reduction and can judge when the reamers and the nail have been inserted past the fracture site.

The bone entrance is made through a longitudinal incision in the patella tendon. A guidewire is not used to determine the proper location because there is no fluoroscopy. The bone entrance is made with a curved awl that is also used to contour the channel anteriorly for 4 cm. This anterior channel created by the curved awl makes posterior penetration of the nail less likely. The fat pad is not disturbed.

The 7 to 9 mm reamers are pointed and the 10 to 14 mm reamers are blunt tipped (**Fig. 3**). The reamers are guided down the canal using tactile sense. If the tibia fracture is in the proximal third, the **Fig. 4**position is used for reaming and placement of the nail. Pressure is placed posteriorly on the proximal fracture if the fracture site is apex anterior. A blocking screw can be used for proximal tibia fractures; however, it is usually not necessary using **Fig. 4** position. After the pointed reamers have been passed, the surgeon passes the blunt-tipped reamer through the fracture site,

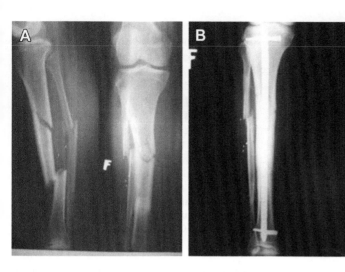

Fig. 2. (*A, B*) Closed tibia fracture reduced by closed reduction. (*Courtesy of* SIGN Fracture Care International; with permission.)

stopping at the subchondral bone. This maneuver is used to determine the length of the nail. Reaming continues until chatter occurs for 4 cm in the canal. The nail chosen is 1 to 2 mm smaller than the largest reamer used. Advantages of hand reaming include

- The bone from the flutes of the reamers is saved and placed in the fracture site if an open reduction is done
- The canal is contoured for a straight nail due to the progressive increasing size of the reamer shaft and tip; 3-point fixation occurs with the straight nail and curved canal.

The SIGN nail is a solid, straight nail made from stainless steel (see **Fig. 4**). If a guide pin and fluoroscopy are not used, there is no reason to use a hollow nail. A solid nail has less surface area on which biofilm can adhere. The SIGN nail reports on the surgical database were queried by Young and colleagues.[3] Studies show that a hollow nail must be 2 mm larger in diameter to equal the strength of a solid nail.[3] The solid nail allows slots to be used instead of than circular holes. This slot allows for slight compression during weightbearing for faster healing. The slots are large enough to accommodate the SIGN interlocking screws,

which have a 4.5 mm shaft. The configuration of the slot is used to mechanically find its location.

The SIGN nail is straight. The 9° proximal bend in the nail provides rotational stability and provides a better canal fit in the proximal tibia. The 1.5° degree distal bend gives better vibratory feedback to the surgeon who rotates the nail as it proceeds down the canal. The same nail is used for left and right sides and for fractures of the tibia and femur, including retrograde, antegrade, and humerus. There is no increase in nail diameter of the proximal end.

Once the nail size has been chosen, it is attached to the L-handle. The target arm is adjusted to align the holes in the target arm with the slots in the nail. The target arm only determines the longitudinal orientation of the nail. If the nail bends during insertion, the nail rotates, which changes the orientation of the slots in relationship to the hole made in the near cortex. The slot finders accommodate for this change in rotation.

The nail is introduced into the bone entrance with enough flexion of the knee to prevent impingement by the patella. The distal 1.5° bend provides more tactile feel as the surgeon rotates the nail during passage down the canal. Rotation of the nail plus the 1.5° degree bend results in less possibility of penetration of the nail through

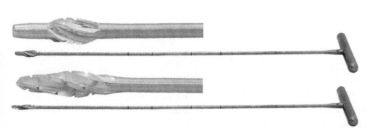

Fig. 3. Hand reamers. (*Courtesy of* SIGN Fracture Care International; with permission.)

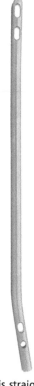

Fig. 4. The SIGN nail is straight and solid with proximal and distal bends. (*Courtesy of* SIGN Fracture Care International; with permission.)

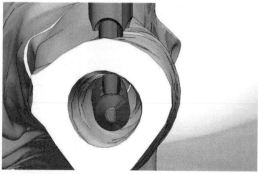

Fig. 5. The solid slot finder placed through the slot of the SIGN nail is guided by tactile sensations. (*Courtesy of* SIGN Fracture Care International; with permission.)

the fracture site. Usually the nail is inserted by axial pressure and rotation. If a mallet is used, the authors suggest 2 small taps followed by rotation of the nail during insertion.

Once the nail has been placed, the target arm is reattached to locate the distal interlocking screw slots. The distal interlocking screws are inserted first so the surgeon can rotate the nail as needed. A cannula is placed on the bone and the drill guide placed through the cannula, which guides the drill through the near cortex. This pilot hole is enlarged by a step drill, which is turned by hand. The hole in the near cortex can be chamfered using the screw-hole broach. Chamfering removes the ring of bone at the bottom of the hole in the near cortex and redirects the direction of the opening. The solid slot finder is then placed in the hole to locate the slot in the nail (**Fig. 5**). If the slot is located, the solid slot finder is replaced by the cannulated slot finder, which guides the location of the hole in the far cortex (**Fig. 6**).

The depth gauge measures the width of the bone. The interlocking screw chosen is 4 mm longer than the measurement so that 2 threads are prominent on both sides of the canal. The SIGN interlocking screw has threads on both ends, with the threads on the near cortex enlarged to accommodate the enlargement of the hole made by the step drill (**Fig. 7**).

The second interlocking screw is then placed in a similar manner. The alignment pin is placed in the hex of the screw to help guide the process.

If the hole is drilled and the solid slot finder does not enter the slot in the nail, the longitudinal alignment between the target arm and the hole in the near cortex is evaluated by determining whether the fracture fragments have changed position or the nail has changed position after the hole has been made. After longitudinal alignment has been confirmed, rotational malalignment is corrected. The target arm is removed, a curved slot finder is placed in the hole, and the nail is rotated, which allows the slot finder to enter the slot in the nail (**Fig. 8**). The hole in the near cortex and the slot in the nail are now aligned and the cannulated slot finder is placed to guide drilling of the hole in the far cortex.

The proximal interlocking screws are placed using the target arm without the slot finders. Slot finders are not needed because the distance between the L-handle and the holes is less and,

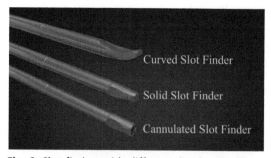

Fig. 6. Slot finders with different distal ends. (*Courtesy of* SIGN Fracture Care International; with permission.)

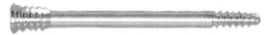

Fig. 7. The SIGN screw has threads at both ends. (*Courtesy of* SIGN Fracture Care International; with permission.)

therefore, more accurate. Rotational malalignment does not occur in the proximal end of the nail.

The authors suggest placing 2 screws when the fracture is within 6 cm of the interlocking slots or when the screws go through the metaphysis. Accurate reduction plays a major role in providing and maintaining stability.

One absolute indication for stabilizing the fibula is if the fibula fracture fragments are overlapping. If they are overlapping, the fracture is in valgus. The authors are assessing other indications by observing follow-up on the SIGN surgical database.[4] There are many variables.

Floating knees, or fracture of tibia and femur in the same patient, is common due to motorcycle injuries. These fractures can be reduced and stabilized at the same time in the supine position. The same incision longitudinally through the patellar tendon for nail insertion can be used, or an incision may be made medial to the patella tendon.[5] A window in the fat pad must be created for the retrograde approach to the femur.

Education

Education regarding fracture care is interconnected. SIGN surgeons all learn from each other. The SIGN surgical database facilitates communication between surgeons. The operating surgeon describes reasons for his or her surgical decisions in the comment section along with preoperative and postoperative radiographs. Many questions are resolved by the follow-up radiographs and reports, which are the orthopedic surgeons' report card. Often these findings lead to clinical studies that are presented at regional conferences throughout the world. Surgeons from developing countries present most of the papers during these conferences and the annual SIGN conference in Washington state in the United States (**Fig. 9**). We strive to engage all attendees.

These discussions result in better decisions regarding technique and indications. New indications for SIGN implants are presented by surgeons throughout the world. The authors have the highest respect for these surgeons who treat high-energy fractures with excellent results.

Validation

The follow-up reports on the SIGN Surgical Database provide validation for SIGN implants, instruments, and surgical skill. The overall average follow-up percentage is 43% for 2014 and continues to increase.

EVOLUTION OF RETROGRADE FEMORAL NAILING WITH THE SURGICAL IMPLANT GENERATION NETWORK SYSTEM

In August 1999, a young woman in Vietnam presented in the emergency room with a segmental fracture of her femur and a fractured tibia, or floating knee. The authors incised the patella tendon longitudinally to place the SIGN nail and interlocking screws to stabilize the tibia. A hole in the fat pad was excised and made the bony entrance through the femoral notch. At that time, the authors were unaware that other surgeons had used this technique to stabilize a fractured femur. We knew Marc Swiontkowski MD had stabilized fractures of the distal femur by placing flexible nails through the lateral and medial side of the distal femur. In retrospect, other surgeons had done retrograde approach to the femur using a similar approach that we used but, at the time, we were unaware of their reports.

The Vietnamese surgeons sent a picture of the patient standing on her fractured leg at 6 weeks (**Fig. 10**). This picture encouraged us to use this approach again because Vietnam patients have many floating knee injuries. The Vietnamese were reluctant to place a nail through the knee because squatting is part of their lifestyle. We studied the patients who had retrograde approach to the knee and found that slowly manipulating the knee at the end of the procedure to gain flexion was important for preventing contractures of the knee. The family is instructed to continue range

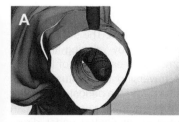
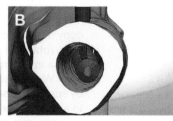

Fig. 8. (*A*) The curved slot finder is used to seek the slot in the nail if the nail bends during insertion. (*B*) The curved slot finder identifies the slot in the nail. (*Courtesy of* SIGN Fracture Care International; with permission.)

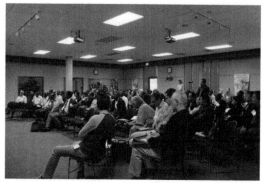

Fig. 9. SIGN conference 2014. (*Courtesy of* SIGN Fracture Care International; with permission.)

of motion exercises after surgery. The patients have had very little residual flexion contracture using this approach.

The retrograde approach to the femur has increased in frequency as SIGN surgeons become used to using this approach. If intercondylar fractures are present, the anterior total knee approach is used to expose the fracture, place intercondylar screws, and then place the nail. The authors recommend the retrograde approach for all distal

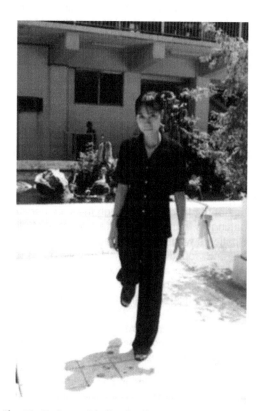

Fig. 10. Patient with floating knee treated with SIGN implants. (*Courtesy of* SIGN Fracture Care International; with permission.)

femur fractures and many midshaft femur fractures.

We avoid placing a nail that ends 6 cm below the lesser trochanter because this is the high-stress area. This high-stress area serves as a stress concentrator. Additional trauma can result in a fracture at the end of the nail or through an interlocking screw hole.

Two months after the first retrograde approach to the femur using the SIGN nail, we received a letter from Dr Han Khoi Quang with the accompanying radiographs of SIGN nail stabilization of a femur through the antegrade approach (**Fig. 11**). At the time, commercial implant companies were developing cephalomedullary nails to treat femur fractures. These nails had increased diameter in the proximal portion to accommodate the large compression screw that entered from the lateral trochanteric wall into the femoral head. Dr Quang taught us a very important technique, "As the nail is being introduced and the proximal bend enters the femur and passes down the bend, allow the nail to rotate freely and place the interlocking screws may be placed anterior to posterior or lateral to medial" (**Fig. 12**). Forced rotation will cause hoop stresses which may fracture the femoral neck. We took Dr Quang's advice and did not increase the diameter of the SIGN nail for antegrade approaches to the femur. By allowing proximal interlocking from anterior to posterior or lateral to medial directions, left and right nails are not necessary and stability is not compromised.

The straight SIGN nail inserted into the curved anterior bow of the femur provides additional stability due to 3 point fixation. The hand reamers have increasing shaft diameter as the reamer tip increases in diameter. This provides a straighter path than a flexible reamer on a guide pin used when fluoroscopy is available.

Technique

The supine position is used for retrograde approach. The lateral position is used for antegrade approach. Similar techniques for reduction, nail, and interlocking screw insertion are used for all femur approaches.

Reduction

Most reductions of the femur done without fluoroscopy must be open reductions. The surgeon controls rotational alignment by aligning the linea aspera in the fragments on each side of the fracture. We suggest traversing the vastus lateralis by spreading the fibers with the periosteal elevator to approach the bone. The perforator vessels can be seen and cauterized or ligated under direct

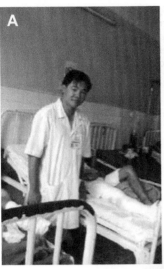
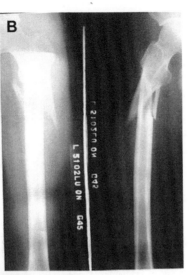
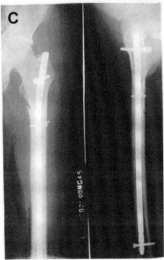

Fig. 11. (*A*) Han Khoi Quang and (*B, C*) the radiographs he provided of the first antegrade approach to femur using SIGN implants. (*Courtesy of* SIGN Fracture Care International; with permission.)

vision. A distractor may be necessary to bring the fragments out to length.

Often the fracture is weeks or months old and, therefore, the canal must be reamed for 6 cm on either side of the fracture site during open reduction. If this is not done, the bone that grew into the canal may not allow the canals of the main fragments to align for passage of the nail. After the reamer is withdrawn, remove the bone from the flutes of the reamer and place it in the fracture site at the end of the procedure. Reaming from the bone entrance hole is then done.

Nail Insertion

The length of the nail is determined by preoperative radiographs. As the nail is being inserted, the surgeon rotates the nail and pushes it down the canal. If the nail must be struck with a mallet, 2 small taps followed by twisting of the nail is recommended. The 1.5° bend at the distal end of the nail is very helpful for determining the position of the end of the nail as well as making the track a little wider.

During insertion of the proximal bend of the nail, the surgeon allows the nail to rotate as it progresses down the femoral canal as previously described.

Placing Interlocking Screws

The distal interlocking technique without fluoroscopy is sometimes affected when the nail bends as it goes through the isthmus. The target arm, which remains straight, lines up anterior to the slots in the nail and sometimes to the femur itself (**Fig. 13**). The degree of bending depends on the nail diameter, arc of radius of the femur, and how

A

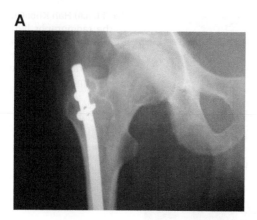

B

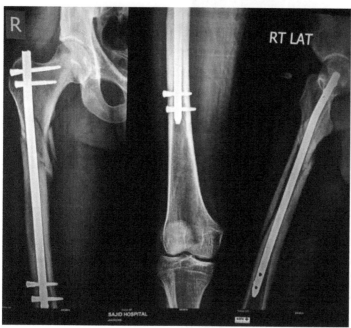

Fig. 12. (*A, B*) Proximal interlocking screws can be placed anterior to posterior or lateral to medial. (*Courtesy of* SIGN Fracture Care International; with permission.)

much force is applied as the nail is being introduced.

If the target arm lines up so the alignment pin is anterior to the femur, the distal aspect of the target arm is loosened, which allows the target arm to swing over the femur and direct the pilot hole in the cortex. The longitudinal orientation of the hole will still be accurate because the target arm has not changed in length from when the nail and target arm were lined up before nail insertion. The bending results in a change in rotational malalignment. This is corrected by rotating the nail as the slot finders are being introduced. The same principle of lining up 2 holes to find the slot in the nail is used with fluoroscopy.

Once the slot finder enters the slot in the nail, the usual technique of placing the interlocking screw

is used. After the cannulated slot finder is placed, the hole is drilled in the far cortex. The interlocking screw is then inserted. The surgeon can be sure the interlocking screw is in the slot of the nail by trying to rotate the nail because the rotation is blocked by the screw.

In summary, longitudinal orientation is directed by the target arm. Rotational orientation is directed by the slot finders.

After the distal interlocking screws are placed, the fracture is back-slapped for compression. The proximal interlocking screws are then placed.

Peritrochanteric Fractures

Peritrochanteric fractures can also be treated using SIGN hip construct without using fluoroscopy.

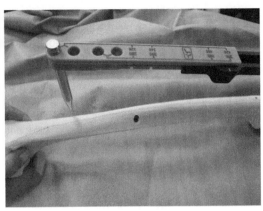

Fig. 13. When the nail bends during insertion, the target arm will direct the alignment pin anterior to the femur. (*Courtesy of* SIGN Fracture Care International; with permission.)

Tactile sense is substituted for fluoroscopy images during placement of the compression screws used to compress the fracture and the interlocking screw. SIGN has designed a pilot to make the track for the screws to traverse. This pilot provides

tactile sensation to the surgeon as it passes through the lateral trochanteric wall, metaphysis, femoral neck, and into the subchondral bone of the femoral head.

Subtrochanteric Fractures

Subtrochanteric and intertrochanteric fractures in which the fracture line is below the interlocking screws may be difficult to hold in reduction. It is important that the fracture be reduced and held reduced while the canal is reamed and the nail inserted. The proximal fragment tends to fall into varus and external rotation, especially if the lesser trochanter is fractured. Once the nail is inserted, a specially designed plate is attached to the distal end of the 2 proximal interlocking screws and passes across the fracture site in a helical fashion to counteract the tendency of the proximal fragment to slip into external rotation and varus (**Fig. 14**).

The combination intertrochanteric fracture and femoral shaft fracture is stabilized by a specially designed hip nail and compression screws to stabilize both fractures.

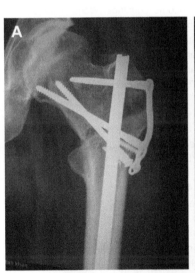
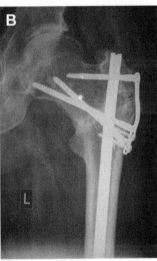
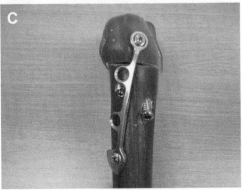

Fig. 14. (*A*) Fresh peritrochanteric fracture. (*B*) 3 months postoperative. (*C*) SIGN hip construct before bench testing. (*Courtesy of* SIGN Fracture Care International; with permission.)

IMPACT OF THE SURGICAL IMPLANT GENERATION NETWORK IN DEVELOPING COUNTRIES

SIGN implants have been a blessing for injured patients in developing countries. These implants have provided successful treatments of more than 1000,000 poor patients who have sustained long bone fractures in motor vehicle accidents, gunshot wounds, bomb blast injuries, and so forth. The unique design of implant has helped to treat fractures of femur, tibia, and humerus in patients of all age groups.

The free-of-cost implant and instrumentation enables the patients to be treated early and saves them from using their precious earnings to buy expensive implants. This helps them in early recovery and return to work, which is very important because most are daily wage earners. Because they are often the sole bread earners of their family, their time off work also has a financial impact.[6]

SIGN implants have a positive impact on the hospitals in which they are being supplied. With provision of free implants, patients are undergoing surgery earlier, compared with before when they used to collect money for their implants and surgery. Early surgery results in early discharge of patients, resulting in decreased length of stay in hospitals and decreased bed occupancy. This is very important, especially in war-struck areas like Afghanistan and northern Pakistan because large numbers of bomb blast casualties can come in at any time.

SIGN has improved quality of fracture care in developing countries by not only providing state-of-the-art instrumentation but also by active and continuous capacity building of surgeons. With regular feedback on every surgery and follow-up visit, the surgeon learns to improve fracture care. This increases surgeons' confidence in treating such fractures. The annual SIGN conference in Richland, WA, USA, provides a platform for surgeons from developing countries to share and learn new techniques in treating difficult fractures of long bones.

SIGN surgeons have contributed to orthopedic literature by providing evidence regarding fracture care in developing countries. Surgeons have looked at the fracture healing in pediatric populations,[7] infection in open fractures, fracture healing and infection in infected nonunions, high-energy open fractures, and so forth. Surgeons in different hospitals in various developing countries use the same implant and that is helpful in conducting multicenter clinical studies.

REFERENCES

1. World Health Organization. World report on road traffic injury prevention - Main messages. From Violence and Injury Prevention. 2004. Available at: http://www.who.int/violence_injury_prevention/publications/road_traffic/world_report/main_messages_en.pdf. Accessed March 24, 2015.
2. United Nations. Hunger – Vital Statistics. From Resources for Speakers on Global Issues. 2010. Available at: http://un.org/en/globalissues/briefingpapers/food/vitalstats.shtml. Accessed March 24, 2015.
3. Young S, Lie SA, Halan G, et al. Risk factors for infection after 46,113 intramedullary nail operations in low and middle income countries. World J Surg 2013; 37(2):349–55.
4. Shahab F, Stephens KR, Galat D, et al. Management Of Distal Metaphyseal Tibia Fractures With The SIGN Intramedullary Nail In Three Developing Countries [abstract 37546]. In: Programs and abstracts of the 23rd SICOT Triennial World Congress. Rio de Janeiro (Brazil): 2014. p. 120.
5. Shahab F, Shahabuddin, Zirkle LG. Treatment of Floating Knee Injuries By SIGN Intramedullary Nails [abstract 37044]. In: Programs and abstracts of the 23rd SICOT Triennial World Congress. Rio de Janeiro (Brazil): 2014. p. 117.
6. Peden M, Seurfield R, Sleet D, et al. World Report on Road Traffic Injury Prevention. Geneva: World Health Organization; 2004. p. xv, 217.
7. Shahabuddin, Shahab F, Zirkle L. Comparison of SIGN Pediatric and FIN Nail in Pediatric Diaphyseal Femur Fractures: Early Clinical Reults. J othop Trauma 2015;29(2):e46–50.

Management of Aseptic Tibial and Femoral Diaphyseal Nonunions Without Bony Defects

Mark R. Brinker, MD[a,b], Daniel P. O'Connor, PhD[c],*

KEYWORDS

- Fractures, Ununited • Exchange nailing • Augmentative plating • Revision surgery • Bone graft

KEY POINTS

- The presence of in situ hardware is a primary determinant of nonunion treatment.
- Aseptic diaphyseal nonunion of the tibia or femur without segmental defect and with an in situ nail are best managed with augmentative plating or exchange nailing.
- Aseptic diaphyseal nonunion of the tibia or femur without segmental defect and with in situ plate and screw fixation are best managed with revision plate and screw fixation and bone graft.
- Various bone graft methods, including intramedullary reaming, autogenous iliac crest bone marrow, and reamer-aspirator-irrigator technique, facilitate healing.
- Biologic implants (eg, recombinant human bone morphogenetic protein, platelet gel) and nonoperative treatments (ultrasound, electrical shock wave therapy) are associated with relatively high healing rates in most reports.

INTRODUCTION

This article describes an evidence-based approach to the treatment of aseptic tibial and femoral diaphyseal nonunions without segmental defects. The evidence for current best practices was obtained by searching the English-language literature for articles published from January 2005 through January 2015. The authors systematically searched Medical Literature Analysis and Retrieval System Online (MEDLINE) using the key terms: "fractures, ununited" or "nonunion" or "nonunions", "tibia" or "tibial" or "femur" or "femoral", and "treatment". The search was limited to adults (age ≥18 years). The results were 860 potential articles. We then reviewed the abstracts of all of these articles to identify the relevant papers.

We excluded articles reporting treatment of only infected nonunions or segmental defects. We excluded case reports, review articles, and technique papers that did not report results of treatment. We excluded papers reporting treatment of failed arthroplasty, failed arthrodesis, tumor resection, nonunions involving the articular surface, metaphyseal or epiphyseal nonunions, nonunions following periprosthetic fracture, and nonunions

Funding Sources: None (Dr M.R. Brinker); Research funding from CDC (U18DP003350), NIH (2R44GM095005), US Department of Education (H133G120192), Joe W. King Orthopedic Institute (Dr D.P. O'Connor).
Conflict of Interest: None (Dr M.R. Brinker); Consultant for Nimbic, Inc (Dr D.P. O'Connor).
a Fondren Orthopedic Group LLP, Texas Orthopedic Hospital, 7401 South Main Street, Houston, TX 77030, USA;
b Department of Orthopaedic Surgery, The University of Texas Medical School at Houston, 6431 Fannin Street, Houston, TX 77030, USA; c Department of Health and Human Performance, University of Houston, 3855 Holman GAR104, Houston, TX 77204-6015, USA
* Corresponding author.
E-mail address: dpoconno@central.uh.edu

Orthop Clin N Am 47 (2016) 67–75
http://dx.doi.org/10.1016/j.ocl.2015.08.009

following pathologic fractures. Finally, we excluded articles that had insufficient detail or contained large variation in the reported nonunion types or treatments. This process left 41 articles (25 femur, 22 tibia, 6 both) that we retrieved and reviewed in full.

FEMUR
Augmentative Plating

Eight articles described the use of augmentative plating, the use of plate and screw fixation in addition to an in situ intramedullary nail, with autogenous bone grafting for aseptic femoral diaphyseal nonunions (**Table 1**).[1–8] All 147 cases reported in these 8 papers healed (100% union rate) with average times to union ranging from 4.3 to 7.5 months.

In 2005, Choi and Kim[1] reported a 100% union rate for 15 aseptic femoral nonunions treated with augmentative plating using an AO plate. In 2009, Birjandinejad and colleagues[2] reported a 100% union rate for 25 aseptic femoral nonunions treated with augmentative plating using a lateral 4.5 mm broad dynamic compression plate (DCP) for midshaft nonunions with bone graft from the ipsilateral iliac crest for cases with less than 50% cortical contact (dynamic condylar screws or blade plates were used for proximal or distal nonunions but these were not reported separately from the overall series). The following year, Chen and colleagues[3] reported a 100% union rate and good-to-excellent functional outcomes for 50 aseptic femoral shaft nonunions treated with augmentative plating using a broad 4.5 mm DCP. Also in 2010, Park and colleagues[4] reported a 100% union rate for 11 aseptic femoral shaft nonunions treated with augmentative plating using compression plates.

Gao and colleagues[5] reported a 100% union rate for 13 aseptic nonisthmic femoral nonunions treated with augmentative plating using locking plates. Hakeos and colleagues[6] reported a 100% union rate for 7 nonunions treated with an augmentative plating technique that included removing the interlocking screws at 1 end of the in situ nail, applying compression intraoperatively via the plate or an articulated tensioning device, and then replacing the interlocking screws before DCP fixation. One subject had a postoperative infected hematoma and 1 had a residual leg length discrepancy. Said and colleagues[7] reported a 100% union rate for 14 aseptic femoral nonunion treated with augmentative plating with a 4.5 mm broad DCP. In 2012, Lin and colleagues[8] reported a 100% union rate for 22 femoral shaft nonunions treated with augmentative plating using a 4.5 mm broad DCP.

Blade Plate Fixation

In 2006, de Vries and colleagues[9] reviewed a consecutive series of 33 aseptic subtrochanteric femoral nonunions that had a variety of prior failed methods of internal and external fixation. The subjects were treated with hardware removal, blade plate, and autologous bone graft (13 cases), or demineralized bone matrix (DBM; 10 cases). Five infected nonunions were included but were not reported separately from the overall series. Union was achieved in 32 of the 33 nonunions (97%).

Intramedullary Nail Fixation

We identified 3 articles reporting the use of intramedullary nailing to treat a total of 70 aseptic femoral shaft nonunions, with an overall union rate of 83% in 4 to 8 months.

In 2007, Niedzwiedzki and colleagues[10] reported on 22 cases of aseptic femoral shaft nonunions treated with locked intramedullary nail fixation using nails 11 to 16 mm in diameter and 0.5 mm over-reaming. Although all cases had undergone 3 to 8 prior surgeries, these surgeries were not described except that 13 had failed at least 1 prior nailing. In addition, several cases were treated with either exchange nailing or with augmentative plating with intramedullary nailing; these cases were not reported separately. The union rate was only 59%. In 2009, Wu[11] reported a union rate of 89% for 18 aseptic, atrophic supracondylar femoral nonunions with in situ plate and screw fixation treated with hardware removal, debridement, a 12 mm diameter retrograde nail with 1 mm over-reaming, dynamic locking, and autogenous bone graft. In 2009, Megas and colleagues[12] reported a 97% union rate for 30 aseptic femoral shaft nonunions (25 atrophic) with an in situ plate treated with hardware removal, debridement, bone grafting in atrophic cases, and antegrade reamed intramedullary nailing with 1.5 mm of over-reaming. The nails were dynamically locked in 22 atrophic cases and statically locked in the 5 hypertrophic cases and in the 3 atrophic cases with 1 to 2 cm of shortening, for which the defect was filled with autogenous iliac crest bone graft at the time of intramedullary nailing.

Exchange Nailing

We located 8 publications reporting results of exchange nailing for a total of 266 aseptic femoral shaft nonunions, with an overall union rate of 89% with time to union ranging from 4 to 8 months.

In 2007, Wu[13] reported a 92% union rate in 74 aseptic nonunions of the femoral diaphysis treated with exchange nailing including over-reaming by at

Table 1
Articles published between 2005 and 2015 reporting treatment of aseptic nonunions of the femoral diaphysis without bone defect

Article	Number	Treatment Details	Union Rate (%)	Time to Union (mo)
Augmentative Plating				
Choi & Kim,[1] 2005	15	Augmentative plating with autograft	100	7.2
Birjandinejad et al,[2] 2009	25	Augmentative plating with autograft if <50% cortical contact	100	4.8
Chen et al,[3] 2010	50	Debridement, decortication, augmentative plating with autograft	100	6.0
Park et al,[4] 2010	11	Debridement, augmentative plating with autograft	100	7.3
Gao et al,[5] 2011	13	Debridement, augmentative plating with screws around nail, and autograft	100	7.5
Hakeos et al,[6] 2011	7	Augmentative plating with autograft; remove interlocking screws at 1 end of the nail, apply compression via the plate or tensioning device, relock the nail	100	5.0
Said et al,[7] 2011	14	Augmentative plating with compression and autograft in 9 cases	100	4.3
Lin et al,[8] 2012	22	Decortication, augmentative plating with autograft	100	5.5
Blade Plate Fixation				
de Vries et al,[9] 2006	33[a]	Hardware removal, blade plate with autograft or DBM in select cases	97	5.0
Intramedullary Nail				
Niedzwiedzki et al,[10] 2007	22	Hardware removal (if present), statically or dynamically locked intramedullary nailing, with reaming 0.5 mm larger than the nail	59	NR
Wu,[11] 2009	18	Hardware removal, debridement, 12 mm retrograde nail with 1 mm over-reaming, autograft	89	4.2
Megas et al,[12] 2009	30	Hardware (plate) removal, debridement, canalization, antegrade nailing with 1.5 mm over-reaming and static locking for hypertrophic cases or dynamic locking for atopic cases	97	7.9
Exchange Nailing				
Wu,[13] 2007	74	Exchange nailing, over-reaming ≥1 mm, statically or dynamically locked	92	4.4
Oh et al,[14] 2008	11	Statically locked exchange nailing (series included 1 infected nonunion)	91	NR
Shroeder et al,[15] 2009	35	Reamed exchange nailing with over-reaming ≥1 mm, new nail ≥2 mm larger than the original nail; statically or dynamically locked	86	4.0
Gao et al,[16] 2009	5	Reamed exchange nailing with nail 1–2 mm larger than the in situ nail	100	7.8
Naeem-ur-Razaq et al,[17] 2010	43	Statically locked exchange nailing	91	5.0
Park et al,[4] 2010	7	Reamed exchange nailing	29	7.0
Yang et al,[18] 2012	41	Reamed exchange nailing, new nail 1–3 mm larger	78	6.8
Swanson et al,[19] 2015	50	Exchange nailing, over-reaming ≥1 mm, statically locked, new nail ≥2 mm larger; subsequent dynamization required in 14 cases (28%)	100	7.0

[a] 28 cases were aseptic and 5 cases were infected; the results of the infected cases were not reported separately.
Data from Refs.[1–19]

least 1 mm. In 2008, Oh and colleagues[14] reported successful union in 10 of 11 cases (91%) of femoral shaft nonunion (1 infected, result not reported separately) treated with reamed, locked exchange nailing with a nail diameter at least 1 mm larger than the removed nail. In 2009, Shroeder and colleagues[15] reported a 91% union rate for 35 cases of aseptic femoral shaft nonunion treated with closed exchange nailing with over-reaming of at least 1 mm and new nail at least 2 mm (mean, 2.65 mm) larger than the initial nail. Gao and colleagues[16] reported a 100% union rate in a mean of 8 months for 5 aseptic femoral shaft nonunions treated with exchange nailing.

In 2010, Naeem-ur-Razaq and colleagues[17] reported on 43 aseptic femoral shaft nonunions treated with statically locked exchange nailing with a union rate of 91%. In 2010, Park and colleagues[4] reported that only 2 of 7 (29%) aseptic femoral nonisthmal diaphyseal nonunions achieved union following exchange nailing with a nail at least 1 mm larger and over-reaming by at least 1 mm. Yang and colleagues[18] reported union in 32 of 41 (78%) cases of aseptic femoral nonunion treated with exchange nailing with a 1 to 3 mm increase in nail diameter. Union was achieved in 27 of 31 (87%) isthmal cases and only 5 of 10 (50%) nonisthmal cases. In 2015, Swanson and colleagues[19] reported a 100% union rate in a consecutive series of 50 aseptic femoral shaft nonunions (all with >50% cortical contact) treated with exchange nailing, including a statically locked nail with a diameter at least 2 mm larger than the removed nail and over-reaming of 1 mm. Nail dynamization was performed in 14 cases (28%) before attaining union.

High union rates can be attained with exchange nailing of aseptic nonunions of the femoral shaft, specifically for nonunions located in the isthmus. The technique includes over-reaming by equal to or greater than 1 mm, inserting a new nail with a diameter equal to or greater than 2 mm larger than the in situ nail, static interlocking using new screw locations to optimize screw purchase (eg, use a nail from a different manufacturer from the in situ nail), and nail dynamization in cases showing slow progression toward healing following exchange nailing.[20]

Ilizarov Method

In 2010, Lammens and colleagues[21] reported on 8 subjects with aseptic femoral shaft nonunion following reamed medullary nailing. The 4 cases with no segmental defect were treated with nail removal and Ilizarov monofocal compression. All subjects achieved union at an average of 7 months.

Other Methods

In 2013, Giannoudis and colleagues[22] reported successful union in 13 of 14 cases (93%) of aseptic subtrochanteric femoral nonunions with an in situ broken intramedullary nail treated with nail removal; revision internal fixation (exchange nail or plate); and the diamond concept, which is combined use of recombinant human bone morphogenetic protein (rhBMP)-7, reamer-aspirator-irrigator (RIA) graft from the contralateral femur, and bone marrow aspirate.

In 2008, Calori and colleagues[23] published a multicenter randomized trial that compared rhBMP-7 to platelet-rich plasma (PRP) for treatment of 113 aseptic long bone nonunions (including tibia, femur, humerus, and radius or ulna). Most subjects also received revision fixation. Results were not reported by bone; however, the overall union rate was 87% at an median of 8 months for the rhBMP-7 group and 68% at a median of 9 months in the PRP group.

In 2009, Cacchio and colleagues[24] compared 2 intensities of extracorporeal shock-wave therapy (ESWT; 4 weekly sessions of 4000 impulses at either 0.4 mJ/mm^2 or 0.7 mJ/mm^2) with surgery (intramedullary nailing or external fixation) to treat long bone nonunions, including 34 femurs. Healing rates were very high ($\geq 92\%$) in all 3 groups but were not reported by bone. Xu and colleagues[25] reported a 64% healing rate among 22 atrophic or hypertrophic femoral nonunions treated with only a single session of ESWT (6000–10,000 impulses, 0.6 mJ/mm^2). In 2012, Roussignol and colleagues[26] reported a healing rate of 92% for 12 femoral shaft nonunions treated by low-intensity (30 mW/cm^2) ultrasound for 20 minutes per day up to 6 months.

Summary for Femoral Nonunions

For aseptic femoral shaft nonunions without segmental defect and with an in situ intramedullary nail, augmentative plating with bone grafting was reported to have a 100% union rate in all 8 articles reviewed (**Fig. 1**). Exchange nailing is also a good treatment option with slightly lower reported union rates ranging from 78% to 100%, with higher rates reported for nonunions in the isthmal region. For aseptic nonunions with an in situ plate, hardware removal followed by blade plate fixation or intramedullary nailing with autogenous bone graft has comparably high success rates ($\geq 89\%$ across 3 reports).

Treatment methods intended to stimulate the local biology and facilitate bone healing may be useful in appropriately selected cases. Bone graft methods and rhBMP biologics are most frequently used adjunctively with surgical fixation to improve

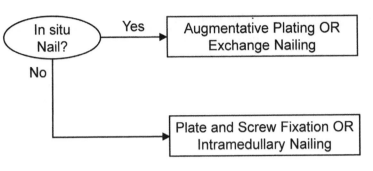

Fig. 1. Evidence-based approach to aseptic nonunion of the femoral diaphysis without segmental defect based on synthesis of 21 scientific articles published between 2005 and 2015.

mechanical stability. Noninvasive treatments to stimulate bone healing, including ESWT and ultrasound, can have high success rates and may be useful for patients unable to receive surgical intervention.

TIBIA
Plate and Screw Fixation

Augmentative plating
Two articles described the use of augmentative plating with autogenous bone grafting for a total

of 41 aseptic tibial diaphyseal nonunions, with a 93% union rate and time to union of 5 months or less (**Table 2**).

In 2009, Birjandinejad and colleagues[2] reported an 85% union rate following augmentative plating in the presence of a medullary nail to treat 13 aseptic tibial nonunions. A minimally invasive plate (4.5 mm narrow DCP) was applied to the medial aspect of the tibia, with the nail left in situ, and bone graft. In 2013, Ateschrang and colleagues[27] reported union in 96% of 28 aseptic tibial nonunions treated with augmentative plating using

Table 2
Articles published between 2005 and 2015 reporting treatment of aseptic nonunions of the tibial diaphysis without bone defect

Article	Number	Treatment Details	Union Rate (%)	Time to Union (mo)
Augmentative Plating				
Birjandinejad et al,[2] 2009	13	Retain in situ nail, augmentative DCP, autograft	85	4.8
Ateschrang et al,[27] 2013	28	Retain in situ nail, augmentative locking compression plate, nail dynamization; 79% had plates removed after union due to pain	96	3.8
Compression Plating				
Gardner et al,[28] 2008	16	Hardware removal, debridement, compression plate, autograft or DBM	100	4.4
Intramedullary Nail				
Faisham et al,[29] 2006	12	Static intramedullary nailing; 3 patients developed postoperative infection	100	4.0
Niedzwiedzki,[30] 2007	33	Reamed intramedullary nailing	94	9.2
Exchange Nailing				
Hsiao et al,[31] 2006	47	Dynamically locked exchange nailing	100	4.7
Gao et al,[16] 2009	7	Reamed exchange nailing with nail 1–2 mm larger than the in situ nail	100	7.8
Swanson et al,[32] 2015	46	Exchange nailing, over-reaming ≥1 mm, statically locked, new nail ≥2 mm larger; subsequent dynamization required in 4 cases (9%)	98	4.8
Oh et al,[14] 2008	12	Statically locked exchange nailing	75	NR

Data from Refs.[2,14,16,27–32]

an anteromedial narrow 4.5 mm locking compression plate and nail dynamization to allow compression. Plate removal was required in 79% cases due to pain.

Compression plating

In 2008, Gardner and colleagues[28] reported a series that included 16 aseptic proximal tibial nonunions at a 100% union rate that were treated with hardware removal, debridement, compression plate fixation, and bone graft (10 autogenous, 6 DBM).

Intramedullary Nail Fixation

In 2006, Faisham and colleagues[29] reported a series of 12 aseptic tibial nonunions treated by reamed statically locked intramedullary nails that had a 100% union rate, although 3 subjects developed a postoperative infection. The following year, Niedzwiedzki[30] reported a union rate of 93.9% (31 of 33 aseptic diaphyseal nonunions) following treatment with reamed intramedullary nailing.

Exchange Nailing

We located 4 publications reporting results of exchange nailing for a total of 112 aseptic femoral shaft nonunions, with an overall union rate of 96% with time to union ranging from 5 to 8 months.

In 2006, Hsiao and colleagues[31] reported a 100% union rate for 47 aseptic tibial shaft nonunions treated with dynamically locked exchange nailing (19 of the 47 subjects had malalignment and underwent acute deformity correction at the time of nailing). In 2008, Oh and colleagues[14] reported on 12 aseptic tibial nonunions (from a larger series of 17 tibial nonunions) that had been treated with statically locked exchange nailing with a larger (≥1 mm) nail. Nine of the 12 cases (75%) achieved union without requiring further surgery. Gao and colleagues[16] reported a 100% union rate in a mean of 8 months for 7 aseptic tibial shaft nonunions treated with exchange nailing. In 2015, Swanson and colleagues[32] published a case series with a 98% union rate for 46 aseptic tibial nonunions treated with exchange nailing, including 1 mm over-reaming, a new nail from a different manufacturer that was at least 2 mm larger in diameter than the in situ nail, and static interlocking.

As in the femur, exchange nailing of aseptic nonunions of the tibial shaft has a high rate of successfully achieving bony healing using a systematic approach (over-reaming by ≥1 mm, new nail diameter ≥2 mm larger than old nail, static interlocking using new screw locations, dynamization in cases with slow progression toward healing).[20]

Other Methods

Bone grafting

In 2013, Breda and colleagues[33] reported on 43 tibial nonunions (30 aseptic) treated with autogenous iliac crest bone along the interosseous membrane between the tibia and fibula following decortication of the nonunion site. Union was achieved in 88%, although residual pain persisted in 37%.

In 2005, Goel and colleagues[34] injected 15 cc of bone marrow aspirated from the iliac crest into the nonunion site, which resulted in union in 15 of 20 (75%) cases at a mean of 14 weeks, although 13 subjects required a repeat injection. That same year, Hernigou and colleagues[35] reported the treatment of 60 aseptic tibial shaft nonunions by pooling many small aliquots of iliac crest bone marrow to obtain 300 cc of aspirate. This aspirate was filtered and centrifuged for 5 minutes at 1200 g, then the buffy coat layer (containing progenitor cells) was removed and injected (~50 cc) into the nonunion site. Union was achieved in 88% of cases at a mean of 12 weeks after injection. Nonunions that healed had a higher number of progenitor cells in the injectate than cases that did not heal. In 2013, Braly and colleagues[36] reported on 11 aseptic distal tibial nonunions with stable in situ plate and screw fixation who were percutaneously injected with 40 to 80 cc of autologous bone marrow from the posterior iliac crest. Nine cases (82%) healed at an average of 4.1 months postinjection, with sustained improvements in function, pain, and health-related quality of life at follow-up ranging from 1 to 8 years after treatment.

Ultrasound

In 2007, Rutten and colleagues[37] published the results of a prospective study of 71 tibial nonunions treatments with 20 minutes per day of low-intensity (30 mW/cm^2) pulsed ultrasound (200-μs burst of 1.5 MHz acoustic sine waves, repeated at modulation frequency of 1 kHz). Solid bony healing occurred in 73% of cases in an average of 184 days, with longer healing times for oligotrophic and atrophic nonunions. In 2011, Hemery and colleagues[38] reported the use of low-intensity (30 mW/cm^2) ultrasound for 20 minutes per day for up to 3 months to treat 5 aseptic tibial nonunions. Union was achieved in 4 of the 5 (80%) cases at an average of 7 months. In 2012, Roussignol and colleagues[26] reported a healing rate of 100% for 23 tibial nonunions treated by low-intensity ultrasound.

Electrical stimulation

In 2012, Assiotis and colleagues[39] reported a 77% union rate in a prospective cohort of 44 aseptic

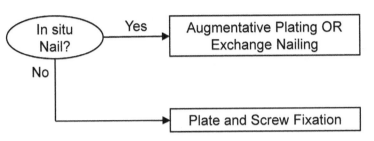

Fig. 2. Evidence-based approach to aseptic nonunion of the tibial diaphysis without segmental defect based on synthesis of 26 scientific articles published between 2005 and 2015.

tibial nonunions or delayed unions that were treated using pulsed electromagnetic fields for 3 hours per day and a median duration of 30 weeks.

In 2009, Xu and colleagues[25] reported an 81% union rate for 26 atrophic or hypertrophic tibial nonunions treated with a single session of ESWT (6000–10,000 impulses, 0.62 mJ/mm²). None of the atrophic nonunions healed. In 2010, Elster and colleagues[40] reported that 80% of 172 subjects with aseptic tibial nonunion who had undergone ESWT (median 4000 pulses at 0.38–0.40 mJ/mm² for 20–60 minutes, 1–3 sessions) achieved union at an average of 5 months. As discussed previously, Cacchio and colleagues[24] published a randomized trial comparing ESWT to surgical treatment with high healing rates in both groups (≥92%) that included 67 tibias; however, results were not reported by bone.

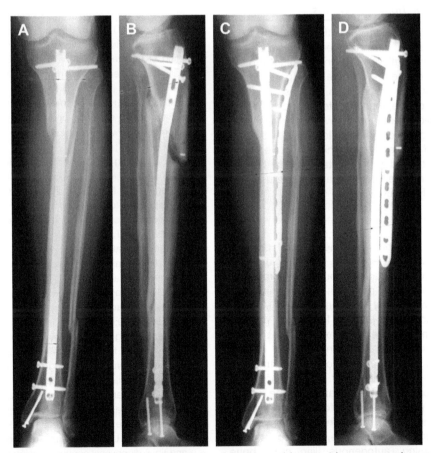

Fig. 3. (A) Anteroposterior and (B) lateral radiographs of a 46-year-old man with a segmental nonunion of the tibia 4 months after a segmental fracture that had been treated with intramedullary nailing. The patient was initially treated with an electrical bone stimulator for 3 months but failed to show any signs of progression toward healing. (C) Anteroposterior and (D) lateral radiographs showing solid bony healing of both nonunion sites 4 months after augmentative plating with autogenous iliac crest bone graft.

Biologics

In 2007, Chiang and colleagues[41] reported that 5 cases of tibial nonunion all healed following treatment with autogenous bone graft augmented by autologous platelet gel and stabilization with internal or external fixation. The gel was created from the subject's blood, which was centrifuged, combined with bovine or autologous thrombin, and stimulated with activator. The gel was sprayed on the graft material, the ends of the bone fragments, and the local soft tissues surrounding the nonunion site. Administration of platelet-leukocyte-rich gel (PLRG) injection for treatment of 9 aseptic tibial nonunions was also reported by Bielecki and colleagues[42] in 2008. The subject's whole blood was centrifuged to extract platelet-leukocyte-rich plasma, which was then mixed with bovine thrombin to form PLRG for injection under fluoroscopic guidance. Six of the 9 (67%) aseptic tibial nonunions healed at an average of 15 weeks.

Summary for Tibial Nonunions

For aseptic tibial nonunions without segmental defects and an in situ intramedullary nail, either augmentative plating with bone grafting (**Figs. 2 and 3**) or reamed exchange nailing results in consistently high union rates. For aseptic nonunions without segmental defects and an in situ plate, revision plate and screw fixation with free flap, bone graft, or other biologic implant has a high rate of success. As in the femur, treatment methods intended to stimulate the local biology and facilitate bone healing may also be useful in appropriately selected cases.

SUMMARY

For aseptic nonunions of the femoral or tibial diaphysis without segmental defect, plate and screw fixation with autogenous bone graft was the most frequently reported treatment method and had consistently high union rates. Aseptic nonunion presenting with an in situ nail may be treated with either reamed exchange nailing or augmentative plating and bone grafting, or with lower union rates for exchange nailing in the non-isthmal regions of the femur. Aseptic nonunion with in situ plate and screw fixation may be treated with revision plate and screw fixation and autogenous bone graft with a very high rate of bony union.

Various bone graft methods, including intramedullary reaming, autogenous iliac crest bone marrow aspirate, and RIA technique, facilitate healing when used in conjunction with surgical fixation. Biologic implants (eg, rhBMP, platelet gel) and nonoperative treatment methods (ultrasound, ESWT) are associated with relatively high healing rates in most reports.

REFERENCES

1. Choi YS, Kim KS. Plate augmentation leaving the nail in situ and bone grafting for non-union of femoral shaft fractures. Int Orthop 2005;29:287–90.
2. Birjandinejad A, Ebrahimzadeh MH, Ahmadzadeh-Chabock H. Augmentation plate fixation for the treatment of femoral and tibial nonunion after intramedullary nailing. Orthopedics 2009;32:409.
3. Chen CM, Su YP, Hung SH, et al. Dynamic compression plate and cancellous bone graft for aseptic nonunion after intramedullary nailing of femoral fracture. Orthopedics 2010;33:393.
4. Park J, Kim SG, Yoon HK, et al. The treatment of non-isthmal femoral shaft nonunions with IM nail exchange versus augmentation plating. J Orthop Trauma 2010;24:89–94.
5. Gao KD, Huang JH, Tao J, et al. Management of femoral diaphyseal nonunion after nailing with augmentative locked plating and bone graft. Orthop Surg 2011;3:83–7.
6. Hakeos WM, Richards JE, Obremskey WT. Plate fixation of femoral nonunions over an intramedullary nail with autogenous bone grafting. J Orthop Trauma 2011;25:84–9.
7. Said GZ, Said HG, el-Sharkawi MM. Failed intramedullary nailing of femur: open reduction and plate augmentation with the nail in situ. Int Orthop 2011;35:1089–92.
8. Lin CJ, Chiang CC, Wu PK, et al. Effectiveness of plate augmentation for femoral shaft nonunion after nailing. J Chin Med Assoc 2012;75:396–401.
9. de Vries JS, Kloen P, Borens O, et al. Treatment of subtrochanteric nonunions. Injury 2006;37:203–11.
10. Niedzwiedzki T, Brudnicki J, Niedzwiedzki L. Treatment of femoral shaft union disturbances with intramedullary nailing. Treatment failure. Ortop Traumatol Rehabil 2007;9:377–83.
11. Wu CC. Retrograde dynamic locked nailing for femoral supracondylar nonunions after plating. J Trauma 2009;66:195–9.
12. Megas P, Syggelos SA, Kontakis G, et al. Intramedullary nailing for the treatment of aseptic femoral shaft non-unions after plating failure: effectiveness and timing. Injury 2009;40:732–7.
13. Wu CC. Exchange nailing for aseptic nonunion of femoral shaft: a retrospective cohort study for effect of reaming size. J Trauma 2007;63:859–65.
14. Oh JK, Bae JH, Oh CW, et al. Treatment of femoral and tibial diaphyseal nonunions using reamed intramedullary nailing without bone graft. Injury 2008;39:952–9.
15. Shroeder JE, Mosheiff R, Khoury A, et al. The outcome of closed, intramedullary exchange

nailing with reamed insertion in the treatment of femoral shaft nonunions. J Orthop Trauma 2009; 23:653–7.

16. Gao KD, Huang JH, Li F, et al. Treatment of aseptic diaphyseal nonunion of the lower extremities with exchange intramedullary nailing and blocking screws without open bone graft. Orthop Surg 2009;1:264–8.

17. Naeem-ur-Razaq M, Qasim M, Sultan S. Exchange nailing for non-union of femoral shaft fractures. J Ayub Med Coll Abbottabad 2010;22:106–9.

18. Yang KH, Kim JR, Park J. Nonisthmal femoral shaft nonunion as a risk factor for exchange nailing failure. J Trauma Acute Care Surg 2012;72:E60–4.

19. Swanson EA, Garrard EC, Bernstein DT, et al. Results of a systematic approach to exchange nailing for the treatment of aseptic femoral nonunions. J Orthop Trauma 2015;29:21–7.

20. Brinker MR, O'Connor DP. Exchange nailing of ununited fractures. J Bone Joint Surg Am 2007;89: 177–88.

21. Lammens J, Vanlauwe J. Ilizarov treatment for aseptic delayed union or non-union after reamed intramedullary nailing of the femur. Acta Orthop Belg 2010;76:63–8.

22. Giannoudis PV, Ahmad MA, Mineo GV, et al. Subtrochanteric fracture non-unions with implant failure managed with the "Diamond" concept. Injury 2013; 44(Suppl 1):S76–81.

23. Calori GM, Tagliabue L, Gala L, et al. Application of rhBMP-7 and platelet-rich plasma in the treatment of long bone non-unions: a prospective randomised clinical study on 120 patients. Injury 2008; 39:1391–402.

24. Cacchio A, Giordano L, Colafarina O, et al. Extracorporeal shock-wave therapy compared with surgery for hypertrophic long-bone nonunions. J Bone Joint Surg Am 2009;91:2589–97.

25. Xu ZH, Jiang Q, Chen DY, et al. Extracorporeal shock wave treatment in nonunions of long bone fractures. Int Orthop 2009;33:789–93.

26. Roussignol X, Currey C, Duparc F, et al. Indications and results for the Exogen ultrasound system in the management of non-union: a 59-case pilot study. Orthop Traumatol Surg Res 2012;98:206–13.

27. Ateschrang A, Albrecht D, Stockle U, et al. High success rate for augmentation compression plating leaving the nail in situ for aseptic diaphyseal tibial nonunions. J Orthop Trauma 2013;27:145–9.

28. Gardner MJ, Toro-Arbelaez JB, Hansen M, et al. Surgical treatment and outcomes of extraarticular proximal tibial nonunions. Arch Orthop Trauma Surg 2008;128:833–9.

29. Faisham WI, Sulaiman AR, Sallehuddin AY, et al. Early outcome of reamed interlocking nail for nonunion of tibia. Med J Malaysia 2006;61:339–42.

30. Niedzwiedzki L. Use of reamed locked intramedullary nailing in the treatment of aseptic diaphyseal tibial non-union. Ortop Traumatol Rehabil 2007;9: 384–96.

31. Hsiao CW, Wu CC, Su CY, et al. Exchange nailing for aseptic tibial shaft nonunion: emphasis on the influence of a concomitant fibulotomy. Chang Gung Med J 2006;29:283–90.

32. Swanson EA, Garrard EC, O'Connor DP, et al. Results of a systematic approach to exchange nailing for the treatment of aseptic tibial nonunions. J Orthop Trauma 2015;29:28–35.

33. Breda R, Rigal S. Attaining tibiofibular union using an inter-tibiofibular autograft. A series of 43 cases. Orthop Traumatol Surg Res 2013;99:202–7.

34. Goel A, Sangwan SS, Siwach RC, et al. Percutaneous bone marrow grafting for the treatment of tibial non-union. Injury 2005;36:203–6.

35. Hernigou P, Poignard A, Beaujean F, et al. Percutaneous autologous bone-marrow grafting for nonunions. Influence of the number and concentration of progenitor cells. J Bone Joint Surg Am 2005;87:1430–7.

36. Braly HL, O'Connor DP, Brinker MR. Percutaneous autologous bone marrow injection in the treatment of distal meta-diaphyseal tibial nonunions and delayed unions. J Orthop Trauma 2013;27:527–33.

37. Rutten S, Nolte PA, Guit GL, et al. Use of lowintensity pulsed ultrasound for posttraumatic nonunions of the tibia: a review of patients treated in the Netherlands. J Trauma 2007;62:902–8.

38. Hemery X, Ohl X, Saddiki R, et al. Low-intensity pulsed ultrasound for non-union treatment: a 14-case series evaluation. Orthop Traumatol Surg Res 2011;97:51–7.

39. Assiotis A, Sachinis NP, Chalidis BE. Pulsed electromagnetic fields for the treatment of tibial delayed unions and nonunions. A prospective clinical study and review of the literature. J Orthop Surg Res 2012;7:24.

40. Elster EA, Stojadinovic A, Forsberg J, et al. Extracorporeal shock wave therapy for nonunion of the tibia. J Orthop Trauma 2010;24:133–41.

41. Chiang CC, Su CY, Huang CK, et al. Early experience and results of bone graft enriched with autologous platelet gel for recalcitrant nonunions of lower extremity. J Trauma 2007;63:655–61.

42. Bielecki T, Gazdzik TS, Szczepanski T. Benefit of percutaneous injection of autologous plateletleukocyte-rich gel in patients with delayed union and nonunion. Eur Surg Res 2008;40:289–96.

Surgical Management of Patellar Fractures

Rafael Kakazu, MD*, Michael T. Archdeacon, MD, MSE

KEYWORDS

- Patella fracture • Extensor mechanism • Tension band • Partial patellectomy
- Surgical management

KEY POINTS

- The patella is a crucial component of the extensor mechanism.
- Modern surgical techniques provide good results with proper indications.
- Management of patella fractures depends on the fracture morphology.
- Symptomatic implants often lead to additional surgery.
- New techniques aim to reduce implant complications.

INTRODUCTION: NATURE OF THE PROBLEM

The patella plays a crucial role in the extensor mechanism to increase the mechanical advantage of the quadriceps. Forces up to 5 times the body weight have been recorded from the extensor mechanism; the patella displaces the quadriceps tendon-patellar tendon link away from the axis of knee rotation, effectively increasing the moment arm of the quadriceps.[1,2]

Every year, roughly 1 in every 100 fractures will involve the patella.[3] Fractures can be classified based on displacement, comminution, and fracture pattern and often involve concurrent injury to the proximal tibia, distal femur, or knee ligaments. Although conservative treatment remains an option, open reduction and internal fixation (ORIF) and/or partial patellectomy have emerged as the preferred treatment options.[4] Numerous biomechanical and long-term studies highlighted the importance of the patella and tempered enthusiasm for total patellectomy as the treatment of choice for all patella fracture.[5-8] In the 1950s, the Arbeitsgemeinschaft für Osteosynthesefragen

(AO) introduced and promoted the use of anterior tension band principles for patella fracture fixation.[9] Subsequent studies validated its stability.[10-12] Modern treatment options include internal fixation using tension bands with Kirschner (K) wires or cannulated screws, lag screw fixation, and partial patellectomy, all with reasonably good clinical results.

INDICATIONS/CONTRAINDICATIONS

Indications for treatment of patellar fractures are largely determined by the type of fracture encountered. However, the goals of treatment remain the same: (1) restoration of the extensor mechanism and (2) maintenance of a congruous articular surface. Thus, the literature often has focused on treatment type rather than fracture type.

Conservative Management

Nondisplaced, closed patellar fractures, including stellate, transverse, and vertical, or fractures with less than 2-mm articular steps can be treated conservatively.[3] Stellate, transverse, and vertical

Disclosures: No disclosures (R. Kakazu); Consultant: Stryker; Speaker: AO North America, Stryker; Royalties: Stryker, Slack, Inc (M.T. Archdeacon).
Funding Source: None.
Department of Orthopaedic Surgery, University of Cincinnati Academic Health Center, PO Box 670212, Cincinnati, OH 45267-0212, USA
* Corresponding author.
E-mail address: Rafael.kakazu@uc.edu

orthopedic.theclinics.com

fractures of the patella often spare the medial and lateral retinaculum, maintaining knee extension.[10,13] Transverse fractures can present with significant displacement, such as 4 to 5 mm. However, if patients are able to extend their leg actively, the retinaculum is likely intact and can be managed conservatively.[10] Because the distal portion of the patella is extra-articular, fractures of the inferior pole can also be managed conservatively.

Conservative management usually includes weight-bearing-as-tolerated (WBAT) ambulation with the knee in fixed extension supported by a splint, knee immobilizer, or hinged knee brace. At 2 to 3 weeks, patients begin passive range of motion (PROM) from 0° to 30°, increasing the arc of motion by 15° per week. At approximately 8 weeks, patients should have nearly a full PROM of the knee and can begin advancing WBAT without immobilization.

SURGICAL TECHNIQUE/PROCEDURE
Surgical Indications

Indications for surgery include open fracture, articular step of 2 mm or greater, and loss of knee extension (**Fig. 1**). Comminuted stellate fractures typically present with intact retinaculum; however, because of the articular incongruity, surgical intervention may be recommended (**Fig. 2**). Highly comminuted and displaced fractures can present as transverse fractures with massive comminution or stellate fractures with massive diastasis. These injuries are often open.

Preoperative Planning

Standard radiographic views for the patella fractures include anteroposterior and lateral radiographs. The patella position and height are readily assessed with this view. A lateral radiograph will often provide an excellent survey of the fracture as well as an opportunity to determine patellar height (**Fig. 3A, B**). Most reliably, this is accomplished using the Insall technique.[14,15] A computed tomography scan can provide more detailed information regarding fracture character and articular step, though it is not routinely obtained (see **Fig. 3C–E**).

Prep and Patient Positioning

In addition to the implants necessary for fixation, a small-fragment instrument and implant set and pointed bone reduction forceps can be useful. Additionally, wire instruments, such as tensioners, wire forceps, and crimpers, can be helpful (**Fig. 4**). Angiocatheters can provide a convenient conduit for passing suprapatellar and infrapatellar wires. Patients are placed supine on the operating table with an optional tourniquet placed on the proximal thigh. Care should be taken to ensure that the tourniquet is placed as high as possible and inflated during knee flexion to avoid quadriceps trapping.

Surgical Approach

A midline longitudinal or lateral para-patellar incision is most frequently used. This approach facilitates reduction and is safe for future arthroplasty. In addition, this approach avoids the saphenous branch of the femoral nerve, which safely lies medial to the incision. Several case series promote arthroscopically assisted reduction and fixation of minimally displaced patellar fractures.[16–18] However, this technique may not be

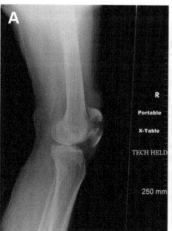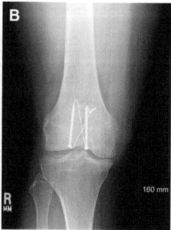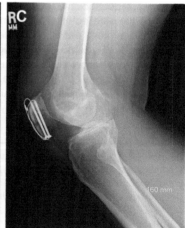

Fig. 1. (*A*) Lateral radiograph of open transverse fracture of the patella with significant displacement. (*B, C*) Anteroposterior and lateral radiographs following fixation with 4.0-mm cannulated lag screws and tension band.

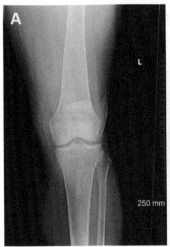
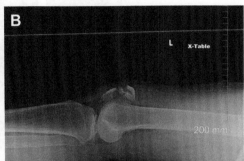

Fig. 2. (*A, B*) Anteroposterior and lateral radiographs of a highly comminuted patella fracture.

appropriate for highly comminuted or displaced fractures.

Surgical procedure (steps)

Cannulated screw fixation with supplemental wiring

1. A midline longitudinal incision is made through skin and bursa.
2. The fracture edges are cleaned, and the joint is irrigated to remove debris.
3. The K wire is passed in a retrograde fashion through the proximal fragment starting within the fracture line, roughly 5 mm from the articular surface of the patella, and at the junction of a line separating the patella into thirds. The K wire is driven proximally until flush with the fracture edge.
4. A second K wire is passed in a similar fashion parallel to the first K wire.
5. The fracture is reduced and held with Weber or patellar reduction clamps.
6. K wires are advanced across the fracture and out through the patellar tendon.
7. A cannulated drill is used to drill over the K wires followed by placement of 3.5- or 4.0-mm cannulated screws.
8. An 18-gauge wire is passed through one cannulated screw and then through an 18-gauge angiocatheter through the patellar tendon. The wire is then loop through the other screw in the opposite direction followed by passing it through the quadriceps tendon. The wire is then tightened on the dorsal surface of the patella.
9. Reduction of the articular surface is examined with the knee in extension by palpation

through the retinacular rent and by fluoroscopy.

Postoperative Care

Following anatomic reduction and stable fixation of the patellar fracture, patients are encouraged to begin careful and protected motion. Use of a continuous passive motion machine can be used; however, caution is recommended to prevent failure of fixation. Starting on postoperative day 1, patients are allowed to begin quadriceps isometric exercises. All drains in place are removed on postoperative day 2. Patients can then be placed in a removable knee brace locked in extension and unlocked for physical therapy targeting range of motion. Physical therapy is instructed not to begin these exercises until the wound is completely healed, typically at 2 to 3 weeks following surgery.

At 6 weeks, radiographic evidence of healing is available and progressive resistance exercises are introduced. Gradually, the brace is weaned and can be discarded at 3 months when fracture healing can be confirmed. Physical therapy may be continued up to 6 months following surgery, at which point restrictions on sport are lifted.

The protocol is modified if operative fixation failed to produce a stable construct. A hinged knee brace is locked in extension, with isometric quadriceps strengthening exercises delayed until 2 weeks following surgery. Flexion is limited to the degree determined during surgery. Active flexion exercises are restricted until there is evidence of fracture healing. Although weight bearing in full extension is permitted as tolerated, weight bearing in flexion is deferred until fracture healing is confirmed. Under these circumstances,

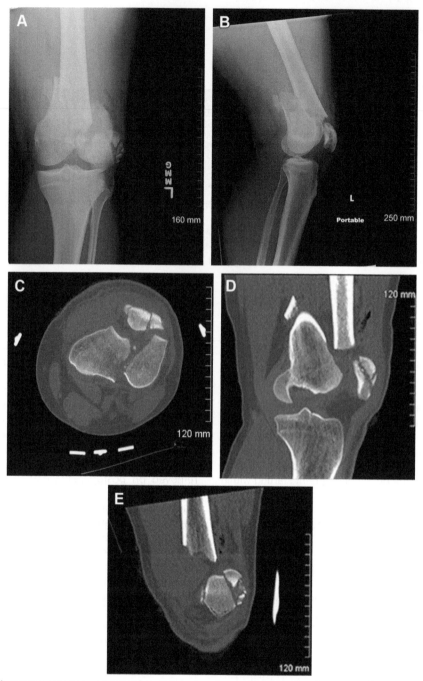

Fig. 3. (*A, B*) Anteroposterior and lateral radiographs of a vertical patellar fracture with comminution. (*C–E*) Computed tomography scan demonstrating comminution along axial, sagittal, and coronal planes.

it is important to counsel patients that these precautions to protect the repair often lead to stiffness and weakness. Once fracture healing is confirmed, aggressive physical therapy is permitted to improve range of motion and strength.

Outcomes

Nondisplaced fractures treated conservatively have good outcomes, defined as no arthrosis, weakness, or pain as well as full range of motion.[10,19,20] Boström[10] examined 422 patellar

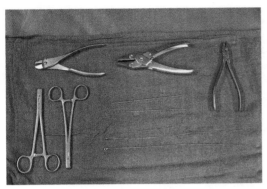

Fig. 4. Recommended instrumentation to be available for surgical treatment of patella fractures.

fractures, of which 219 were treated nonoperatively. All had less than 4-mm articular incongruity, and 98% exhibited good or excellent results. Other studies agree with these findings.[19,20]

Surgeons often allow the type of fracture to dictate the surgical technique used. Therefore, many report results based on fracture type and surgical technique, seldom with direct comparison. Modified anterior tension band wiring currently gives the best results, with 85% of patients reporting good or excellent outcomes according to 2 studies providing a combined cohort of 59 patients.[11,21] The same studies also compared it with cerclage wiring, showing only 19 of 31 (61%) with good or excellent outcomes. Additionally, Weber and colleagues[12] reported the biomechanical superiority of tension band wiring compared with cerclage wiring. However, the high occurrence of symptomatic fixation implants has spurred the development of novel constructs. Chen and colleagues[22] proposed a transosseous suturing technique indicated for transverse or comminuted fractures of the patella. They reported good results with lower complication rates compared with tension bands; however, their case series was only 25 patients. Hoshino and colleagues[23] compared the use of K wires with cannulated screws in the tension band construct. They found cannulated screws to have a higher rate of failure (7.5% vs 3.5%) but a much lower rate of elective implant removal (23% vs 37%). Other constructs that have been biomechanically tested include locking plate with tension band, fixed-angle plate, and compressive cannulated locking bolt and nut, though rigorous studies evaluating clinical results have not been published.[24–26] A recent Cochrane review identified 5 randomized controlled trials and concluded that evidence overall is limited for guiding the management of patellar fractures in adults.[27]

More recent reports have evaluated outcomes using validated outcome instruments.[28–30] LeBrun and colleagues[28] evaluated 40 patients with isolated patellar fractures treated with ORIF or partial patellectomy. On the Knee Injury and Osteoarthritis Outcome Score, all showed significant disability, with longitudinal anterior banding with cerclage scoring the highest in the small sample size. Lazaro and colleagues[29] evaluated 30 patients with low-energy patellar fractures treated with ORIF. Using the Knee Outcome Survey–Activities of Daily Living Scale, they reported that significant deficit persists at 1 year. Bonnaig and colleagues[30] retrospectively compared ORIF with partial patellectomy and found both methods resulted in similar functional scores and complication rates. However, higher-energy injuries were more likely to have received a partial patellectomy compared with ORIF in their system, complicating the data.

Because of the important role played by the patella in the extensor mechanism, patellectomy would seem to significantly decrease function. In fact, the literature supports this notion.[9–11,31–33] Einola and colleagues[6] reported outcomes of 28 patients an average 7.5 years following patellectomy. Only 6 patients reported good results (21%), with the most predominant complaint being weakness and pain on movement and exertion. Quadriceps atrophy was also a problem, with power being within 75% of the normal knee in only 7 cases (25%). Another study by Scott[19] reported that out of 71 patients, only 4 (6%) were happy with their long-term outcome following patellectomy. Nearly everyone experienced aching in the joint, and 60% complained of weakness. All patients exhibited quadriceps wasting. Given the poor outcomes, patellectomy should be considered only in massive comminution in which repair is futile. There are no studies to provide guidance on how much patella should be saved to preserve function.

Complications and Management

The most common complications are related to fixation implants and postoperative pain. Often, an additional surgery is necessary to remove the symptomatic implant. Lazaro and colleagues[29] reported 11 of 30 (37%) patients with patellar fracture requiring removal of symptomatic implants. Additionally, 24 (80%) of the patients reported anterior knee pain.[29] Functionally, decreases in strength, power, and endurance of knee extension by about 40% persisted at 1 year. Lebrun and colleagues[28] reported 14 of 27 patients (52%) requiring removal of symptomatic implants and 5 of 13 (38%) with retained implants reporting anterior knee pain.

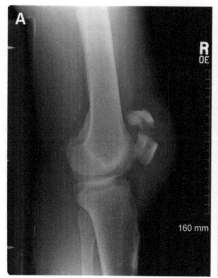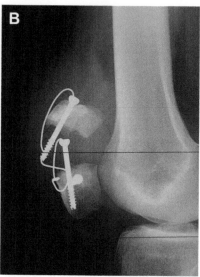

Fig. 5. (*A*) Lateral radiograph of a transverse fracture with displacement. (*B*) Lateral radiographs demonstrating failure of fixation requiring revision.

Other complications of patellar fracture treatment include infection, fixation failure, delayed union and malunion, loss of motion, osteoarthritis, and tendon rupture.[34] Infection can be treated by standard protocols depending on the soft tissue involvement. If severe osteomyelitis develops, a total patellectomy may be required. Tension band failure may occur with premature motion and requires revision if the fracture fragments are displaced by more than 3 mm or the articular surface has a step of more than 3 mm (**Fig. 5**). With modern surgical techniques, nonunion is rare. However, if detected, a period of restricted motion will often unite the fracture. Loss of knee motion is uncommon because of the early motion therapy protocols; however, if flexion is restricted several months following fixation, aggressive physical therapy to restore motion is recommended. In severe cases, manipulation under anesthesia may be beneficial, exercising extra caution in patients with a patellectomy. Arthroscopy to lyse intra-articular adhesions is also a reasonable option. If no improvement is noted after 12 months, a quadricepsplasty may be necessary. Osteoarthritis may develop and can be associated with an incongruous joint surface. Rarely, the extensor mechanism may rupture following total patellectomy, usually occurring at the proximal edge of the patellar tendon.

SUMMARY

1. The patella is a crucial component of the extensor mechanism.

2. Modern surgical techniques provide good results with proper indications.
3. Management of patella fractures depends on the fracture morphology.
4. Symptomatic implants often lead to additional surgery.
5. New techniques aim to reduce implant complications.

REFERENCES

1. Huberti HH, Hayes WC, Stone JL, et al. Force ratios in the quadriceps tendon and ligamentum patellae. J Orthop Res 1984;2(1):49–54.
2. Lieb FJ, Perry J. Quadriceps function. An anatomical and mechanical study using amputated limbs. J Bone Joint Surg Am 1968;50(8):1535–48.
3. Galla M, Lobenhoffer P. Patella fractures. Chirurg 2005;76(10):987–97 [quiz: 998-9]; [in German].
4. Blodgett W, Fairchild R. Fractures of the patella. JAMA 1936;20:2121–5.
5. Depalma AF, Flynn JJ. Joint changes following experimental partial and total patellectomy. J Bone Joint Surg Am 1958;40-A(2):395–413.
6. Einola S, Aho AJ, Kallio P. Patellectomy after fracture. Long-term follow-up results with special reference to functional disability. Acta Orthop Scand 1976;47(4):441–7.
7. Haxton H. The function of the patella and the effects of its excision. Surg Gynecol Obstet 1945;9:177–248.
8. Jakobsen J, Christensen KS, Rasmussen OS. Patellectomy–a 20-year follow-up. Acta Orthop Scand 1985;56(5):430–2.

9. Muller M, Allgower M, Schneider R. Manual of internal fixation: techniques recommended by the AO group. Berlin: Springer-Verlag; 1979. p. 248–53.

10. Boström A. Fracture of the patella. A study of 422 patellar fractures. Acta Orthop Scand Suppl 1972; 143:1–80.

11. Levack B, Flannagan JP, Hobbs S. Results of surgical treatment of patellar fractures. J Bone Joint Surg Br 1985;67(3):416–9.

12. Weber MJ, Janecki CJ, McLeod P, et al. Efficacy of various forms of fixation of transverse fractures of the patella. J Bone Joint Surg Am 1980;62(2): 215–20.

13. Griswold AS. Fractures of the patella. Clin Orthop 1954;4:44–56.

14. Carson WG, James SL, Larson RL, et al. Patellofemoral disorders: physical and radiographic evaluation. Part II: radiographic examination. Clin Orthop Relat Res 1984;(185):178–86.

15. Insall J, Goldberg V, Salvati E. Recurrent dislocation and the high-riding patella. Clin Orthop Relat Res 1972;88:67–9.

16. Makino A, Aponte-Tinao L, Muscolo DL, et al. Arthroscopic-assisted surgical technique for treating patella fractures. Arthroscopy 2002;18(6):671–5.

17. Tandogan RN, Demirors H, Tuncay CI, et al. Arthroscopic-assisted percutaneous screw fixation of select patellar fractures. Arthroscopy 2002;18(2):156–62.

18. Turgut A, Günal I, Acar S, et al. Arthroscopic-assisted percutaneous stabilization of patellar fractures. Clin Orthop Relat Res 2001;389:57–61.

19. Scott JC. Fractures of the patella. J Bone Joint Surg Br 1949;31B(1):76–81.

20. Sorensen KH. The late prognosis after fracture of the patella. Acta Orthop Scand 1964;34:198–212.

21. Böstman O, Kiviluoto O, Santavirta S, et al. Fractures of the patella treated by operation. Arch Orthop Trauma Surg 1983;102(2):78–81.

22. Chen C-H, Huang H-Y, Wu T, et al. Transosseous suturing of patellar fractures with braided polyester - a prospective cohort with a matched historical control study. Injury 2013;44(10):1309–13.

23. Hoshino CM, Tran W, Tiberi JV, et al. Complications following tension-band fixation of patellar fractures with cannulated screws compared with Kirschner wires. J Bone Joint Surg Am 2013;95(7):653–9.

24. Banks KE, Ambrose CG, Wheeless JS, et al. An alternative patellar fracture fixation: a biomechanical study. J Orthop Trauma 2013;27(6):345–51.

25. Thelen S, Schneppendahl J, Jopen E, et al. Biomechanical cadaver testing of a fixed-angle plate in comparison to tension wiring and screw fixation in transverse patella fractures. Injury 2012;43(8): 1290–5.

26. Domby B, Henderson E, Nayak A, et al. Comparison of cannulated screw with tension band wiring versus compressive cannulated locking bolt and nut device (CompresSURE) in patella fractures-a cadaveric biomechanical study. J Orthop Trauma 2012; 26(12):678–83.

27. Sayum Filho J, Lenza M, Teixeira de Carvalho R, et al. Interventions for treating fractures of the patella in adults. Cochrane Database Syst Rev 2015;(2):CD009651.

28. LeBrun CT, Langford JR, Sagi HC. Functional outcomes after operatively treated patella fractures. J Orthop Trauma 2012;26(7):422–6.

29. Lazaro L, Wellman D, Sauro G. Outcomes after operative fixation of complete articular patellar fractures: assessment of functional impairment. J Bone Joint Surg Am 2013;96(1):1–8.

30. Bonnaig NS, Casstevens C, Archdeacon MT, et al. Fix it or discard it? A retrospective analysis of functional outcomes after surgically treated patella fractures comparing ORIF with partial patellectomy. J Orthop Trauma 2015;29(2):80–4.

31. Duthie HL, Hutchinson JR. The results of partial and total excision of the patella. J Bone Joint Surg Br 1958;40-B(1):75–81.

32. Thompson J. Comminuted fractures of the patella. J Bone Joint Surg Am 1935;17:431–4.

33. Thompson J. Fracture of the patella treated by removal of the loose fragments and plastic repair of the tendon. Surg Gynecol Obstet 1942;74:860–6.

34. Archdeacon M, Sanders R. Patella fractures and extensor mechanism injuries. In: Browner BD, Jupiter JB, Levine AM, et al, editors. Skeletal trauma: basic science, management, and reconstruction volume 2. 4th edition. Philadelphia: Saunders; 2009. p. 2131–66.

Management of Distal Femur Fractures in Adults
An Overview of Options

Anup K. Gangavalli, MD*, Chinenye O. Nwachuku, MD

KEYWORDS

- Supracondylar • Femur fracture • Adult • Distal femur • Trauma • Options

KEY POINTS

- The incidence of distal femur fractures among all orthopedic injuries is less than 1% and follows a bimodal distribution between low-energy mechanisms and high-energy trauma.
- Articular involvement, alignment of the meta-diaphyseal region, comminution, construct stability/rigidity, and the bone quality are parameters that must be accounted for.
- Current treatment options broadly include conservative management, external fixation, locked and nonlocked plating with or without augmentation (plate, wire, or graft), fixed-angle devices (blade or sliding barrel options), intramedullary nailing, and arthroplasty.
- Complications primarily include nonunion, malunion, hardware failure, infection, and reoperation.

BACKGROUND

Supracondylar femur fractures are severe injuries that can be technically challenging to operatively treat. Although they account for less than 1% of all fractures and between 3% and 6% of femur fractures, their incidence is likely to increase with the rising geriatric populations and the increasing number of peri-prosthetic injuries.[1] Injuries to the distal femur follow a bimodal distribution between geriatric low energy fractures and high-energy trauma.[1,2] As with all fractures involving periarticular metaphyseal bone, treatment invariably includes understanding the fracture characteristics, careful preoperative planning, assessment of patient goals and health, bone quality, surgeon experience and implant selection.

In the early 1960s, most distal femur fractures were managed conservatively with fracture bracing and traction, achieving acceptable results in 67% to 90% of patients.[3] However, with the advent of new surgical techniques and implants, the pendulum shifted from conservative management to surgical stabilization of these injuries.

Through historical review, Henderson and colleagues[3] chronicled the increasing success rates with operative fixation from 52% to 54% in the 1960s, 73.5% to 75% in the 1970s, to 74% to 80% in the 1980s. Steady advances in our understanding of distal femoral anatomy and fracture biology have heralded various implant designs that further optimized successful treatment of these injuries. These modalities, each with their own merits and drawbacks, range broadly from external fixation, fixed-angle device (blade or sliding barrel implants), plate fixation (locked and unlocked), intramedullary nailing, arthroplasty, and distal femoral replacement (DFR) (**Box 1**). The authors intend to review these modalities and examine their success and pitfalls to provide a primer for the current clinical care of adult supracondylar femur fractures.

ANATOMY AND CLASSIFICATION

The distal femur is descriptively divided into a supracondylar region encompassing the region between the meta-diaphyseal junction and the

---

Disclosures: The authors have nothing to disclose.
Department of Orthopaedic Surgery, St. Luke's University Health Network, 801 Ostrum Street, PPHP2, Bethlehem, PA 18015, USA
* Corresponding author.
E-mail address: anup.gangavalli@gmail.com

Orthop Clin N Am 47 (2016) 85–96
http://dx.doi.org/10.1016/j.ocl.2015.08.011
0030-5898/16/$ – see front matter © 2016 Elsevier Inc. All rights reserved.

Box 1
Treatment options

Splinting and casting

Skin or skeletal traction

External fixation

Plate fixation (locked and unlocked)

Intramedullary nail

Arthroplasty/DFR

condyles and an intercondylar region that encompasses the condyles and articular surfaces. The periarticular/supracondylar region enjoys a better blood supply than that of the distal shaft, enabling adequate healing when stabilized. The normal anatomic axis of the femoral shaft is oriented between 6° and 11° of valgus in relation to the joint line (**Fig. 1A**). Restoration of this mechanical axis and prevention of varus collapse is a crucial factor in the success of distal femoral reconstruction and ultimate longevity of the joint. The medial and lateral cortices of the distal femur also taper anteriorly toward the midline at angles of approximately 25° and 10°, respectively (see **Fig. 1B**). This taper must be taken into account when selecting screw lengths and confirmed with internal rotation views to prevent hardware irritation from prominent screws medially. Knowledge of anatomy is crucial during placement of plates, which are often designed to be positioned along the anterior distal femur, approximating the border of the articular surface while avoiding intra-articular penetration of screws within the notch posteriorly or the trochlea anteriorly. Care must be taken during patient positioning and prep to allow for satisfactory imaging to be obtained intraoperatively in

order to avoid such pitfalls. Other considerations during the preoperative setup include obesity, body habitus, other prostheses, and wounds.

The distal femur is spanned by several muscle groups that can create deformities across fractures. Depending on the fracture plane and comminution, the quadriceps typically cause shortening,[1] whereas in the coronal plane varus/valgus deformity can be imparted by the adductors or iliotibial (IT) band.[4] Additionally, the distal segment can be deformed by the two heads of the gastrocnemius, causing an apex posterior deformity best seen on lateral radiographs or in the form of a "paradoxic notch view" on an anteroposterior (AP) image.[5]

The most commonly used classification system for distal femur fractures is the AO/Orthopedic Trauma Association (OTA) system (**Fig. 2**). Fractures are broadly classified into types A, B, and C corresponding to extra-articular, partial articular, and intra-articular injuries, respectively. They are further subclassified (1–3) based on pattern and degree of comminution. Type B1 involves sagittal splits of the lateral condyle; B2 involves sagittal splits of the medial condyle; B3 involves coronal patterns commonly known as Hoffa fractures. Type C fractures are divided into C1 (simple articular, simple metaphyseal), C2 (simple articular, multi-fragmentary metaphyseal), and C3 (multi-fragmentary). Careful scrutiny of radiographs and additional studies may be needed to accurately describe fracture patterns.

DIAGNOSIS AND IMAGING

Initial evaluation of patients begins with an accurate history and physical examination to identify the mechanism and time course of the injury. Identification of high- versus low-energy mechanism

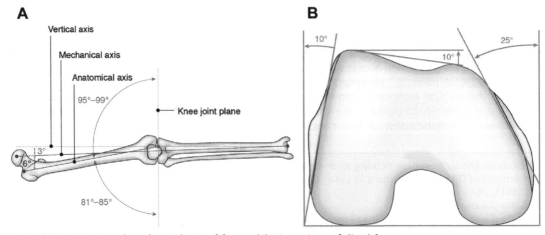

Fig. 1. (*A*) Anatomic and mechanical axis of femur. (*B*) Dimensions of distal femur.

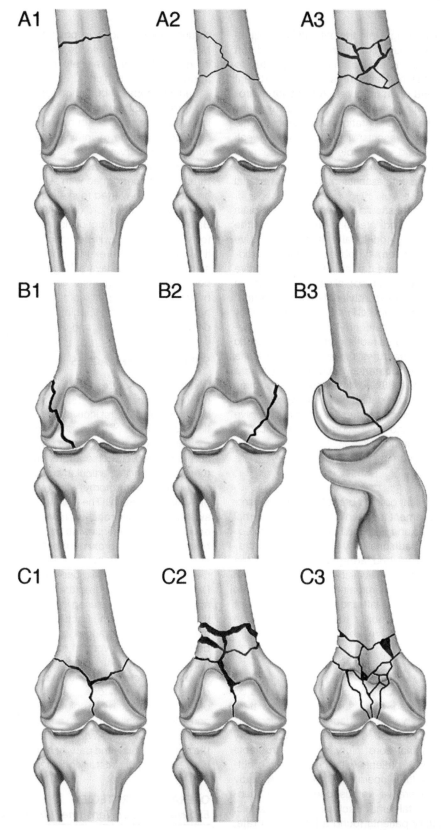

Fig. 2. AO/OTA classification for distal femoral fractures. (*Adapted from* Gwathmey FW Jr, Jones-Quaidoo SM, Kahler D, et al. Distal femoral fractures: current concepts. J Am Acad Orthop Surg 2010;18(10):597–607.)

may also allow insight into the patients' bone quality and general health condition. Swelling and soft tissue condition should be critically evaluated to identify effusions/hemarthrosis, compartment syndrome, and open fractures. A baseline neurovascular examination of both lower extremities can aid in the documentation of prior neurologic compromise or vascular insufficiency. If weak pulses are found, a Doppler probe should be used and ankle brachial index should be performed to aid in assessing possible arterial compromise.

Imaging studies should always begin with plain radiographs (AP and lateral) of the knee and the hip to rule out any additional trauma. If excessive shortening or deformity obscures initial radiographs, traction views can aid in the preoperative visualization. Although not always necessary in extra-articular supracondylar femur fractures,[4] computed tomography (CT) scans can play a key role in identifying intercondylar extension in patients with inadequate radiographs or osteoporotic bone. Type B3 fractures or coronal plane Hoffa fractures of the posterior femoral condyle are prevalent in up to 38% of intercondylar fractures and may elude initial detection on orthogonal plain films. These injuries can often be open and involve both condyles, and evaluation with a CT scan is strongly recommended.[6]

MANAGEMENT

Current treatment options broadly include conservative management (cast/splint, traction), external fixation, locked and unlocked plating, lateral fixed-angle device (blade or sliding barrel options), intramedullary nailing, and arthroplasty. Despite the myriad of techniques available, the primary goal of surgical treatment remains: restoration of the articular unit to the shaft and anatomic alignment while maintaining stability to enable early range of motion (ROM) and rehabilitation.

NONOPERATIVE

Although most distal femoral fractures tend to be operatively treated, there still exists a consistent role for conservative management. Indications include nondisplaced fracture, nonambulatory patients or spinal cord injury, unreconstructable injuries, or those patients with multiple comorbidities that preclude operative fixation.[1,4] A study comparing operative versus conservative management of distal femur fractures in myelopathic, nonambulatory patients found a 90% union rate, with complications including skin and wound issues in patients treated conservatively and no

wound complications in patients treated operatively.[7] Surgeon experience and implant availability must also be taken into consideration when approaching such injuries.

Various methods of immobilization include long leg splints, casts, or skin/skeletal traction. Splinting or casting paired with non–weight-bearing restrictions must be maintained for 4 to 6 weeks[8] with routine interval radiographs to monitor healing progress. Initial stabilization of supracondylar fractures may be performed with skin or Buck traction and may be converted to skeletal traction through the insertion of a proximal tibial traction pin. Balanced skeletal traction is advised in patients for whom traction will be definitive treatment, as it avoids excessive exertion of force through the skin and soft tissue layers. Regardless of modality, conservative management with prolonged immobilization has inherent complications: joint stiffness, decubitus ulcers, pulmonary complications, deep vein thrombosis, and deconditioning.[1,7]

SURGICAL APPROACHES

Distal femur fractures can be operatively treated through minimally invasive submuscular techniques involving small lateral incisions or through conventional exposures performed anteriorly, laterally, or medially based on the fracture pattern and surgeon comfort. The workhorse approach proven in fractures involving the articular surface is the lateral para-patellar arthrotomy with varying degrees of proximal extension. The swashbuckler and mini swashbuckler approaches have been described, enumerating techniques to extend the laterally based arthrotomy proximally between the IT band and vastus lateralis by following the lateral intermuscular septum to expose the distal femur.[9,10] Depending on the fracture pattern, a medial approach may also be used in conjunction to the arthrotomy to access the fracture for reduction or fixation purposes. This accessory approach may also be used to secure vertical or coronal fractures in type B injuries with interfragmentary screws if necessary. Retrograde intramedullary nailing requires astute knowledge of anatomy and selection of an optimal starting point. Many investigators agree that a small 3- to 4-cm arthrotomy positioned medial to the patellar tendon allows best access to the notch, because the patellar tendon and tibial tubercle are slightly laterally oriented structures.[1,11]

OPERATIVE STRATEGIES
External Fixation/Tensioned Ring Fixation

In patients with severe soft tissue injury, application of a knee-spanning external fixator can allow for temporization and implementation of damage control protocols. Careful planning of pin placement outside the zone of injury will reduce the risk of infection and maintain the integrity of the soft tissue for a staged formal surgical approach.[12] Severely comminuted fractures can also be treated definitively with tensioned external fixation devices such as the Ilizarov fixator. Arazi and colleagues[13] evaluated 14 complex fractures (type A and C) treated in this manner and found that union occurs around 16 weeks with a mean ROM of 105° at the knee. With the only complication being an infected nonunion, they concluded that the fixator is a safe option that provides adequate stability. Subsequently, Kumar and colleagues[14] examined the outcomes of the Ilizarov fixator in open supracondylar fractures and found that union occurred much later at 39 weeks, with at least 4 cm of shortening noted in 40% of fractures and pin-track infections in 21% of patients. Clinical outcomes were also fraught with complaints of pain and loss of ROM.

Open Reduction Internal Fixation with Fixed-Angle Blade Plate and Dynamic Condylar Screws

The advent of the fixed-angle blade plate transformed the care of distal femur fractures by providing a construct with polyaxial stability and inherent rigidity. The early designs constituted an angled side plate that could be impacted into the distal femur and held rigidly in place by means of the precontoured region of the plate that laid along the metaphyseal flare of the distal femur. The angle of the blade was commonly 95°, and careful implantation ensured that length and alignment could be restored even in injuries with metaphyseal comminution. The drawbacks of this design include the large exposure needed, inadequate fixation in osteoporotic bone, and the inability to address coronal plane fractures.[1] When compared with locked plates in a cadaveric biomechanical study, fixed-angle blade plates were a significantly weaker construct, tolerating less load to failure and resulting in more subsidence during cyclic stress.[15]

The fixed-angle concept was further developed into a sliding screw with a side-plate design to allow compression between intercondylar splits. This implant, commonly known as the dynamic condylar screw (DCS), was rapidly incorporated for its ease of application and smaller exposure. Drawbacks are similar to those of the fixed-angle blade plates in that the DCS remains incapable of securing coronal fractures and incurs large amounts of bone loss during insertion of the screw. Additionally, biomechanical studies showed that DCS implants bent at the plate-barrel junction when cyclically loaded causing varus fracture deformity. When compared with locked plates, the DCS was also noted to be weaker in axial stiffness and cyclic loading but similar in torsional stiffness.[16] Although fixed-angle blade plates and DCS implants have both had satisfactory results in long-term follow-up with 82% and 81% good to excellent results, respectively,[17,18] other options should also be considered.

Open Reduction Internal Fixation with Plate Fixation

When the decision has been made for operative intervention, knowledge of the fracture pattern and the use of the AO classification can help determine the optimal use of plate fixation. Broadly, type A fractures with a simple pattern should be plated in compression, whereas those with comminution should be bridged, ensuring uniform callus formation. Type B fractures typically require compression across the fracture site or a buttress-type construct (**Fig. 3**). Low-profile lag screw placement perpendicular to the fracture is imperative, especially in Hoffa-type fractures. Type C fractures require anatomic reduction of the articular surface in addition to attaining appropriate anatomic alignment and rotation (**Fig. 4**).

With the advances in options for plate osteosynthesis and screw design, precontoured locking plates have quickly become the most commonly used implant in modern orthopedics. Several minimally invasive plating systems are commercially available that can be applied submuscularly through small incisions with the use of radiolucent outriggers and guides. Although locking plate technology allows for the preservation of periosteal blood supply by circumventing a tight plate-bone interface, they also inherently create very stiff constructs that have been known to suppress fracture healing.[19] Granted, techniques that confer added rigidity may in some instances positively influence bony union; making a construct too rigid can conversely be detrimental to healing callus formation.[20] Biological motion across a fracture site has long been known to be both stimulatory and necessary for healing across comminuted segments of bone and remains the premise for bridge plating techniques.

Important considerations when plating include the material composition of the plates. Given that stainless steel is roughly twice as rigid as a comparable titanium plate, the use of titanium and associated alloys confers more flexibility and

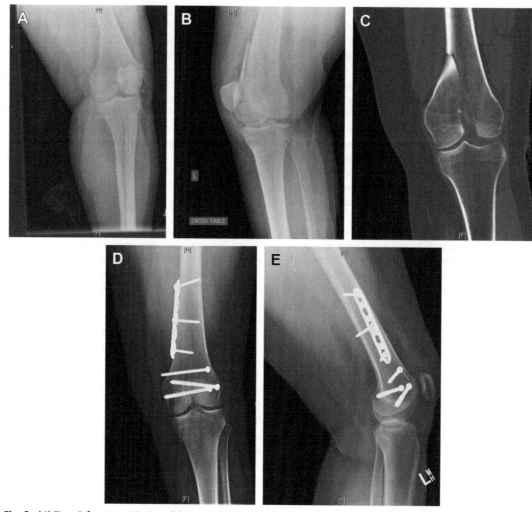

Fig. 3. (A) Type B fracture, AP view. (B) Type B fracture, oblique view. (C) Type B fracture, coronal CT. (D) Type B fracture; buttress plate and interfragmentary screw fixation, AP view. (E) Type B fracture; after fixation, lateral view.

aids in the formation of more callus.[19] Screw selection and placement also play a significant role in the biomechanics of the planned construct. Placement of locking screws at the terminal ends of the plate has been correlated with increasing thigh pain[11,21] and risk of periprosthetic fractures due to excess stiffness and stress concentration.[22] Although omission of screws in the holes immediately adjacent to the fracture site has been recommended in the past to increase the bridging zone and reduce stiffness,[23] this technique has not been consistently shown to be sufficient in modern locked plate designs.[19] Plates with polyaxial screw capability allow the surgeon to apply screws in various angles with the use of locking caps, providing fixed-angle stability. A biomechanical comparison showed that these configurations are mechanically sound and superior, with torsional stiffness and load to failure

both greater than their uniaxial/traditional counterparts.[24]

In addition to techniques, numerous implants have also been developed to impart varying degrees of motion at the fracture site, allowing a more physiologic healing environment. Considering the necessary balance between stability and fracture motion, new concepts such as far cortical locking (FCL) screws were introduced that combine locking technology with elastic materials to yield a dynamic plating solution. Using flexible locked screws that engage only the far diaphyseal cortex, symmetric compression is allowed across the entire fracture when loaded. The sliding near cortex forms a motion envelope enabling symmetric callus formation and axial motion around the fracture, while evenly distributing the load between FCL screws, preventing stress risers.[19,25] A prospective observational study

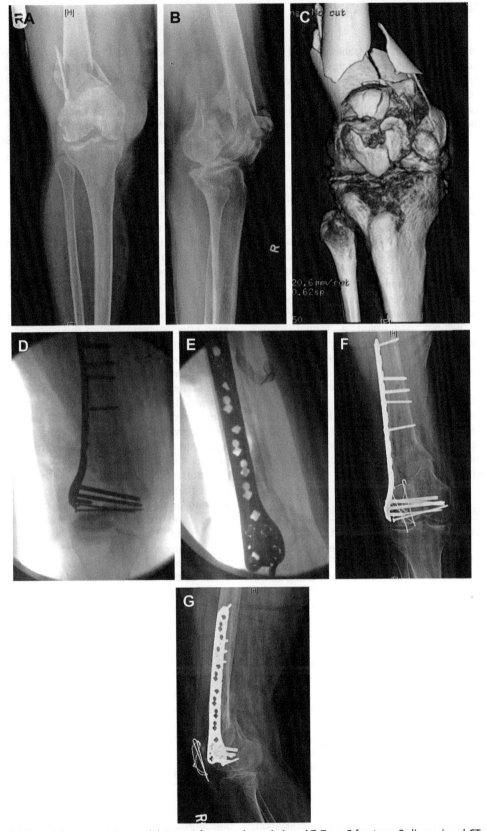

Fig. 4. (*A*) Type C fracture, AP view. (*B*) Type C fracture, lateral view. (*C*) Type C fracture, 3-dimensional CT reconstruction. (*D*) Type C fracture, intraoperative AP view. (*E*) Type C fracture, intraoperative lateral view. (*F*) Type C fracture; after fixation, AP view. (*G*) Type C fracture; after fixation, lateral view.

conducted on a cohort of 31 patients found that on average between 3 and 5 FCL screws were used in the shaft (125 total screws), yet there was no screw breakage and only 2 patients required revision surgery.[25] Complications included varus collapse, infection, and hypertrophic nonunion. Based on these findings, the investigators asserted that the use of FCL screws is a safe and effective method to stabilize fractures of the distal femur.

Locked lateral plate constructs, although biologically friendly, may not always impart adequate stability in light of severe medial comminution. Composite plating techniques, such as medial endosteal plate augmentation, allows for bicolumnar support in poor bone through a single lateral incision. Patients with extensive medial compromise or soft tissue injury would be ideal candidates for the insertion of a surrogate medial cortex, without performing a formal medial approach. A biomechanical study found that the insertion of an interlocked medial endosteal plate to augment a lateral plate imparted a significant increase in rigidity (decreased motion in torsion and axial loading) when compared with a lateral buttress plate alone. The applicability of this technique is limited to a few unstable fracture types, with potential disadvantages including prolonged surgical time, blood loss, and difficulty with future implant removal or arthroplasty.[26]

Retrograde Intramedullary Nailing

Improvement in implant design and insertion techniques has gradually led to the increase in applications for intramedullary nails. With careful consideration of fracture reduction, starting point, and reaming, nailing options offer a relatively soft-tissue friendly modality of fracture care performed through a small incision. Additionally, the use of an intramedullary device can offer earlier weight bearing and motion in the injured extremity because the implant can be load sharing. This advantage prevents the occurrence of deconditioning and complications due to prolonged immobilization in older patients or patients with polytrauma (**Fig. 5**).

As with all nailing techniques, it is paramount that the desired fracture reduction is obtained before reaming and nail insertion. Various techniques may be used to decrease deformity, including sterile triangles and bumps, intraoperative traction or distal femoral distractor, small incisions to apply clamps or bone hooks, application of Schanz pin joysticks, blocking screws, and so forth. Careful radiographic assessment is critical at each step to ensure proper rotation and alignment, which may be readily compared with images of the contralateral limb and the profile of the lesser trochanter of the injured limb.[11,27] Fractures with intraarticular extension may be safely stabilized with nails once the articular block has been reconstructed with interfragmentary screws. Of course, this must be done in consideration with the nail's intended trajectory as well as placement of interlocking screws.

Once the fracture is adequately reduced and the intended lag screws have been secured, the process of nail insertion can be planned. The starting point should be found fluoroscopically just anterior to the distal extent of the Blumensaat line on the lateral view. The guide wire is inserted in the intercondylar notch, just anterior to the footprint of the posterior cruciate ligament on the femur. Using soft-tissue friendly methods, the notch may be opened and reaming may be initiated after ensuring secure reduction. Preoperative and intraoperative planning with radiographs and fluoroscopy by placing nail templates beside the fracture can aid in the planning of proposed lag screws in conjunction with interlocking screws. The length of the nail must also be considered, ensuring that there are enough interlocking slots above and below the fracture, for adequate fixation while also confirming that the nail does not protrude within the joint. Long nails are often recommended as they prevent periprosthetic fractures at the nail tip and increase the working length of the nail (enabling biologic micromotion) and to obtain an isthmic fit for optimal stability and load distribution.[11] A recent biomechanical study comparing the combination of a retrograde nail and locking plate against either of the implants in isolation found that the combination was more resistant in axial, torsional, and load-to-failure tests.[28] When compared with dynamic condylar screws and locking condylar plates, intramedullary nails demonstrated 47.5% and 77.0% greater axial stability, respectively, and were found to have less micromotion.[29] A long-term study of 23 fractures with around 80 months of follow-up comparing plates with nails showed that nails required less bone grafting (67% vs 9%) and had lower malunion rates (42% vs 0%), respectively.[30]

Arthroplasty and Distal Femoral Replacement

Fractures in elderly patients can be challenging when there is extensive comminution of the articular surface. Despite anatomic reconstruction and rehabilitation, posttraumatic arthritis and knee pain are complaints that commonly arise in addition to any baseline osteoarthritis. Often, the

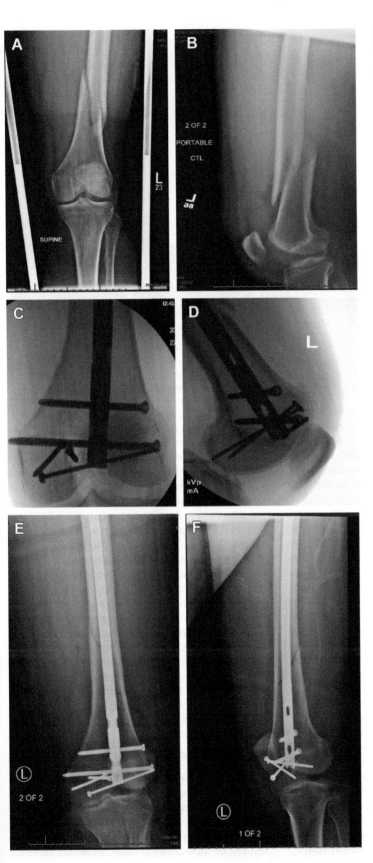

Fig. 5. (*A*, *B*) Preoperative intramedullary nailing. (*C*, *D*) Intraoperative intramedullary nailing. (*E*, *F*) Postoperative intramedullary nailing.

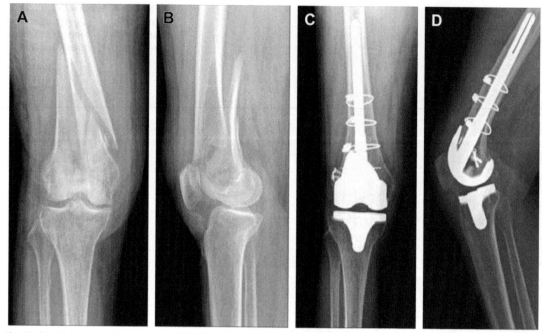

Fig. 6. (*A, B*) Preoperative primary TKA. (*C, D*) Postoperative primary stemmed TKA augmented with cerclage wires and screws. (*From* Choi NY, Sohn JM, Cho SG, et al. Primary total knee arthroplasty for simple distal femoral fractures in elderly patients with knee osteoarthritis. Knee Surg Relat Res 2013;25(3):141–6; with permission.)

treatment algorithm overlooks primary arthroplasty and DFR as a treatment option in younger patients; but it can be a valuable alternative in older patients with baseline osteoarthritis, metaphyseal bone loss, and extensive intra-articular involvement.

Several investigators have proposed arthroplasty as a primary means of treating distal femoral injuries and avoiding issues of nonunion while allowing early weight bearing. Careful preoperative planning and imaging of the contralateral limb are important to gauge and use as a template for implants. Based on the fracture pattern, implant options can include unstemmed total knee arthroplasty (TKA) for simple fractures, stemmed TKA for fractures with metaphyseal extension, hinged prostheses for injuries likely to have ligamentous instability, and DFR for fractures with extensive metaphyseal comminution and bone loss. All the aforementioned prostheses may be augmented with the adjunctive use of interfragmentary screws, cabled and cement when necessary for stability. Bell and colleagues[31] reported excellent results in a series of 14 patients with supracondylar or intercondylar femur fractures treated with primary TKA. Rosen and colleagues[32] followed a series of 24 patients who underwent primary DFR TKA for 11 months, with 71% of them returning to their preinjury level of ambulation. This group of patients had an average range of motion from 1°

to 103° and did not have any surgical complications. In a recent study in 2013, Choi and colleagues[33] evaluated the use of TKA in 8 patients with distal femur fractures and underlying osteoarthritis. The investigators used the medial pivot knee model with and without the use of a stem depending on the fracture type. They found that all patients united around 15 weeks with good clinical results (**Fig. 6**). They concluded that TKA combined with limited internal fixation is a good option for patients with simple fracture types and adequate bone stock. Arthroplasty has also been studied as a salvage option in the event of failed internal fixation or nonunion. A series of 17 patients had TKA performed and were followed for 5 years, with significant improvements in their Knee Society score and mean functional scores. Although the procedure provided reliable pain relief in most patients, the investigators remarked that the surgeries were difficult and fraught with complications.[34]

SUMMARY

With the increasing active and geriatric population, supracondylar femur fractures will continue to be a common occurrence. A thorough scrutiny of patients and their long-term health and goals will aid and guide in the treatment of their injury. The results of operative fixation have consistently improved and continue to have a decreasing biological impact on patients using minimally invasive techniques and soft-tissue friendly strategies. As with all injuries, careful planning and consideration of the fracture biomechanics and biology render even the most complex supracondylar femur fracture a treatable malady.

REFERENCES

1. Gwathmey FW Jr, Jones-Quaidoo SM, Kahler D, et al. Distal femoral fractures: current concepts. Review. J Am Acad Orthop Surg 2010;18(10):597–607.
2. Martinet O, Cordey J, Harder Y, et al. The epidemiology of fractures of the distal femur. Injury 2000; 31(Suppl 3):C62–3.
3. Henderson CE, Kuhl LL, Fitzpatrick DC, et al. Locking plates for distal femur fractures: is there a problem with fracture healing?. Review. J Orthop Trauma 2011;25(Suppl 1):S8–14.
4. Agarwal A. Open reduction and internal fixation of the distal femur. In: Wiesel SW, editor. Operative techniques in orthopaedic surgery, vol. 1. Philadelphia: Lippincott Williams & Wilkins; 2011. p. 582–4.
5. Suk M, Desai P. Supracondylar femur fractures. In: Archdeacon MT, editor. Prevention and management of common fracture complications. Thorofare (NJ): Slack; 2012. p. 236.
6. Nork SE, Segina DN, Aflatoon K, et al. The association between supracondylar-intercondylar distal femoral fractures and coronal plane fractures. J Bone Joint Surg Am 2005;87:564–9.
7. Cass J, Sems SA. Operative versus nonoperative management of distal femur fracture in myelopathic, nonambulatory patients. Orthopedics 2008;31(11): 1091.
8. Kancherla VK, Nwachuku CO. The treatment of periprosthetic femur fractures after total knee arthroplasty. Review. Orthop Clin North Am 2014;45(4): 457–67.
9. Starr AJ, Jones AL, Reinert CM. The "swashbuckler": a modified anterior approach for fractures of the distal femur. J Orthop Trauma 1999;13:138–40.
10. Beltran MJ, Blair JA, Huh J, et al. Articular exposure with the swashbuckler versus a "mini-swashbuckler" approach. Injury 2013;44:189–93.
11. Beltran MJ, Gary JL, Collinge CA. Management of distal femur fractures with modern plates and nails: state of the art. J Orthop Trauma 2015;29(4):165–72.
12. Haidukewych GJ. Temporary external fixation for the management of complex intra- and periarticular fractures of the lower extremity. J Orthop Trauma 2002;16(9):678–85.
13. Arazi M, Memik R, Ogün TC, et al. Ilizarov external fixation for severely comminuted supracondylar and intercondylar fractures of the distal femur. J Bone Joint Surg Br 2001;83(5):663–7.
14. Kumar P, Singh GK, Singh M, et al. Treatment of Gustilo grade III B supracondylar fractures of the femur with Ilizarov external fixation. Acta Orthop Belg 2006;72(3):332–6.
15. Higgins TF, Pittman G, Hines J, et al. Biomechanical analysis of distal femur fracture fixation: fixed-angle screw-plate construct versus condylar blade plate. J Orthop Trauma 2007;21:43–6.
16. Singh AK, Rastogi A, Singh V. Biomechanical comparison of dynamic condylar screw and locking compression plate fixation in unstable distal femoral fractures: an in vitro study. Indian J Orthop 2013;47(6):615–20.
17. Kolb K, Grützner P, Koller H, et al. The condylar plate for treatment of distal femoral fractures: a long-term follow-up study. Injury 2009;40(4):440–8.
18. Huang HT, Huang PJ, Su JY, et al. Indirect reduction and bridge plating of supracondylar fractures of the femur. Injury 2003;34(2):135–40.
19. Lujan TJ, Henderson CE, Madey SM, et al. Locked plating of distal femur fractures leads to inconsistent and asymmetric callus formation. J Orthop Trauma 2010;24(3):156–62.
20. Henderson CE, Lujan TJ, Kuhl LL, et al. 2010 mid-America Orthopaedic Association Physician in Training Award: healing complications are common after locked plating for distal femur fractures. Clin Orthop Relat Res 2011;469(6):1757–65.
21. Bottlang M, Doornink JK, Fitzpatrick DC, et al. Non-locked end screws improve the fixation strength of locked plating constructs in the osteoporotic diaphysis. Presented as a poster presentation at the Annual Meeting of the Orthopaedic Trauma Association. Denver (CO), 2008.
22. Bottlang M, Doornink J, Byrd GD, et al. A nonlocking end screw can decrease fracture risk caused by locked plating in the osteoporotic diaphysis. J Bone Joint Surg Am 2009;91(3):620–7.
23. Stoffel K, Dieter U, Stachowiak G, et al. Biomechanical testing of the LCP–how can stability in locked internal fixators be controlled? Injury 2003;34(Suppl 2):B11–9.
24. Wilkens KJ, Curtiss S, Lee MA. Polyaxial locking plate fixation in distal femur fractures: a biomechanical comparison. J Orthop Trauma 2008;22(9):624–8.
25. Bottlang M, Lesser M, Koerber J, et al. Far cortical locking can improve healing of fractures stabilized with locking plates. J Bone Joint Surg Am 2010; 92(7):1652–60.
26. Prayson MJ, Datta DK, Marshall MP. Mechanical comparison of endosteal substitution and lateral plate fixation in supracondylar fractures of the femur. J Orthop Trauma 2001;15(2):96–100.
27. Jaarsma RL, Verdonschot N, van der Venne R, et al. Avoiding rotational malalignment after fractures of the femur by using the profile of the lesser trochanter: an in vitro study. Arch Orthop Trauma Surg 2005;125:184–7.

28. Başcı O, Karakaşlı A, Kumtepe E, et al. Combination of anatomical locking plate and retrograde intramedullary nail in distal femoral fractures: comparison of mechanical stability. Eklem Hastalik Cerrahisi 2015; 26(1):21–6.

29. Heiney JP, Barnett MD, Vrabec GA, et al. Distal femoral fixation: a biomechanical comparison of trigen retrograde intramedullary (i.m.) nail, dynamic condylar screw (DCS), and locking compression plate (LCP) condylar plate. J Trauma 2009;66(2): 443–9.

30. Thomson AB, Driver R, Kregor PJ, et al. Long-term functional outcomes after intra-articular distal femur fractures: ORIF versus retrograde intramedullary nailing. Orthopedics 2008;31(8):748–50.

31. Bell KM, Johnstone AJ, Court-Brown CM, et al. Primary knee arthroplasty for distal femoral fractures in elderly patients. J Bone Joint Surg Br 1992; 74(3):400–2.

32. Rosen AL, Strauss E. Primary total knee arthroplasty for complex distal femur fractures in elderly patients. Clin Orthop Relat Res 2004;(425):101–5.

33. Choi NY, Sohn JM, Cho SG, et al. Primary total knee arthroplasty for simple distal femoral fractures in elderly patients with knee osteoarthritis. Knee Surg Relat Res 2013;25(3):141–6.

34. Haidukewych GJ, Springer BD, Jacofsky DJ, et al. Total knee arthroplasty for salvage of failed internal fixation or nonunion of the distal femur. J Arthroplasty 2005;20(3):344–9.

Management of Adult Elbow Fracture Dislocations

John D. Jennings, MD[a],*, Alexander Hahn, BS[b,1],
Saqib Rehman, MD[a], Christopher Haydel, MD[a]

KEYWORDS

• Elbow dislocation • Elbow fracture • Surgical management • Complications • Adult elbow

KEY POINTS

• Complex elbow dislocations are typically high-energy injuries that present a challenge to the treating physician, almost always require surgery, and are commonly burdened with complications.
• Advanced imaging is often helpful to assess the extent of injury and to determine the approach and type of fixation necessary.
• A methodological surgical approach results in improved outcomes. The authors use an inside-out technique beginning with addressing any coronoid injuries if present, then proceed to the radial head, lateral ligament structures, and finally medial ligaments, if necessary.
• If elbow stability is in question after all bony and lateral ligamentous structures have been addressed, an external fixator may be applied with or without the repair of the medial ligaments.
• Early motion is crucial in avoiding postoperative stiffness and contractures; however, maintenance of a stable reduction is paramount.

INTRODUCTION

Adult elbow fracture dislocations present a significant challenge to the treating surgeon and are associated with a high complication rate.[1] The elbow is a highly congruent trochoginglymoid joint with a significant amount of stability conferred from its bony structures. The elbow joint is comprised of articulations between the radial head and humeral capitellum, the olecranon and humeral trochlea, and the proximal radius and ulna. This construct is enhanced by the medial and lateral soft tissue constrains, which must also be addressed at the time of surgery.[2]

Functional range of motion at the elbow is classically described as 50° of pronation and supination with a 100° arc of flexion, ranging from 30° to 130°.[3] Contemporary studies using 3-D tracking techniques have found that required functional motion may be greater than previously reported.[4] An important goal of treatment is to preserve or restore functional use of the elbow.

Dislocations of the elbow may be simple or complex, with simple dislocations representing a purely soft tissue injury of the elbow resulting in the dislocation. Complex dislocations are associated with a combination of fractures and soft

Disclosures: Royalties from Jaypee Medical Publishing, Speaking fees from AO North America and Depuy Synthes, Committee member on Orthopedic Trauma Association, Editorial for Orthopedic Clinics of North America (Dr S. Rehman); Dr C. Haydel: Speaking fees from Depuy Synthes.
[a] Department of Orthopedic Surgery and Sports Medicine, Temple University Hospital, 3501 North Broad Street, Philadelphia, PA 19140, USA; [b] Department of Orthopedic Surgery and Sports Medicine, Temple University School of Medicine, 3501 N. Broad St, Philadelphia, PA 19102, USA
[1] 1535 Pine Street, Apartment 1F, Philadelphia, PA 19102.
* Corresponding author.
E-mail address: john.jennings2@tuhs.temple.edu

tissue injuries, and for this reason may also be termed *fracture dislocations*.

In general, complex dislocations are described as anterior or posterior based on the translation of the ulna with respect to the distal humerus. Posterior dislocations are typically the result of an axial load applied through a supinated elbow with valgus stress.[5] Conversely, anterior dislocations occur in the setting of a posterior force applied to the elbow in a flexed position or hyperextension trauma.[1] The Horii circle, described by O'Driscoll and colleagues,[6] outlines the typical pattern of soft tissue injury for elbow dislocations proceeding from lateral to medial (**Fig. 1**).

Several classification systems have been proposed to group these fracture dislocations and guide treatment. Ring and Jupiter[7] noted 4 common patterns of injury:

1. Posterior dislocation of the elbow with fracture of the radial head
2. Posterior dislocation with fracture of both the radial head and coronoid, described by Hotchkiss as the "terrible triad"[2,8]
3. Anterior transolecranon fracture dislocation

4. Proximal Monteggia posterior fracture dislocations

Morrey[9] further classified these injuries with the inclusion of soft tissue injury. Classification systems also exist for the patterns of injury to the individual components of the elbow, including radial head, coronoid, and olecranon fractures.

The most commonly used classification for radial head fractures was initially described by Mason in 1954, further modified by Broberg and Morrey in 1987, and finally Hotchkiss in 1997.[10,11] Although the full details of the modified Mason classification are presented in **Table 1**, generally, type 1 represents nondisplaced fractures, type 2 is a displaced (>2 mm) fractures, and type 3 is reserved for severely comminuted radial head fractures.[12]

Coronoid fractures are described using the Regan and Morrey classification, where type 1 involves the tip of the coronoid process, type 2 is a fracture of less than 50% of the coronoid height, and type 3 fractures include greater than 50% of the coronoid.[13,14] The O'Driscoll classification describes coronoid fracture fragments of the tip, anteromedial, and basal region.[15]

Finally, olecranon fractures are most commonly classified with the Schatzker, Mayo, or AO classification system. The Schatzker classification describes the pattern and location (intra/extra-articular) and is organized by mechanical construct needed for fixation.[16] The Mayo classification simplifies the fracture pattern into type 1 nondisplaced stable fractures, type 2 displaced stable fractures, and unstable type 3 fractures, which are commonly comminuted.[17]

INDICATIONS/CONTRAINDICATIONS

Simple elbow dislocations should be managed with concentric reduction as soon as possible. Stable range of motion should be assessed immediately after reduction and any subluxation or dislocation with extension or valgus stress documented. Typically, stable reductions are successfully managed nonoperatively with close monitoring and early range of motion. In patients who are morbidly obese, mentally impaired, or intubated, frequent examination and interval radiographs may be required to ensure that the initial closed reduction has not been lost.

Elbow dislocations with associated periarticular fractures (ie, complex dislocations); however, frequently necessitate surgical intervention, and the indications are predicated on the specific fracture pattern. For this reason, CT scan is often helpful in preoperative planning (**Fig. 2**). With exception

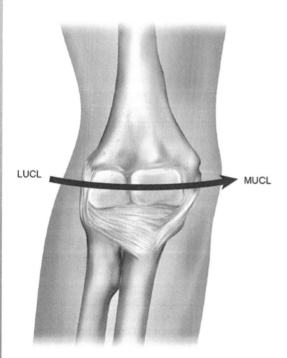

Fig. 1. Progression of soft tissue injury as the elbow dislocates, which begins with the LUCL and finally involves the MUCL, which can be partially (stage 3a) or completely (stage 3b) disrupted. (*Modified from* O'Driscoll SW, Morrey BF, Korinek S, et al. Elbow subluxation and dislocation. A spectrum of instability. Clin Orthop Relat Res 1992;(280):186–97.)

Table 1
Modified Mason classification for radial head fractures

Type	Description
1	Nondisplaced or minimally displaced fracture of head or neck; forearm rotation is limited only by acute pain and swelling, intra-articular fracture <2 mm, or marginal lip fracture.
2	Displaced (>2 mm) fracture of head or neck. Motion may be mechanically blocked or incongruous, without severe comminution (possible to repair by ORIF), or fracture involving more than marginal lip of radial head.
3	Severely comminuted fracture of head and neck that is nonreconstructible, usually requiring excision and/or replacement.

Data from Hotchkiss RN. Displaced fractures of the radial head: internal fixation or excision? J Am Acad Orthop Surg 1997;5(1):1–10.

of a select pattern of injuries, nearly all fracture dislocations require some level of operative intervention.[18]

1. Radial head fractures: posterior elbow dislocations with associated isolated fracture of the radial head are rare injuries and a relative indication for surgical fixation.[19,20] These injuries can be managed in a long arm cast, although conservative management may be associated with joint arthrosis and blocks to forearm rotation.[7] When operative fixation is chosen, open reduction and internal fixation or acute radial head replacement are recommended because radial head excision in the presence of a traumatic elbow dislocation is contraindicated due to the risk of proximal migration.[7,21,22] Elbow dislocation with a radial head fracture and a concomitant coronoid fracture (**Fig. 3**) is nearly always an indication for surgery. Nonoperative treatment is reserved only for cases where concentric reduction is

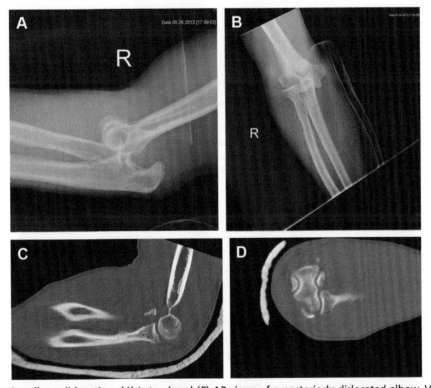

Fig. 2. Posterior elbow dislocation. (*A*) Lateral and (*B*) AP views of a posteriorly dislocated elbow. Visualization and assessment of small periarticular fractures is difficult on plain film imaging; however, CT images clearly demonstrate fractures of the (*C*) coronoid and (*D*) lateral epicondyle.

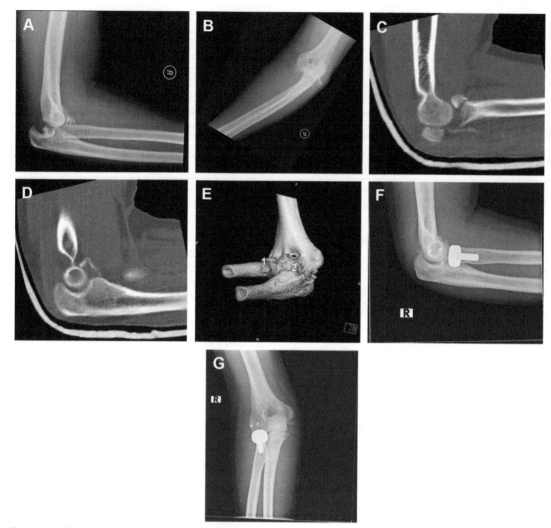

Fig. 3. Terrible triad (*A*) Lateral and (*B*) AP radiographs of a complex elbow dislocation. CT imaging demonstrates associated (*C*) radial head and (*D*) coronoid fractures. (*E*) A 3-D reconstruction again showing (1) radial head and (2) coronoid fractures after reduction of the elbow. Postoperative (*F*) lateral and (*G*) posteroanterior radiographs showing radial head replacement and suture anchors at the LUCL origin maintaining a stable reduction. The coronoid was fixed with a suture lasso placed through the capsular attachments and tied at the base of the ulna through 2 drill holes.

achieved, there are no blocks to motion, and fracture fragments are small and nondisplaced.[23]

2. Coronoid fracture: elbow dislocation with isolated fracture of the coronoid is rare and surgical intervention is, to some extent, based on the size and location of the coronoid fragment. Some investigators conservatively manage isolated fractures involving less than 10% of the coronoid height with a long arm cast.[20] Surgical fixation is indicated for elbow dislocations with fractures greater than 10% of coronoid height as well as the well-known terrible triad injury of simultaneous elbow dislocation with coronoid and radial head fractures (see **Fig. 3**).[7,12,20,24]

3. Olecranon fracture: anterior transolecranon fracture dislocation necessitates operative intervention. The ulnar articular surface must be anatomically restored and any associated injuries to the coronoid, distal humerus, or radial head addressed at the time of fixation. Unlike a Monteggia fracture dislocation, the proximal radioulnar joint is not compromised with these injuries (**Fig. 4**).[20]

4. Soft tissues: O'Driscoll and colleagues[25] described the disruption of soft tissue structures from lateral to medial in elbow

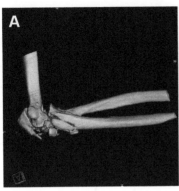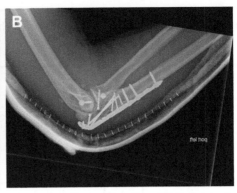

Fig. 4. (*A*) 3-D reconstruction of a transolecranon, or anterior elbow dislocation. (*B*) Postoperative radiograph demonstrate fixation of the olecranon with a proximal ulna plate, LUCL repair with suture anchors, and MUCL repair of bony avulsion with a screw and washer and fixation of the coronoid.

dislocations originating at the lateral ulnar collateral ligament (LUCL) and, in cases of high energy trauma, progressing to disruption of the medial ulnar collateral ligament (MUCL). After bony anatomy is restored, attention should be turned to the soft tissue structures for reconstruction. The annular ligament and LUCL should be repaired, because rotatory instability ensues with any deficit in the lateral collateral ligament (LCL) complex.[7,26,27] The medial collateral ligament (MCL), however, needs only to be restored if the elbow remains unstable after all other fractures and soft tissue structures have been addressed. An alternative option is to place a hinged external fixator in this situation.[28–31]

SURGICAL TECHNIQUE/PROCEDURE
Preoperative Planning

Preoperative planning begins with a thorough history, physical examination, and complete imaging, including standard anteroposterior (AP), lateral, and oblique views of the elbow. For elbow fracture dislocations, CT scanning is often helpful in recognizing complex intra-articular fracture patterns and can guide the surgical approach and treatment. MRI has limited utility in the acute setting, although it may prove helpful in cases of chronic elbow instability. Preoperative neurologic deficits must be carefully noted. All dislocations should be reduced and splinted at 90° until operative intervention.

A decision-making algorithm is demonstrated in **Fig. 5**. Regardless of the fracture pattern, the surgeon should be prepared for several contingencies. A hinged external fixator should be available if the final reduction is deemed unstable. If the radial head is involved, the surgeon should be prepared to replace the radial head acutely.

Preparation and Patient Positioning

There are several options for positioning of the patient for adequate access to the elbow, which vary to some extent with the surgical approach chosen but are mostly based on surgeon preference. The procedure is typically performed under general anesthesia and adjunctive nerve blocks before or after surgery can assist in reducing postoperative pain.

The patient may be positioned supine with the arm adducted across the body to allow access to the posterior elbow (**Fig. 6**). A bump placed under the ipsilateral scapula can assist arm positioning. Another option is to position the patient in the lateral decubitus position with the affected arm supported by bone foam or a bolster so that the elbow rests in a flexed position (**Fig. 7**).

Regardless of the position chosen, the authors typically mark the ulnar and radial side of the elbow as well as the position of the ulnar nerve (see **Figs. 6** and **7**), because the surgeon can easily become disoriented when approaching the posterior elbow in this manner. A sterile tourniquet is applied after draping.

Surgical Approach

The approach to the elbow typically begins with a universal posterior skin incision, which provides circumferential access by raising full-thickness skin flaps while avoiding creating skin bridges.[32,33] Some surgeons curve this incision around the olecranon to avoid postoperative pain with direct pressure on the subcutaneous bone. The posterior approach allows a panoramic view of the elbow, is convenient if a hinged external fixator is applied later in the procedure, and is conveniently accessed in the lateral decubitus position.[34] Alternatively, separate medial and lateral skin incisions

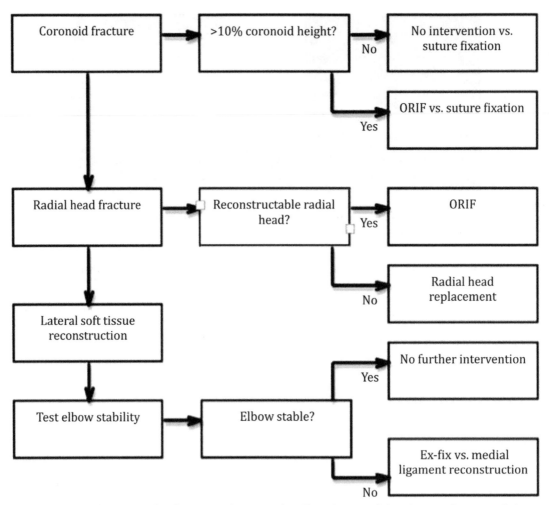

Fig. 5. Decision-making algorithm for approaching complex elbow fracture dislocations. Ex-fix, External Fixator; ORIF, Open Reduction and Internal Fixation.

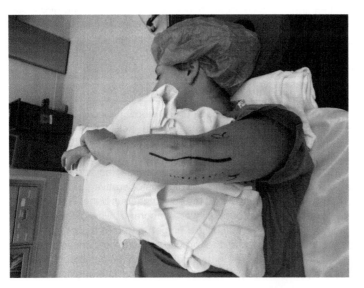

Fig. 6. When supine positioning is chosen, the patient's operative arm is draped freely across the body with blankets used as a bolster. Ulnar and radial sides are marked for orientation as well as the location of the ulnar nerve (*dotted line*). The planned posterior incision is shown (*solid line*).

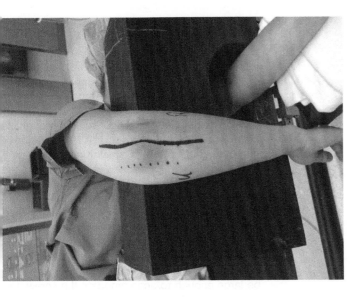

Fig. 7. Lateral positioning is shown with a beanbag to maintain position. Bone foam is used to support the operative arm. Ulnar and radial sides are marked for orientation and the ulnar nerve (*dotted line*) is demonstrated as well.

may be used that are beneficial in cases of medial soft tissue repair that must be performed, of an ulnar nerve that needs to be explored, or when visualization is not adequate through the posterior incision.[34]

The lateral column can be approached through several deep intervals regardless of the skin incision chosen. The posterolateral (Kocher) approach (**Fig. 8**) occurs between the extensor carpi ulnaris (ECU) and the anconeus, which provides direct access to the joint capsule; however, there is increased risk of injury to the LUCL. Alternatively the direct lateral (Kaplan) approach (**Fig. 9**) accesses the joint at the muscular interval between the extensor digitorum communis (EDC) and the extensor carpi radialis brevis (ECRB). Although iatrogenic injury to the LUCL is less common, if the LUCL has been damaged, this approach does not allow for visualization for repair or reconstruction. In cases of elbow

fracture dislocation, the soft tissues are often disrupted. Regardless of the interval chosen, dissection should be carried out with the elbow in pronation to reduce risk of injury to the posterior interosseous nerve (PIN).

Medially, an anteromedial interval between the pronator teres and brachialis may be used to access the anterior capsule. The posteromedial (flexor carpi ulnaris [FCU]-splitting) exposure necessitates anterior ulnar nerve transposition and the FCU is divided between the 2 heads of the muscle.[35,36] The Hotchkiss over-the-top approach (**Fig. 10**) splits the flexor-pronator mass and the pronator teres is released from the epicondyle to provide access to the coronoid and medial elbow structures.[2,35] Access to olecranon fractures can typically be approached between the ECU and FCU at the subcutaneous border of the ulna. Subperiosteal dissection frequently provides adequate exposure for hardware placement.

A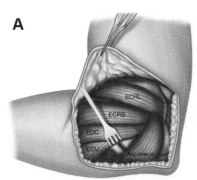

B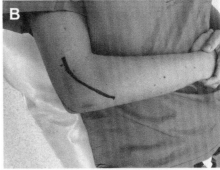

Fig. 8. The Kocher approach. To the right is the planned surgical incision approaching the radial elbow if separate incisions are to be used. ECRL, extensor carpi radialis longus. Planned surgical incision (*A*) and the deep dissection (*B*).

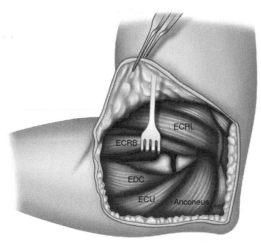

Fig. 9. The Kaplan approach. ECRL, extensor carpi radialis longus.

Surgical Procedure

The surgical procedure is highly dependent on the specific pattern of injury to the elbow structures. Most commonly, the injuries are addressed in an inside-out fashion, addressing any injury to the coronoid first, then progressing to the radial head, olecranon, lateral soft tissues, and finally the medial soft tissue structures.

Coronoid

The size and position of the coronoid fracture govern the fixation, if any, that is required. For type 1 fractures, nonoperative management is usually successful, although some surgeons have recommended suture fixation. Suture fixation may also be used for type 2 fractures if adequate screw fixation is not possible due to fracture size or bone quality or to augment internal fixation.

The coronoid can frequently be approached through the lateral approach, because the radial-sided structures are commonly already interrupted. If suture fixation is chosen (see **Fig. 3**F, G; **Fig. 11**), 2 drill holes are created along the subcutaneous border of the ulna to serve as tunnels for the suture, directed toward either side of the coronoid footprint.[37] Typically the coronoid fragment is too small to accommodate drill holes and, therefore, is most commonly captured by passing a number-1 braided suture through its anterior capsular attachment.[36–38] The fragment may be held in place by small Kirschner wires if needed and the suture is tied at the border of the ulna after other injuries have been addressed.

Types 2 and 3 fractures often require a medial-sided approach because they are commonly fixed with formal open reduction and internal fixation. Smaller fractures can be fixed with a headless screw that can be augmented with the addition of suture fixation. In this case, the fragment must be large enough to accommodate the screw and the bone must be of adequate quality.[39] The screw should be placed in the posterior to anterior direction to achieve greater fixation strength and to reduce the risk of injury to anterior neurovascular structures.[36]

For larger fragments, anteromedial buttress plating can be used with or without combined headless compression screws (**Fig. 12**). Occasionally, a surgeon is faced with multiple coronoid fragments that may necessitate separate medial and dorsal plates, which again may be augmented with suture or screw fixation.[39]

Radial head

After any potential coronoid injury is addressed, attention is then turned to the radial head and neck, which are carefully evaluated. Fracture extension into the neck that necessitates more proximal dissection should prompt identification and isolation of the PIN to avoid iatrogenic injury.[34,40] Commonly, the level of fracture comminution and displacement is greater than

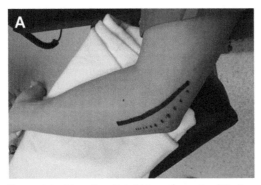
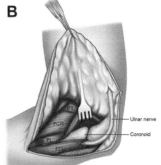

Fig. 10. (A) Planned incision for Hotchkiss approach. (B) demonstrates the deep dissection. The Hotchkiss approach to the medial elbow. Also shown is the planned medial incision (*solid line*) and the course of the ulnar nerve (*dotted line*). FCR, flexor carpi radialis; PL, palmaris longus; PT, pronator teres.

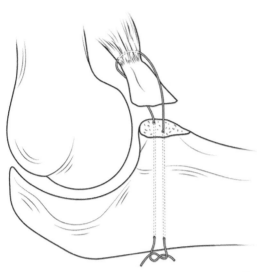

anticipated and, therefore, the surgeon should always be prepared to replace the radial head if necessary. In the context of complex elbow dislocations, excision of the head is contraindicated due to loss of stability and should not be attempted.[34]

If a few large fragments exist and bone is healthy enough to achieve secure fixation, headless compression screws may be used. The radial head articular surface is anatomically restored and maintained with pointed reduction forceps. Kirschner wires are placed and cannulated headless compression screws are implanted over their respective pins. If standard screws are used, it is important to place these implants in the nonarticulating safe zone of the radius to avoid any symptoms with pronation or supination (**Fig. 13**).[41] Fracture extension into the neck is treated with a buttress plate, again placed in the safe zone of the proximal radius to avoid impingement (**Fig. 14**). It is important to restore anatomic alignment and length to avoid future instability.[34]

Fig. 11. Suture fixation of the olecranon. Suture fixation of coronoid fracture through 2 drill holes created at the ulnar border with suture capturing the coronoid fragment through its soft tissue attachments.

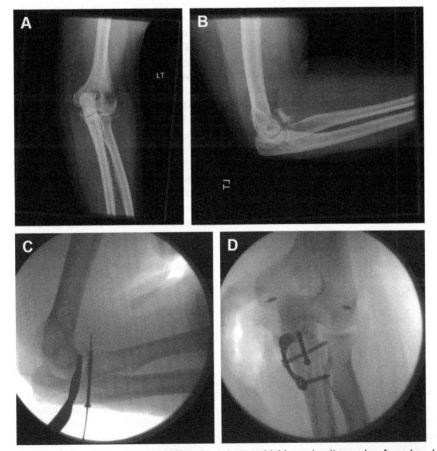

Fig. 12. Coronoid open reduction and internal fixation. (*A*) AP and (*B*) lateral radiographs of a reduced elbow fracture dislocation with a large coronoid fragment. The coronoid fragment was fixed with a (*C*) cannulated screw over a guide wire and (*D*) a medial buttress plate. Suture anchors were used to reattach the LUCL and MUCL to their origins.

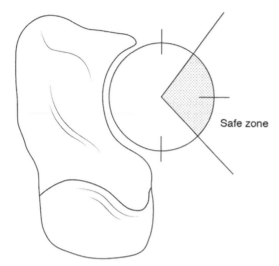

Fig. 13. Safe zone for placement of hardware in the radial head with the wrist in neutral rotation.

If the radial head is extensively comminuted or osteopenic, internal fixation may not be ideal. In this situation, radial head replacement is advisable and has demonstrated good results. The native radial head is removed and pieced together on the back table to estimate the dimensions of the radial head replacement. Options for arthroplasty are extensive, including various materials, modular or monoblock, and monopolar or bipolar implants.[42] The authors prefer the use of uncemented monoblock prosthesis, which may be inserted in a loose fashion if desired.[43]

The most important aspects of replacement are appropriate sizing and positioning of the prosthesis. Although the native head may guide size selection, trials of various-sized components with elbow range of motion and rotation are important because intraoperative imaging may be misleading.[42] Importantly, the radial head must not be overstuffed, which inevitably leads to increased radiocapitellar contact pressures, elbow pain, loss of range of motion, and component failure.[44–47]

Lateral soft tissues

Posterior fracture dislocations of the elbow invariably have some degree of soft tissue damage to the lateral elbow and are the most common cause of injury to the LCL.[48,49] Due to the critical role of the LCL as the primary lateral elbow stabilizer, soft tissue repair is mandatory at the time of surgery because failure to address this injury is a significant cause for recurrent instability.[49–52] Most commonly, the LCL and posterolateral capsule are avulsed as a sleeve from the lateral condyle, leaving a characteristic bare spot.[49]

Surgical repair with suture anchors or bone tunnels placed at the origin of the LCL at the bare area on the epicondyle. The LCL may be reapproximated with its neighboring capsule, fascia, and muscular structures.[40] Some investigators advocate repair with the elbow in supination to prevent overtensioning of the ligament complex.[2]

Complications and Management

Surgical treatment of complex elbow dislocations and proper postoperative therapy can improve elbow function; however, despite proper technique and follow-up, patients still are susceptible to the several sequelae of a traumatic injury to the elbow. Postoperative complications, such as heterotopic ossification (HO), recurrent joint instability, ulnar neuropathy, recurrent joint stiffness, and elbow osteoarthritis can compromise both early and late outcomes after surgery.

Heterotopic ossification

HO is a commonly observed complication seen in the posttraumatic elbow that can cause pain and decreased joint mobility. Radiologic evidence of HO may be seen in up to 37% of surgically treated elbow fractures.[53] Significant HO is associated with terrible triad injury, transolecranon fracture dislocation, and Monteggia fracture dislocation. Other factors, such as joint instability, severe chest trauma, and delay in definitive surgical treatment, were also associated with a higher prevalence of HO.[53,54]

Excision of ossification is the mainstay of surgical management for symptomatic HO to restore function and range of motion (**Fig. 15**).[55–57] Both single-fraction radiation therapy (RT) and indomethacin have been used for HO prophylaxis in complex elbow fracture surgery. Acceptable results and low rates of recurrent HO after prophylactic RT have been reported; however, the rate of nonunion may be significantly increased.[58–60] A systematic review of the literature on RT for prevention of HO in the elbow yielded weak evidence mostly from case series to support its use, and the investigators recommended against its use as first-line prophylaxis against HO.[61] Further studies are needed to elucidate the effectiveness of HO prophylactic measures.

Recurrent joint instability

Recurrent elbow instability presents with repeated painful dislocations or subluxations after an initial traumatic dislocation. O'Driscoll[62] detailed the timing, involved anatomy, direction and degree of displacement, and presence or absence of associated fractures in his description of this complication. Due to the variety of injury patterns,

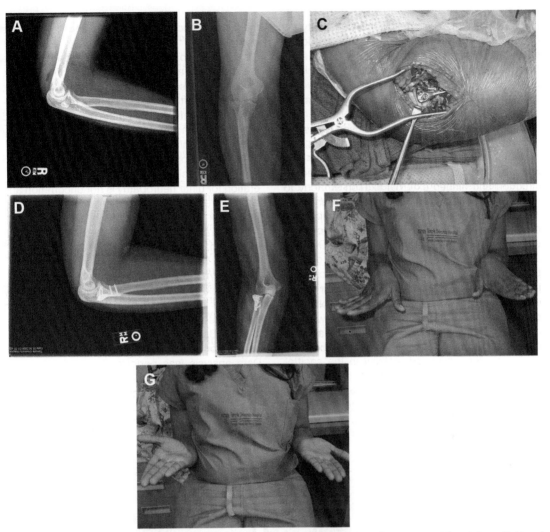

Fig. 14. Radius fixation. (*A*) Lateral and (*B*) posteroanterior (PA) radiographs of a woman with a right radial head fracture with extension into the neck. (*C*) An intraoperative photograph of the proximal radius plate fixation is shown. Postoperative (*D*) lateral and (*E*) PA demonstrate the plate fixation combined with headless compression screws. Near-complete restoration of (*F*) pronation and (*G*) supination compared with the contralateral side.

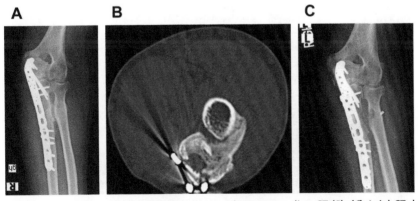

Fig. 15. (*A*) Xray demonstrating synostosis/HO formation with corresponding CT (*B*). (*C*) Axial CT demonstrating bridging bone from the ulna to the radius. AP film showing the after-synostosis excision. This patient suffered an iatrogenic biceps tendon avulsion that was repaired by tenodesis. It is important keep the instruments on the ulna to avoid this complication.

management of recurrent joint instability is directed by the characteristics of each particular case, but surgical correction is usually the definitive treatment. Elbow function and stability have been restored by using ligament and tendon allografts to reconstruct chronically unstable elbows.[63–65]

External fixators have also been used to restore and stabilize a congruent elbow articulation and facilitate early motion (**Fig. 16**).[66,67] Sørensen and Søjbjerg[68] used a combination of anatomic reconstruction and hinged external fixation strategy to treat recurrent dislocated elbows and found that mobility and flexion were restored in a majority of elbows treated. They also advocate for treatment within 6 weeks of acute injury for superior results.

Ulnar neuropathy

Ulnar neuropathy manifests as sensory or motor deficits in the hand and can be a debilitating complication of treatment of complex elbow dislocations. Reports of postoperative neuropathy as high as 11.1% to 18.2% after repair of terrible triad injuries reflect the significance of this complication.[69]

Ulnar neuropathy can present secondary to the initial trauma, as iatrogenic injury during surgery, or due to the sequelae of inflammation, scarring, or nonunion after surgery. For this reason, a thorough preoperative examination is crucial, followed by careful handling of the nerve intraoperatively and close monitoring after surgery.

Although prophylactic ulnar nerve transposition or decompression is not routinely practiced, reoperation for ulnar neuropathy is not uncommon and some investigators advocate addressing this at the index surgery.[70] Decompression in situ or anterior transposition typically results in symptom resolution, and early treatment is recommended.[71]

Elbow stiffness/contractures

The etiology of elbow stiffness is typically anatomic in nature, frequently associated with soft tissue contracture, HO, or incongruous articulation.[72] Basic science research on the pathogenesis of contractures at the cellular and molecular

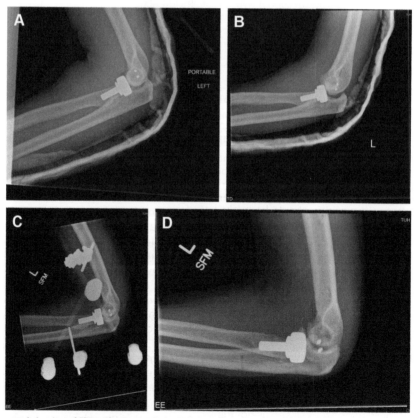

Fig. 16. Recurrent joint instability. The immediate postoperative images of a left elbow after radial head replacement with ligament reconstruction (*A*) in a patient, who subsequently experienced recurrent instability and subluxation (*B*). The patient was taken back to the operating room for reduction and external fixation (*C*), and ex-fix was subsequently removed (*D*) with maintenance of stable reduction.

levels has shown that dysregulation of myofibro-blasts and alpha-smooth muscle actin may play a role in this disease; therapeutic applications of this knowledge have yet to be developed.[73,74]

Nonoperative management with dynamic splint-ing, serial casting, continuous passive motion, and formal therapy have been successful in restoring arc of motion.[75–77] A study of static progressive and dynamic splints demonstrated no difference in outcome, although both improved range of mo-tion.[75] After a trial of conservative management, surgical intervention may be necessary to restore elbow range of motion. Both arthroscopic and open techniques have been described, although, in the setting of significant contracture, caution should be used if arthroscopy is attempted.[78–82]

Posttraumatic osteoarthritis

Osteoarthritis is a common sequela of elbow trauma that can be seen on radiographs in up to 80% of patients at long-term follow-up; however, the correlation with patient symptoms has not been elucidated.[83] For patients undergoing sur-gery for repair of displaced and unstable elbow fractures, 10% to 80% develop moderate to se-vere arthrosis. Multiple studies failed to correlate findings of arthrosis on imaging with clinical exam-ination, and, therefore, treatment is not recom-mended based on radiograph findings alone.[83,84]

Nonoperative treatment with therapy and nonsteroidal anti-inflammatory drugs (NSAIDs) is often successful. Although viscosupplementation has been advocated by some investigators, long-term results are lacking.[85] Surgical treatment op-tions may be guided by the degree and location of structural damage, severity of stiffness, and age of the patient.[86] Surgical options include re-surfacing and débridement to total elbow arthro-plasty or even arthrodesis. Outcomes from these surgeries have demonstrated some improvement in various elbow functions scales and are indi-cated based on the degree and location of arthritis.

POSTOPERATIVE CARE

Postoperative care begins with an initial period of elbow immobilization in a posterior splint at 90° of flexion and neutral rotation. Active range of mo-tion under the supervision of a therapist are initi-ated at approximately 1 week postoperatively to avoid stiffness. Shoulder abduction is avoided to prevent undue valgus stress on the elbow. HO pro-phylaxis with NSAIDs or radiation may be used as well. There are no well-designed studies that have compared postoperative protocols, so at this time the specifics of postoperative care are highly variable.[87] At 6 weeks after surgery, patients who plateau or regress in therapy are placed into a static stretching splint to treat early stiffness.

OUTCOMES

Elbow fracture dislocations nearly always require surgical intervention, with intervention directed at the specific pattern of injury.[50] Although a wide va-riety of presentations and treatments exist, a com-mon theme is the subpar outcomes and frequent complications that plague these injuries.[7,30,88,89]

Complications of chronic instability and stiffness are the most common and are difficult to avoid. Egol and colleagues[88] reported a series of 29 pa-tients with terrible triad injuries and noted improve-ment when a systematic approach is used. In the setting of complex elbow dislocation, radial head fractures are treated with internal fixation or acute replacement. Duckworth and colleagues[90] demonstrated a significant rate of revision or removal with acute radial head replacement and recommended careful consideration before choosing replacements in younger patients. Other investigators, however, have demonstrated equiv-ocal short-term results for radial head replacement versus internal fixation.[91]

Recommendations vary for treatment of coro-noid fractures associated with elbow dislocation. At a mean 31-month follow up, Park and col-leagues[92] demonstrated good or excellent results in maore than 90% of patients with collateral liga-ment repair alone in the treatment of O'Driscoll type 1 coronoid fractures. Optimal results for types 2 and 3 fractures were obtained when internal fix-ation was combined with ligamentous repair. Gar-rigues and colleagues[37] compared anchor or screw fixation with a lasso suture technique, demonstrating superior results with fewer compli-cations when the lasso technique was used for Re-gan and Morrey type 1 and 2 fractures.

For the so-called terrible triad injuries, many in-vestigators describe disappointing results even with a methodical surgical approach, necessi-tating reoperation in up to 28% of patients.[2,7,88] Treatment within 2 weeks of injury may produce better range of motion and slightly improved clin-ical outcomes.[71]

Most investigators prefer to fix the MCL or place a hinged external fixator for elbows that remain un-stable after intra-articular fractures and the lateral ligament complex is addressed.[1,30,66,93] Forthman and colleagues[70] reported on a series of 34 pa-tients with a posterior elbow fracture dislocation without MCL repair or external fixator and found good or excellent results in 74% of their patients. The investigators submit that these results are comparable to general outcomes for terrible triad injuries and obviate a separate incision, dissection, or ulnar nerve transposition.

SUMMARY

Complex elbow dislocations are a notoriously challenging injury to treat due to the technical difficulty of the operation, the high variability of fracture patterns and soft tissue injuries, and the large rate of subpar outcomes with frequent complications. Immediate treatment consists of urgent concentric reduction of the elbow if possible followed by CT scan. If reduction cannot be immediately achieved, temporary elbow-spanning external fixation may be necessary and, in this scenario, CT should be delayed until after surgery.

Surgical treatment is most successful with thorough evaluation of preoperative imaging and a structured algorithm to address any injury encountered intraoperatively. The authors begin with evaluation of the coronoid, followed by the radial head, lateral soft tissues, and finally the medial soft tissue structures. If instability persists after addressing the coronoid and lateral structures, the authors commonly apply a hinged elbow-spanning external fixator for 4 to 6 weeks.

Above all else, restoration of the articular surface must be achieved with concentric reduction. Early motion is important in preventing postoperative complications; however, this should not take precedence over maintenance of the reduction. Stiffness, HO, posttraumatic osteoarthritis, and ulnar nerve complications are, unfortunately, common with these injuries and may require further surgical intervention. Despite the challenges of treating this injury, many aspects of surgical intervention have been well documented and good outcomes certainly can be achieved.

REFERENCES

1. Lill H, Korner J, Rose T, et al. Fracture-dislocations of the elbow joint–strategy for treatment and results. Arch Orthop Trauma Surg 2001;121(1–2):31–7.
2. Bohn K, Ipaktchi K, Livermore M, et al. Current treatment concepts for "terrible triad" injuries of the elbow. Orthopedics 2014;37(12):831–7.
3. Morrey BF, Askew LJ, Chao EY. A biomechanical study of normal functional elbow motion. J Bone Joint Surg Am 1981;63(6):872–7.
4. Sardelli M, Tashjian RZ, MacWilliams BA. Functional elbow range of motion for contemporary tasks. J Bone Joint Surg Am 2011;93(5):471–7.
5. Englert C, Zellner J, Koller M, et al. Elbow dislocations: a review ranging from soft tissue injuries to complex elbow fracture dislocations. Adv Orthop 2013;2013:951397.
6. O'Driscoll SW, Morrey BF, Korinek S, et al. Elbow subluxation and dislocation. A spectrum of instability. Clin Orthop Relat Res 1992;(280):186–97.
7. Ring D, Jupiter JB. Fracture-dislocation of the elbow. Hand Clin 2002;18(1):55–63.
8. Mathew PK, Athwal GS, King GJ. Terrible triad injury of the elbow: current concepts. J Am Acad Orthop Surg 2009;17(3):137–51.
9. Morrey BF. Current concepts in the management of complex elbow trauma. Surgeon 2009;7(3):151–61.
10. Iannuzzi NP, Leopold SS. In brief: the Mason classification of radial head fractures. Clin Orthop Relat Res 2012;470(6):1799–802.
11. Lapner M, King GJ. Radial head fractures. J Bone Joint Surg Am 2013;95(12):1136–43.
12. Hotchkiss RN. Displaced fractures of the radial head: internal fixation or excision? J Am Acad Orthop Surg 1997;5(1):1–10.
13. Regan W, Morrey B. Fractures of the coronoid process of the ulna. J Bone Joint Surg Am 1989;71(9):1348–54.
14. Wells J, Ablove RH. Coronoid fractures of the elbow. Clin Med Res 2008;6(1):40–4.
15. Tashjian RZ, Katarincic JA. Complex elbow instability. J Am Acad Orthop Surg 2006;14(5):278–86.
16. Hak DJ, Golladay GJ. Olecranon fractures: treatment options. J Am Acad Orthop Surg 2000;8(4):266–75.
17. Morrey BF. Current concepts in the treatment of fractures of the radial head, the olecranon, and the coronoid. Instr Course Lect 1995;44:175–85.
18. Chan K, MacDermid JC, Faber KJ, et al. Can we treat select terrible triad injuries nonoperatively? Clin Orthop Relat Res 2014;472(7):2092–9.
19. van Riet RP, Morrey BF, O'Driscoll SW, et al. Associated injuries complicating radial head fractures: a demographic study. Clin Orthop Relat Res 2005;441:351–5.
20. Tarassoli P, McCann P, Amirfeyz R. Complex instability of the elbow. Injury 2013. [Epub ahead of print].
21. Winter M, Chuinard C, Cikes A, et al. Surgical management of elbow dislocation associated with non-reparable fractures of the radial head. Chir Main 2009;28(3):158–67.
22. O'Driscoll SW, Bell DF, Morrey BF. Posterolateral rotatory instability of the elbow. J Bone Joint Surg Am 1991;73(3):440–6.
23. Guitton TG, Ring D. Nonsurgically treated terrible triad injuries of the elbow: report of four cases. J Hand Surg Am 2010;35(3):464–7.
24. Ring D, Jupiter JB, Zilberfarb J. Posterior dislocation of the elbow with fractures of the radial head and coronoid. J Bone Joint Surg Am 2002;84-A(4):547–51.

25. O'Driscoll SW, Jupiter JB, King GJ, et al. The unstable elbow. Instr Course Lect 2001;50:89–102.

26. O'Driscoll SW, Jupiter JB, Cohen MS, et al. Difficult elbow fractures: pearls and pitfalls. Instr Course Lect 2003;52:113–34.

27. Nestor BJ, O'Driscoll SW, Morrey BF. Ligamentous reconstruction for posterolateral rotatory instability of the elbow. J Bone Joint Surg Am 1992;74(8): 1235–41.

28. Giannicola G, Greco A, Sacchetti FM, et al. Complex fracture-dislocations of the proximal ulna and radius in adults: a comprehensive classification. J Shoulder Elbow Surg 2011;20(8):1289–99.

29. Jupiter JB, Ring D. Treatment of unreduced elbow dislocations with hinged external fixation. J Bone Joint Surg Am 2002;84-A(9):1630–5.

30. Pugh DM, Wild LM, Schemitsch EH, et al. Standard surgical protocol to treat elbow dislocations with radial head and coronoid fractures. J Bone Joint Surg Am 2004;86-A(6):1122–30.

31. Iordens GI, Den Hartog D, Van Lieshout EM, et al. Good functional recovery of complex elbow dislocations treated with hinged external fixation: a multicenter prospective study. Clin Orthop Relat Res 2015;473(4):1451–61.

32. Cheung EV, Steinmann SP. Surgical approaches to the elbow. J Am Acad Orthop Surg 2009;17(5): 325–33.

33. Ring D, Jupiter JB. Fracture-dislocation of the elbow. J Bone Joint Surg Am 1998;80(4):566–80.

34. Pugh DM, McKee MD. The "terrible triad" of the elbow. Tech Hand Up Extrem Surg 2002;6(1):21–9.

35. Huh J, Krueger CA, Medvecky MJ, et al. Medial elbow exposure for coronoid fractures: FCU-split versus over-the-top. J Orthop Trauma 2013;27(12): 730–4.

36. Budoff JE. Coronoid fractures. J Hand Surg Am 2012;37(11):2418–23.

37. Garrigues GE, Wray WH, Lindenhovius AL, et al. Fixation of the coronoid process in elbow fracture-dislocations. J Bone Joint Surg Am 2011; 93(20):1873–81.

38. Doornberg JN, van Duijn J, Ring D. Coronoid fracture height in terrible-triad injuries. J Hand Surg Am 2006;31(5):794–7.

39. Ring D. Fractures of the coronoid process of the ulna. J Hand Surg Am 2006;31(10):1679–89.

40. Dyer G, Ring D. My approach to the terrible triad injury. Oper Tech Orthop 2010;20(1):11–6.

41. Smith GR, Hotchkiss RN. Radial head and neck fractures: anatomic guidelines for proper placement of internal fixation. J Shoulder Elbow Surg 1996;5(2 Pt 1):113–7.

42. Charalambous CP, Stanley JK, Mills SP, et al. Comminuted radial head fractures: aspects of current management. J Shoulder Elbow Surg 2011; 20(6):996–1007.

43. Ring D. Radial head fracture: open reduction-internal fixation or prosthetic replacement. J Shoulder Elbow Surg 2011;20(Suppl 2):S107–12.

44. Alolabi B, Studer A, Gray A, et al. Selecting the diameter of a radial head implant: an assessment of local landmarks. J Shoulder Elbow Surg 2013; 22(10):1395–9.

45. Bachman DR, Thaveepunsan S, Park S, et al. The effect of prosthetic radial head geometry on the distribution and magnitude of radiocapitellar joint contact pressures. J Hand Surg Am 2015;40(2):281–8.

46. Delclaux S, Lebon J, Faraud A, et al. Complications of radial head prostheses. Int Orthop 2015;39(5): 907–13.

47. King GJ. Management of comminuted radial head fractures with replacement arthroplasty. Hand Clin 2004;20(4):429–41, vi.

48. Reichel LM, Milam GS, Sitton SE, et al. Elbow lateral collateral ligament injuries. J Hand Surg Am 2013; 38(1):184–201 [quiz: 201].

49. McKee MD, Schemitsch EH, Sala MJ, et al. The pathoanatomy of lateral ligamentous disruption in complex elbow instability. J Shoulder Elbow Surg 2003;12(4):391–6.

50. Lee DH. Treatment options for complex elbow fracture dislocations. Injury 2001;32(Suppl 4):SD41–69.

51. Cohen MS, Hastings H. Rotatory instability of the elbow. The anatomy and role of the lateral stabilizers. J Bone Joint Surg Am 1997;79(2):225–33.

52. Dunning CE, Zarzour ZD, Patterson SD, et al. Ligamentous stabilizers against posterolateral rotatory instability of the elbow. J Bone Joint Surg Am 2001;83-A(12):1823–8.

53. Foruria AM, Augustin S, Morrey BF, et al. Heterotopic ossification after surgery for fractures and fracture-dislocations involving the proximal aspect of the radius or ulna. J Bone Joint Surg Am 2013;95(10):e66.

54. Wiggers JK, Helmerhorst GT, Brouwer KM, et al. Injury complexity factors predict heterotopic ossification restricting motion after elbow trauma. Clin Orthop Relat Res 2014;472(7):2162–7.

55. Salazar D, Golz A, Israel H, et al. Heterotopic ossification of the elbow treated with surgical resection: risk factors, bony ankylosis, and complications. Clin Orthop Relat Res 2014;472(7):2269–75.

56. Koh KH, Lim TK, Lee HI, et al. Surgical treatment of elbow stiffness caused by post-traumatic heterotopic ossification. J Shoulder Elbow Surg 2013;22(8): 1128–34.

57. Baldwin K, Hosalkar HS, Donegan DJ, et al. Surgical resection of heterotopic bone about the elbow: an institutional experience with traumatic and neurologic etiologies. J Hand Surg Am 2011; 36(5):798–803.

58. Strauss JB, Wysocki RW, Shah A, et al. Radiation therapy for heterotopic ossification prophylaxis afer

high-risk elbow surgery. Am J Orthop (Belle Mead NJ) 2011;40(8):400–5.

59. Robinson CG, Polster JM, Reddy CA, et al. Postoperative single-fraction radiation for prevention of heterotopic ossification of the elbow. Int J Radiat Oncol Biol Phys 2010;77(5):1493–9.

60. Hamid N, Ashraf N, Bosse MJ, et al. Radiation therapy for heterotopic ossification prophylaxis acutely after elbow trauma: a prospective randomized study. J Bone Joint Surg Am 2010;92(11):2032–8.

61. Ploumis A, Belbasis L, Ntzani E, et al. Radiotherapy for prevention of heterotopic ossification of the elbow: a systematic review of the literature. J Shoulder Elbow Surg 2013;22(11):1580–8.

62. O'Driscoll SW. Classification and evaluation of recurrent instability of the elbow. Clin Orthop Relat Res 2000;(370):34–43.

63. Baghdadi YM, Morrey BF, O'Driscoll SW, et al. Revision allograft reconstruction of the lateral collateral ligament complex in elbows with previous failed reconstruction and persistent posterolateral rotatory instability. Clin Orthop Relat Res 2014; 472(7):2061–7.

64. van Riet RP, Bain GI, Baird R, et al. Simultaneous reconstruction of medial and lateral elbow ligaments for instability using a circumferential graft. Tech Hand Up Extrem Surg 2006;10(4):239–44.

65. Olsen BS, Søjbjerg JO. The treatment of recurrent posterolateral instability of the elbow. J Bone Joint Surg Br 2003;85(3):342–6.

66. Ruch DS, Triepel CR. Hinged elbow fixation for recurrent instability following fracture dislocation. Injury 2001;32(Suppl 4):SD70–8.

67. McKee MD, Bowden SH, King GJ, et al. Management of recurrent, complex instability of the elbow with a hinged external fixator. J Bone Joint Surg Br 1998;80(6):1031–6.

68. Sørensen AK, Søjbjerg JO. Treatment of persistent instability after posterior fracture-dislocation of the elbow: restoring stability and mobility by internal fixation and hinged external fixation. J Shoulder Elbow Surg 2011;20(8):1300–9.

69. Chen NC, Jupiter JB, Steinmann SP, et al. Nonacute treatment of elbow fracture with persistent ulnohumeral dislocation or subluxation. J Bone Joint Surg Am 2014;96(15):1308–16.

70. Forthman C, Henket M, Ring DC. Elbow dislocation with intra-articular fracture: the results of operative treatment without repair of the medial collateral ligament. J Hand Surg Am 2007;32(8):1200–9.

71. Lindenhovius AL, Jupiter JB, Ring D. Comparison of acute versus subacute treatment of terrible triad injuries of the elbow. J Hand Surg Am 2008;33(6): 920–6.

72. Evans PJ, Nandi S, Maschke S, et al. Prevention and treatment of elbow stiffness. J Hand Surg Am 2009; 34(4):769–78.

73. Hildebrand KA, Zhang M, Befus AD, et al. A myofibroblast-mast cell-neuropeptide axis of fibrosis in post-traumatic joint contractures: an in vitro analysis of mechanistic components. J Orthop Res 2014;32(10):1290–6.

74. Doornberg JN, Bosse T, Cohen MS, et al. Temporary presence of myofibroblasts in human elbow capsule after trauma. J Bone Joint Surg Am 2014;96(5):e36.

75. Lindenhovius AL, Doornberg JN, Brouwer KM, et al. A prospective randomized controlled trial of dynamic versus static progressive elbow splinting for posttraumatic elbow stiffness. J Bone Joint Surg Am 2012;94(8):694–700.

76. Ulrich SD, Bonutti PM, Seyler TM, et al. Restoring range of motion via stress relaxation and static progressive stretch in posttraumatic elbow contractures. J Shoulder Elbow Surg 2010;19(2):196–201.

77. Myden C, Hildebrand K. Elbow joint contracture after traumatic injury. J Shoulder Elbow Surg 2011; 20(1):39–44.

78. Ehsan A, Huang JI, Lyons M, et al. Surgical management of posttraumatic elbow arthrofibrosis. J Trauma Acute Care Surg 2012;72(5):1399–403.

79. Cefo I, Eygendaal D. Arthroscopic arthrolysis for posttraumatic elbow stiffness. J Shoulder Elbow Surg 2011;20(3):434–9.

80. Lindenhovius AL, van de Luijtgaarden K, Ring D, et al. Open elbow contracture release: postoperative management with and without continuous passive motion. J Hand Surg Am 2009;34(5):858–65.

81. Capo JT, Shamian B, Francisco R, et al. Fracture pattern characteristics and associated injuries of high-energy, large fragment, partial articular radial head fractures: a preliminary imaging analysis. J Orthop Traumatol 2015;16(2):125–31.

82. Tan V, Daluiski A, Simic P, et al. Outcome of open release for post-traumatic elbow stiffness. J Trauma 2006;61(3):673–8.

83. Guitton TG, Zurakowski D, van Dijk NC, et al. Incidence and risk factors for the development of radiographic arthrosis after traumatic elbow injuries. J Hand Surg Am 2010;35(12):1976–80.

84. Doornberg JN, van Duijn PJ, Linzel D, et al. Surgical treatment of intra-articular fractures of the distal part of the humerus. Functional outcome after twelve to thirty years. J Bone Joint Surg Am 2007;89(7): 1524–32.

85. van Brakel RW, Eygendaal D. Intra-articular injection of hyaluronic acid is not effective for the treatment of post-traumatic osteoarthritis of the elbow. Arthroscopy 2006;22(11):1199–203.

86. Chammas M. Post-traumatic osteoarthritis of the elbow. Orthop Traumatol Surg Res 2014;100(Suppl 1):S15–24.

87. Harding P, Rasekaba T, Smirneos L, et al. Early mobilisation for elbow fractures in adults. Cochrane Database Syst Rev 2011;(6):CD008130.

88. Egol KA, Immerman I, Paksima N, et al. Fracture-dislocation of the elbow functional outcome following treatment with a standardized protocol. Bull NYU Hosp Jt Dis 2007;65(4):263–70.

89. Fitzgibbons PG, Louie D, Dyer GS, et al. Functional outcomes after fixation of "terrible triad" elbow fracture dislocations. Orthopedics 2014; 37(4):e373–6.

90. Duckworth AD, Wickramasinghe NR, Clement ND, et al. Radial head replacement for acute complex fractures: what are the rate and risks factors for revision or removal? Clin Orthop Relat Res 2014;472(7): 2136–43.

91. Watters TS, Garrigues GE, Ring D, et al. Fixation versus replacement of radial head in terrible triad: is there a difference in elbow stability and prognosis? Clin Orthop Relat Res 2014;472(7):2128–35.

92. Park SM, Lee JS, Jung JY, et al. How should anteromedial coronoid facet fracture be managed? A surgical strategy based on O'Driscoll classification and ligament injury. J Shoulder Elbow Surg 2015; 24(1):74–82.

93. Maniscalco P, Pizzoli AL, Brivio LR, et al. Hinged external fixation for complex fracture-dislocation of the elbow in elderly people. Injury 2014;45(Suppl 6):S53–7.

Management of the Morel-Lavallée Lesion

Dustin Greenhill, MD*, Christopher Haydel, MD, Saqib Rehman, MD

KEYWORDS

- Closed degloving injury • Morel Lavallée lesion • Soft tissue injury • Hematoma • Sclerodesis

KEY POINTS

- Diagnosis of Morel-Lavallée lesions is often missed or delayed.
- The presence of a lesion over operative fractures increases the risk of postoperative infection.
- Advanced imaging may help determine the best methods of treatment.
- Treatment options include compression, aspiration, percutaneous or open surgical treatment, and sclerotherapy. Additionally, postoperative management plays an equal role in treatment success.
- Specific treatment should be individualized for each patient based on a surgeon's thorough understanding of Morel-Lavallée lesions.

INTRODUCTION

In 1863, a French physician named Maurice Morel-Lavallée[1] first described a unique posttraumatic fluid collection that developed in a patient who fell from a moving train. More than a century later, while Letournel and Judet[2] compiled their well-known series of acetabular fractures, they also witnessed the same characteristic lesions develop over the greater trochanter and named them *Morel-Lavallée* (ML) lesions. Such lesions have been described by other terms in the literature, such as ML effusion or hematoma, posttraumatic pseudocyst, posttraumatic soft tissue cyst, closed degloving injury, or chronic expanding hematoma.[2,3] If a lesion occurs, it is almost always after direct trauma to the pelvis, thigh, or knee. A hypovascular suprafascial space develops in which fluid easily accumulates. Posttraumatic hematoma formation increases the risk of infection, and a unique combination of physical properties inhibits physiologic dead space closure.[4]

Such lesions are rare, and diagnosis is often delayed or missed. As a result, their natural history is not yet clearly established. In a series of approximately 1100 consecutive pelvic fractures, Tseng and Tornetta[5] reported that 19 (1.7%) patients developed ML lesions. However, the actual incidence is higher because lesions can occur without an underlying fracture and a small portion likely persist subclinically.[6] Letournel and Judet[2] published an incidence of 8.3% after trauma to the greater trochanter.[2] Consequently, the true incidence is unknown. The current body of available literature consists entirely of case series composed of heterogeneous groups of patients. Therefore, no standard treatment algorithms exist. This article helps physicians understand the currently accepted surgical indications, techniques, and controversies when managing patients with an ML lesion.

CAUSE

Individuals are at risk for developing an ML lesion after sustaining a significant blow or sudden shearing force to any area with strong underlying fascia, most often around the pelvis or lower

The authors have nothing to disclose.
Department of Orthopaedic Surgery & Sports Medicine, Temple University Hospital, 3401 North Broad Street, Zone B 5th Floor, Philadelphia, PA 19140, USA
* Corresponding author.
E-mail address: dustin.greenhill2@tuhs.temple.edu

Orthop Clin N Am 47 (2016) 115–125
http://dx.doi.org/10.1016/j.ocl.2015.08.012
0030-5898/16/$ – see front matter © 2016 Elsevier Inc. All rights reserved.

limb. Motor vehicle collisions tend to be responsible for most of these lesions, and more than 50% are due to high-energy mechanisms.[7,8] However, a low-energy mechanism does not rule out the possibility. ML lesions have been reported to occur after sports injuries or, very rarely, less violent mechanisms.[9–11] The lower limb is involved in greater than 60% of cases, with most involving the greater trochanter.[12] This area of the body is predisposed given the increased mobility of soft tissue, limited anterolateral perforator vessels to the subdermal vascular plexus originating from the lateral femoral circumflex vessels, subcutaneous nature of bone, and strength of the fascia lata as it attaches to the iliotibial band.[13–15] A substantial number of these lesions will occur with underlying osseous fractures and injuries to other organ systems.[14] Female sex and a body mass index of 25 or greater are proposed risk factors, presumably because of the increased fat in predisposed regions.[12,16] However, more recent studies have brought these risk factors into question.[8]

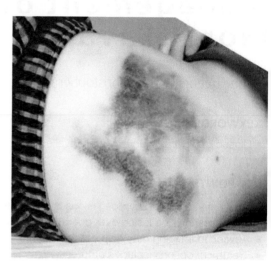

Fig. 1. Clinical appearance of an ML lesion 7 days after the patient sustained a shearing force to the greater trochanter while snowboarding. After the initial injury, the patient resumed sporting activities until a discolored, fluctuant area developed 4 days later.

PATHOGENESIS

As a result of violent shear, a thick layer of subcutaneous fat and skin is ripped from its underlying, firmly secured fascia. During this process, lymphatic channels and perforating vessels from underlying muscle are torn and release their contents into the newly created cavity. The fluid mixture now contains blood, fat, and necrotic debris within a relatively hypovascular space that is ill equipped to drain internally because of the intact underlying fascia. As lesions progress beyond the acute phase, blood is reabsorbed and replaced by serosanguineous and lymphatic fluid, which has low coagulation ability and high molecular weight.[17] A sustained inflammatory reaction eventually leads to a cystic mass surrounded by a fibrous capsule that forms as a result of peripheral deposition of hemosiderin, granulation tissue, and fibrin.[3,18] Exact timing of the aforementioned mechanisms is unknown, but MRI classifications detecting lesions in various phases suggest that lesions are altered with age.[19]

CLINICAL MANIFESTATIONS

A large swollen bruised area whereby a hematoma develops in a delayed fashion should alert practitioners to the possibility of a closed degloving injury (**Fig. 1**). Clinical manifestations of ML lesions include soft tissue swelling with or without ecchymosis, skin contour asymmetry and hypermobility, and soft fluctuance with minimal or absent tenderness. Lesions can occur anywhere but are most often located around the peritrochanteric or peripelvic region. Skin will often have decreased sensation and may appear dry, cracked, or discolored in more chronic lesions (**Fig. 2**). Lesions may not be apparent at the time of initial trauma. Either they are masked by more serious injuries or it takes some time for the hematoma to develop. Reported delays to diagnosis occur in approximately one-third of patients.[12] Depending on the study, the average time to diagnosis ranges between 3 days and 2 weeks.[8,12,20] Patients have even presented complaining of chronic contour deformities up to 13 years after injury.[12] Because ML lesions are a result of trauma, they can present at any age. The youngest documented case was in a child aged 28 months.[21] Those caring for pediatric trauma patients should be especially vigilant when managing soft tissue wounds given the decreased clarity with which children communicate their symptoms.

IMAGING

Standard radiographs can confirm the presence of a soft tissue mass without calcifications.[22] They can also be used to determine whether or not the lesion has underlying fractures, which may significantly affect further management.

Ultrasound is useful as both a diagnostic and therapeutic modality. Neal and colleagues[23] observed ultrasound characteristics in 21 ML lesions. Acute lesions are heterogeneous and lobular with irregular margins. Lesions older than 8 months

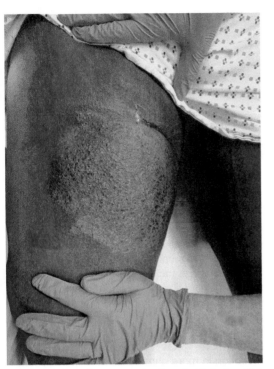

Fig. 2. Clinical appearance of a chronic ML lesion. This 16-year-old boy first presented as an outpatient with a painless slow-growing mass 3 months after sustaining a blow to his inner thigh on the handlebar of a motocross bike.

are homogeneous and flat. Lesions greater than 18 months old have smooth margins. All lesions were compressible and none had vascularity. All lesions were either hypoechoic or anechoic, and there was no relationship between echogenicity and age. This finding was presumed to be a result of repeat hemorrhage or fatty remnants. However, fat can appear as hyperechoic nodules.[24]

Computed tomography is often obtained in trauma patients with ML lesions. Lesions are often differentiated from hematomas by fluid-fluid levels due to sedimentation of blood components.[24] Lesions less than 1 month old will have irregular margins (**Fig. 3**). More chronic lesions will be homogenous and have smooth margins, and a capsule may be appreciated.[21] The average Hounsfield unit for a hematoma is 75, whereas it is 17 for an ML lesion.[17]

MRI is considered the preferred method of imaging to determine lesion characteristics and chronicity.[18] Findings correlate with classic hemorrhage and magnetic properties of blood breakdown products. Within hours of injury, oxygen-rich hemoglobin yields a homogeneous collection that is hypointense on T1-weighted (T1W) images and hyperintense on T2-weighted (T2W) images. Days to weeks after injury, oxidation of iron within heme to its ferric state results in lesions appearing hyperintense on both T1W and T2W images. In more chronic lesions, a peripheral capsule containing hemosiderin appears hypointense on T1W and T2W images.[25] Furthermore, fibrous septations and calcified fat nodules may be present within the lesion (**Fig. 4**).

CLASSIFICATION

No standard classification system exists for ML lesions. Carlson and colleagues[16] classified lesions as acute (<3 weeks old) or chronic (>3 weeks old). However, the choice of 3 weeks was arbitrary and not consistent with the remaining available literature. Multiple investigators have defined acute versus chronic based on the presence or absence of a capsule, and this method does have limited ability to guide treatment.[26,27] Mellado and Bencardino[19] created a classification based on MRI appearance, which does help determine the age of the lesion but has not been used to guide treatment.

DIFFERENTIAL DIAGNOSIS

An extensive list of differential diagnoses exists for ML lesions, especially when they present as chronic lesions with an unclear cause. MRI and physical exam can be used to differentiate almost all confounding diagnoses. Abscess, contusion, or hematoma can be differentiated from ML lesions based on tenderness, firmness, cutaneous sensation, and the condition of the overlying skin. Contusions will have increased skin tension and less fluctuance.[9] In the knee, ML lesions have been misdiagnosed as prepatellar bursitis for as long as 7 months.[28] Extension of fluctuance beyond the anatomic boundaries of the prepatellar bursa is the main distinguishing characteristics of ML lesions of the knee. Prepatellar bursae have been shown to terminate before the midthigh proximally and before the midcoronal plane medially and laterally.[9] Furthermore, ML lesions (as opposed to prepatellar bursitis) do not respond to steroid injections because they lack a synovial lining.[3] ML lesions may also be easily mistaken for soft tissue tumors, especially when they present in the subacute to chronic phase as a painless slow-growing mass. MRI can distinguish benign lesions from sarcomas if contrast reveals internal enhancement of the tumor.[18]

PRINCIPLES OF MANAGEMENT

There is currently no universally accepted treatment algorithm for the management of ML lesions.

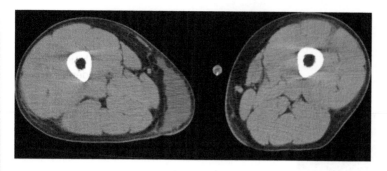

Fig. 3. Computed tomography scan obtained during an initial trauma evaluation identified an acute ML lesion of the right medial thigh. This patient also sustained severe visceral injuries, a closed acetabular fracture, and an open tibia fracture.

However, the available literature does establish the following guidelines. For acute lesions, some form of treatment should be initiated as early as possible. Benign neglect of an acute lesion may predispose patients to develop a chronic hematoma without any reduction in dead space. Theoretically, this further compromises the blood supply to the skin and increases the likelihood of recurrence. Furthermore, hematoma formation in polytrauma patients predisposes the wound to bacterial colonization.[29] In lesions overlying a planned surgical approach to displaced fractures, the potential for bacterial colonization justifies prophylactic surgical debridement. Uncomplicated subacute or chronic lesions should undergo imaging in order to determine the extent and characteristics of the lesion. Presence of a fibrous capsule implies that the lesion will likely recur without surgical intervention.

Absolute indications for surgical intervention include deep infection, severe skin necrosis, or association of a lesion with an open fracture. Relative indications for surgical management include unsuccessful nonsurgical treatment, symptomatic lesions, and those overlying a planned surgical approach for acute fixation of a closed fracture.

Conservative management options include compression dressings and aspiration. Surgical options include debridement of necrotic material through either small percutaneous or large open incisions. Large incisions were originally recommended in order to adequately debride necrotic components. They improve visualization and allow intraoperative dead space closure at the risk of further impairing subdermal vascularity. Furthermore, they allow complete capsular resection in more chronic lesions. More recently, less invasive treatment has been described with superior outcomes. The decision to perform less invasive treatment depends on several factors to include lesion characteristics, approach to underlying fractures, and need for capsular resection. Adjuncts to surgical debridement include sclerodesis and drain placement. Investigators have used the aforementioned treatment options in various combinations. A thorough understanding of lesion pathophysiology and specific lesion characteristics (such as acuity, location, size, symptoms, and absence or presence of underlying operative fracture) will allow surgeons to individualize treatment plans. **Fig. 5** provides the authors' recommended treatment

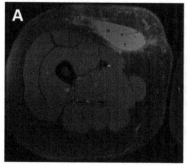
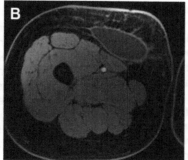
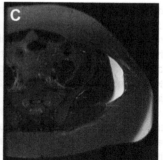

Fig. 4. (A, B) Short tau inversion recovery sequence MRI depicting a chronic ML lesion measuring 8.2 × 6.8 × 3.2 cm with characteristic internal septations, calcified fat globules, and a fibrous capsule. (C) T2-weighted fast spin echo sequence MRI depicting an ML lesion in the gluteal region in a patient who presented 3 years after initial injury with a painless contour deformity.

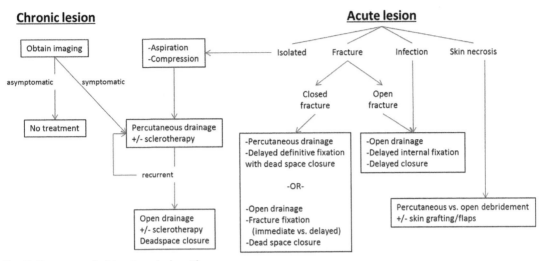

Fig. 5. Recommended treatment algorithm.

algorithm based on a thorough review of the literature.

PREOPERATIVE PLANNING

Timing of definitive fixation for fractures with associated ML lesions is an important aspect of preoperative planning. Both immediate and staged treatment have been described with varied success. Investigators uniformly agree that surgical debridement before internal fixation is necessary to avoid postoperative hematoma.[2,4] Additionally, the increased prevalence of bacterial colonization in acute lesions among trauma patients may indicate staged treatment. In opposition, fractures that undergo delayed open reduction are at risk for increased operative time, blood loss, and difficulty obtaining anatomic reduction. Whether or not to delay definitive fixation should depend on the factors discussed earlier. Also, external fixator pins through the lesion should be avoided if possible.[30] Hak and colleagues[6] treated 15 pelvic fractures at the time of initial debridement with concerning results, but this may have resulted from incisions being left open to heal by secondary intention. By contrast, Carlson and colleagues[16] emphasized strict dead space closure during initial debridement while performing fracture osteosynthesis directly through 6 lesions and had no postoperative infections. These investigators warned that any signs of clinical infection during the index procedure should warrant staged treatment. Tseng and Tornetta[5] delayed definitive fixation until 24 hours after drain removal following percutaneous debridement with excellent results. Surgeons should use their best clinical judgment when scheduling definitive fixation of underlying fractures.

CONSERVATIVE TREATMENT

Nonoperative treatment methods mainly consist of compression bandaging with or without fluid aspiration. In general, investigators suggest that small lesions are more amenable to conservative treatment methods.[28,31] Conservative management was estimated by Shen and colleagues[27] to be successful less than 50% of the time, but this statistic may actually be much higher or lower depending on lesion characteristics. Compression bandaging is a well-documented, necessary adjunct to both conservative and postsurgical treatment in order to allow fibrous adhesions within the preexisting lesion. As expected, its efficacy may depend on lesion location. Among 13 lesions identified in a systematic review that were treated conservatively, all those not receiving compression failed conservative measures, whereas 62.5% of those receiving compression healed successfully.[27] Harma and colleagues[31] reported 5 acute lesions of which 4 healed with conservative management alone after an average of 6.8 ± 3.96 weeks. Those investigators did not mention the size of the lesions and only aspirated one of them. Parra and colleagues[7] treated 2 out of 3 large thigh lesions successfully with compression alone. Multiple investigators have attributed their treatment failures to inadequate compression bandaging.[12,31]

Risk of iatrogenic inoculation via simple aspiration is also a common concern given the increased prevalence of these closed lesions to be culture positive. However, data from some of the larger case series suggest that aspiration under sterile conditions carries an acceptable risk and should be performed when indicated. Among the reported cases of sclerodesis, almost all included patients had at least one aspiration without developing infection.[18,32] The 16 patients reported by Bansal and colleagues[33] averaged 3.4 aspirations before doxycycline sclerodesis within at least a 6-month period and remained free of infection. Zero of 13 uncomplicated knee lesions averaged 2.7 aspiration attempts without any subsequent infections.[9] In a series of 87 lesions whereby 25 underwent simple aspiration, there was one infection in the aspiration group.[8] This finding was not statistically different than the nonoperative and operative group infection rates. One case report describes the clinical course of a patient who underwent 10 aspirations over a 7-month period without developing infection.[28] Another case report describes a patient who underwent multiple repeated aspirations for 10 months without developing infection.[34]

SURGICAL TREATMENT: TECHNIQUES AND OUTCOMES
Open Debridement

In 1976, Ronceray[26] described the first formal open surgical technique aimed at preventing lesion recurrence whereby aponeurotic fenestrations were created deep to the lesion in order to allow internal drainage and healing. This method was primarily applied to abdominal lesions, and the results with respect to injured extremities are not reported. Coulibaly and colleagues[35] reported success rates with this method as low as 40%. Currently described open treatment includes a longitudinal incision across the lesion along a palpable midpoint, removal of necrotic fat, irrigation and debridement of the deep fascial layer (using a plastic brush or electrocautery scratch pad) to encourage revascularization, and dead space closure by sealing healthy fat to fascia with an absorbable suture. If the lesion is chronic and a capsule is present, complete removal of the fibrous capsular tissue should be performed (**Fig. 6**). Additionally, a sclerosing agent may be added at the surgeon's discretion. Outcomes after open treatment have been reported with variable results.

In a landmark article, Hak and colleagues[6] emphasized the challenges of managing an ML lesion over a fractured pelvis. In hopes of preventing hematoma formation over a planned surgical approach, closed degloving lesions in 24 hospitalized polytrauma patients were treated with open surgical debridement before or during internal fixation of pelvic fractures. The duration between injury and initial debridement averaged 13.1 days (range 2–60 days). Fascia was closed but the

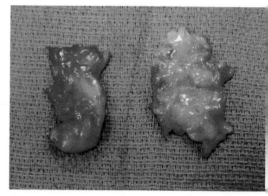

Fig. 6. Specimens obtained during open capsular resection of a chronic ML lesion. The pathology report confirmed fragments of nodular, benign adipose tissue with necrosis, fibrin, and chronic inflammation.

degloved portion was left open to drain and heal by secondary intention. Intraoperative fluid from 11 lesions (46%) yielded positive cultures, although patients did not necessarily exhibit symptoms of infection. Culture results did not correlate with the time between injury and surgical debridement. All wounds eventually healed, but the postoperative course for some patients was alarming. Three patients developed deep bone infections; 2 patients required split-thickness skin grafting; one patient developed a chronic soft tissue infection that needed a posterior thigh flap; 2 patients underwent elective cosmetic surgery after their wounds healed.

The aforementioned outcomes led to subsequent modifications of open surgical technique to encourage meticulous dead space closure by sealing healthy fat to fascia with an absorbable suture.[16,36] If minimal fat remains after debridement, a nonabsorbable suture can be used to join the skin and fascia. Carlson and colleagues[16] reported zero postoperative infections in their series of 24 lesions treated with open debridement and dead space closure.

It is presumed that circulating bacteria in polytrauma patients predisposed acute lesions to have positive cultures. Most patients in the series reported by Hak and colleagues[6] had significant injuries to include 4 open pelvic fractures, numerous visceral organ injuries, and injuries to the peripheral and central nervous system. Of note, only 2 of 9 lesions in this series cultured after 2 weeks had positive cultures. Therefore, clinicians should interpret the aforementioned results with respect to the acuity of the lesion and the trauma patient population that was studied. The likelihood of bacterial colonization in an isolated closed wound may not be as high as that of acutely injured patients with polytrauma. Carlson and colleagues[16] included details for 13 of 14 closed degloving injuries of which zero were clinically infected before initial debridement. Furthermore, Bansal and colleagues[33] cultured fluid from 16 chronic lesions after excluding those with prior surgery or underlying fractures. None of their lesions produced positive cultures.

Limited Incision

Concerns about infection risk and flap survival following open treatment led to the description of minimally invasive techniques as the current gold standard for appropriate lesions. The first mention in the English literature that specifically addressed treatment of closed degloving injuries via a limited incision occurred in 1991. Hudson[12] reported 16 patients who underwent irrigation and debridement through a small incision, appropriately sized to allow evacuation of necrotic products. If displaced fat created a contour deformity, the incision was extended across the entire lesion. All lesions healed successfully except one extensive gluteal lesion over a fractured pelvis in which compression could not be maintained. No lesions within their series occurred over a displaced fracture.

In order to address the treatment of acute lesions over displaced pelvic fractures, Tseng and Tornetta[5] described a new technique using small percutaneous incisions. They reported encouraging results among a series of 19 consecutive patients. Their technique included irrigation and drainage of hematoma through two small 2-cm incisions (one each at the proximal and distal extent of the lesion). The proximal incision was placed posterosuperiorly to ensure the entire cavity was influenced. A plastic brush was used to debride necrotic fat before the lesion was again irrigated with pulse lavage until exiting fluid was clear. Finally, a suction drain was left within the lesion until output was less than 30 mL per day. Intravenous antibiotics were discontinued 24 hours after drain removal.

All lesions were debrided within 3 days of injury, and drain removal took place between 3 and 8 days after debridement. The injury profile of these polytrauma patients was similar to that of the series reported by Hak and colleagues.[6] However, only 3 of 16 (19%) of patients had positive fluid cultures at the time of initial debridement. Fifteen patients underwent surgical fixation of displaced pelvic or acetabular fractures. Percutaneous fixation of the posterior pelvic ring was performed immediately following initial debridement (during the same procedure) in 7 patients. One of these patients had a positive fluid culture but no

sequelae. Open reduction and internal fixation in the remaining 8 patients was delayed until 24 hours after drain removal. Three open reductions were performed directly through the lesion without infectious complications.

Subsequent investigators have reproduced similar satisfactory results after percutaneous debridement. Zhong and colleagues[20] performed the procedure described by Tseng and Tornetta[5] on 8 lesions after an average time to diagnosis of 11.9 days. Lesions healed in an average time of 3.25 weeks after debridement without recurrence or infection, although 2 patients required skin grafting for associated flap necrosis. Additionally, Matava and colleagues[37] performed the aforementioned procedure on an extensive peritrochanteric lesion whereby 500 mL of fluid was aspirated. The patient returned to playing professional football without recurrence 22 days after debridement.

Sclerodesis

Introduction of various sclerosing agents into more chronic lesions has been successfully described as an adjunct to percutaneous surgical treatment. A systematic review reports a success rate for percutaneous sclerodesis of chronic lesions to be 95.7%.[27] Once inside the lesion, sclerosing agents activate an inflammatory cascade that encourages scar formation and fusion of subdermal membranes. Especially in the presence of a chronic or recurring lesion, sclerodesis potentially avoids the need for a more extensive and painful surgical incision wide enough to allow capsular resection and dead space closure. If necessary, sclerodesis can be repeated and does not interfere with future surgical options.

The concept of injecting a sclerosing agent into an ML lesion was derived from its application in malignant pleural effusions, whereby talc and doxycycline are commonly used.[38] In 2006, Luria and colleagues[17] were the first to use sclerodesis in 4 ML lesions that failed prior aspiration. After defining the cavity with contrast fluid under fluoroscopic guidance, they evacuated all contents and instilled 5 g of sterile talc diluted in 50 mL sterile saline, removed the mixture after 5 minutes, and left a drain in until the output was less than 30 mL per day. Three patients had drains removed after 1 week and enjoyed an uncomplicated postprocedural course. One patient with a nonoperative pelvic fracture and bilateral lesions developed subsequent infection treated with only antibiotics and simple drainage.

In 2013, Bansal and colleagues[33] reported their results after using doxycycline as a sclerosing agent in 16 chronic lesions. All lesions were present more than 6 months and failed prior intervention. They inserted 21-gauge needles into the proximal and distal extent of the lesion, drained all fluid from the cavity, instilled 500 mg of doxycycline powder (obtained from 100-mg capsules and mixed with 25 mL of saline solution), had the patients maneuver themselves once every 10 minutes for 1 hour, aspirated the mixture, then applied a compression dressing for 4 weeks. No drains were used. The average volume aspirated was 387 mL (range 150–700 mL). All lesions resolved without recurrence in an average time of 5 weeks and were followed for more than 2 years. Subsequent investigators have also described their use of doxycycline for recurrent lesions with similar success.[9]

Other sclerosing agents proposed for use include alcohol, bleomycin, and tetracycline. Penaud and colleagues[32] described 5 chronic lesions treated with pure ethanol, all of which had confirmation of a capsule via MRI. Postprocedural imaging 6 months later confirmed complete absence of a capsule in 4 patients and a small asymptomatic cavity in one patient. Bleomycin has been used in malignant pleural and pericardial effusions but is less popular because of higher costs.[39] The low postoperative infection rates after sclerodesis have been anecdotally attributed to the antibacterial effects of sclerosing agents.

POSTOPERATIVE CARE

Drains are almost universally described as part of all surgical procedures. In general, surgeons leave them in until the output is less than 30 mL per day. Postoperative drains were generally removed within 1 week for acute lesions and up to several weeks for more chronic lesions.[5,6,16,17,20] Compression is also of utmost importance, and investigators have directly blamed its absence for treatment failure.[33] For patients with acute lesions managed as inpatients, antibiotics were also used until 24 hours after drain removal.[5,16]

COMPLICATIONS
Postoperative Infection

Treating displaced fractures through ML lesions at the time of initial debridement may increase the risk of infection. The study by Hak and colleagues,[6] whereby 46% of closed lesions were culture positive during initial debridement, made the orthopedic community distressingly aware of the potential disaster that might exist within these lesions. Fifteen of 24 patients underwent open reduction and internal fixation at the time of initial

debridement, after which the skin was left to heal by secondary intention. Three patients subsequently developed deep bone infections, and several others had wound complications. There is further concerning evidence that acute ML lesions harbor infectious potential if opened. In a series of 20 patients with vertically unstable sacral fractures, 2 of 5 patients with ML lesions became infected postoperatively. However, none of the 15 patients without an ML lesion developed a postoperative infection.[40] In a case series of 4 patients with spinopelvic dissociation and lesions overlying the approach used for internal fixation, 2 patients developed postoperative infections and one patient developed skin necrosis that led to infection and extensive soft tissue reconstruction.[41]

Most literature highlights the potential risk of bacterial colonization within planned surgical incisions for underlying displaced fractures. However, this risk is not to be confused with that of nonoperative or surgically decompressed lesions. In the series of 19 patients by Tseng and Tornetta,[5] internal fixation was delayed until 24 hours after percutaneous debridement and no patients developed postoperative infections. In 2007, Carlson and colleagues[16] highlighted 6 fractures treated directly through ML lesions after thorough debridement and meticulous dead space closure with no subsequent infections. When sclerodesis is used, the infection risk seems to be low. Doxycycline sclerodesis in 16 patients and alcohol sclerodesis in 5 patients did not result in any postoperative infections.[32,33] Talc sclerodesis in 5 lesions led to one postoperative infection.[17] Conservative management via aspiration and compression dressings in 4 patients by Harma and colleagues[31] led to one sacral ulcer that became infected. In a systematic review by Shen and colleagues,[27] almost all postoperative infections were managed with antibiotics alone. In summary, surgeons should not allow the risk of bacterial colonization in trauma patients to prohibit appropriately staged surgical debridement when necessary.

Recurrence

Lesion recurrence is a primary concern when treating ML lesions. It is thought to occur because of the decreased capability of lesions to evacuate fluid combined, the persistent introduction of blood and lymph, and squamous cells within a more chronic lesion's serosal lining.[17] Persistent fluid collection is a cosmetic and symptomatic nuisance for patients; allows time for a pseudocapsule to develop, thus, making definitive treatment more detailed; and places the overlying soft tissue at risk for ulceration and subsequent infection. Methods used to prevent recurrence aim to enhance fluid drainage and close dead space. Recurrence rates are different with regard to conservative versus operative management. Actual rates of lesion recurrence are unknown. A recent systematic review reports that open treatment exhibited a 4.2% rate of recurrence, whereas less invasive drainage yielded a recurrence rate of 17.4%; but those figures had no statistically significant difference.[27]

Given the widely heterogeneous lesion characteristics within the available literature, it is difficult to determine which lesions have the highest risk of recurrence. The most obvious risk factor for recurrence is the presence of a fibrous capsule. After simple aspiration of an encapsulated lesion, fluid collections are almost guaranteed to recur without capsular resection or sclerodesis. Lesion location has also been suggested as a risk factor for recurrence, as compression bandaging around the hip or buttock region is more difficult to maintain than around the knee and distal thigh.[33] Surgical technique similarly affects recurrence rates. For example, among the 24 patients reported by Carlson and colleagues[16] in which meticulous dead space closure was a main priority, zero lesions recurred.

Lesion size may be a risk factor for recurrence after conservative treatment, and some investigators even modify their surgical indications based on this belief. However, establishing a numerical cutoff value to differentiate small from large lesions is controversial. Ronceray[26] suggested in 1976 that small lesions are more amenable to conservative treatment, whereas operative management should be considered for larger lesions. Nonetheless, he did not define what constitutes a small versus large lesion. Nickerson and colleagues[8] retrospectively reviewed their treatment of 87 lesions and recommended that aspirating more than 50 mL indicates operative intervention because of a statistically higher risk of recurrence. Several statistical flaws confound their conclusion. First, the aspiration group in this study consisted of 25 patients with significantly larger lesions ($P = .006$) and longer diagnostic delays ($P = .001$) than the operatively treated group. Secondly, aspirated lesions were not categorized by location. This point is important because subsequent compression therapy in certain locations, such as the gluteal folds, is more difficult to maintain. Lastly, 75% of the lesions that recurred after aspiration were a result of high-energy trauma. These confounders suggest that other factors may have been responsible for the increased rate of recurrence noted in lesions whereby an initial aspiration yielded greater than 50 mL of fluid. Tejwani and colleagues[9] reported good results after 27 knee lesions were treated with nonoperative measures. Their reported aspirated quantities were relatively low compared with other studies, averaging between 46 and 77 mL (range 12–300 mL).

Skin Necrosis

Soft tissue compromise remains a concern before and after operative management. Limited blood supply to the skin during hematoma formation, combined with increased mechanical friction and shear, predispose these lesions to ulceration and subsequent skin necrosis or infection. Operative intervention with larger incisions may place the skin at more risk for necrosis than less invasive techniques.[5] Skin necrosis should be subsequently managed with further debridement and skin grafting or soft tissue flaps as necessary.

Contour Deformity

Displacement of fat during the initial injury often leads to asymptomatic, asymmetric, and nonfluctuant displacement of the skin when compared with the contralateral extremity.[3] This displacement is primarily a cosmetic concern. Slight skin hypermobility may also be present. By contrast, sclerodesis of chronic lesions leads to skin immobility in a subset of patients that is only symptomatic during persistent high-level athletic activity.[9,33]

SUMMARY

ML lesions represent a serious soft tissue injury, although their diagnosis is often missed or delayed. These lesions are known to be associated with high rates of recurrence, skin necrosis, and infection. In the case of underlying pelvic fractures, lesions have the ability to create treacherous outcomes after open treatment of underlying displaced fractures. Clinicians should remain suspicious when managing patients after shearing injuries or direct blows to the greater trochanter. Early recognition and optimal management can save patients from undesirable morbidity and consequent need for more complex surgical management.

ACKNOWLEDGMENTS

We wish to thank Dr. Alison Gattuso, St. Christopher's Hospital for Children, Philadelphia, PA for her contributions to this article.

REFERENCES

1. Morel-Lavallee M. Decollements traumatiques de la peau et des couches sous-jacentes. Arch Gen Med 1863;1:20–38, 172-200, 300-332.

2. Letournel E, Judet R. Fractures of the acetabulum. 2nd edition. Berlin: Springer; 1993.

3. Li H, Zhang F, Lei G. Morel-Lavallee lesion. Chin Med J (Engl) 2014;127(7):1351–6.

4. Helfet DL, Schmeling GJ. Complications. In: Tile M, editor. Fractures of the pelvis and acetabulum. 2nd edition. Baltimore (MD): Williams and Wilkins; 1995. p. 451–67.

5. Tseng S, Tornetta P. Percutaneous management of Morel-Lavalee lesions. J Bone Joint Surg Am 2006;88(1):92–6.

6. Hak DJ, Olson SA, Matta JM. Diagnosis and management of closed internal degloving injuries associated with pelvic and acetabular fractures: the Morel-Lavallée lesion. J Trauma 1997;42(6): 1046–51.

7. Parra JA, Fernandez MA, Encinas B, et al. Morel-Lavallée effusions in the thigh. Skeletal Radiol 1997;26(4):239–41.

8. Nickerson TP, Zielinski MD, Jenkins DH, et al. The Mayo Clinic experience with Morel-Lavallée lesions: establishment of a practice management guideline. J Trauma Acute Care Surg 2014;76(2): 493–7.

9. Tejwani SG, Cohen SB, Bradley JP. Management of Morel-Lavallee lesion of the knee: twenty-seven cases in the national football league. Am J Sports Med 2007;35(7):1162–7.

10. Moriarty JM, Borrero CG, Kavanagh EC. A rare cause of calf swelling: the Morel–Lavallee lesion. Ir J Med Sci 2011;180(1):265–8.

11. Van Gennip S, Van Bokhoven SC, Van den Eede E. Pain at the knee: the Morel-Lavallée lesion, a case series. Clin J Sport Med 2012;22(2):163–6.

12. Hudson DA. Missed closed degloving injuries: late presentation as a contour deformity. Plast Reconstr Surg 1996;98(2):334–7.

13. Cormack GC, Lamberty BG. The blood supply of thigh skin. Plast Reconstr Surg 1985;75(3): 342–54.

14. Kottmeier SA, Wilson SC, Born CT, et al. Surgical management of soft tissue lesions associated with pelvic ring injury. Clin Orthop Relat Res 1996;(329):46–53.

15. Dawre S, Lamba S, Sreekar H, et al. The Morel-Lavallee lesion: a review and a proposed algorithmic approach. Eur J Plast Surg 2012;35:489–94.

16. Carlson DA, Simmons J, Sando W, et al. Morel-Lavalée lesions treated with debridement and meticulous dead space closure: surgical technique. J Orthop Trauma 2007;21(2):140–4.

17. Luria S, Applbaum Y, Weil Y, et al. Talc sclerodhesis of persistent Morel-Lavallée lesions (posttraumatic pseudocysts): case report of 4 patients. J Orthop Trauma 2006;20(6):435–8.

18. Bonilla-Yoon I, Masih S, Patel DB, et al. The Morel-Lavallée lesion: pathophysiology, clinical presentation, imaging features, and treatment options. Emerg Radiol 2014;21(1):35–43.

19. Mellado JM, Bencardino JT. Morel-Lavallée lesion: review with emphasis on MR imaging. Magn Reson Imaging Clin N Am 2005;13(4):775–82.

20. Zhong B, Zhang C, Luo CF. Percutaneous drainage of Morel-Lavallée lesions when the diagnosis is delayed. Can J Surg 2014;57(5):356–7.

21. Rha EY, Kim DH, Kwon H, et al. Morel-Lavallée lesion in children. World J Emerg Surg 2013;8(1):60.

22. Bomela LN, Basson H, Motsitsi NS. Morel-Lavallée lesion: a review. SA Orthopaedic J 2008;7(2):34–41. Available at: http://www.scielo.org.za/scielo.php?script= sci_arttext&pid=S1681-150X2008000200007&lng= en&nrm=iso. Accessed March 24, 2015.

23. Neal C, Jacobson JA, Brandon C, et al. Sonography of Morel-Lavallée lesions. J Ultrasound Med 2008; 27:1077–81.

24. Nair AV, Nazar P, Sekhar R, et al. Morel-Lavallée lesion: a closed degloving injury that requires real attention. Indian J Radiol Imaging 2014;24(3): 288–90.

25. Liu PT, Leslie KO, Beauchamp CP, et al. Chronic expanding hematoma of the thigh simulating neoplasm on gadolinium-enhanced MRI. Skeletal Radiol 2006; 35:254–7.

26. Ronceray J. Active drainage by partial aponeurotic resection of Morel-Lavallée effusions. Nouv Presse Med 1976;5(20):1305–6 [in French].

27. Shen C, Peng JP, Chen XD. Efficacy of treatment in peri-pelvic Morel-Lavallee lesion: a systematic review of the literature. Arch Orthop Trauma Surg 2013;133(5):635–40.

28. Vanhegan IS, Dala-ali B, Verhelst L, et al. The Morel-Lavallée lesion as a rare differential diagnosis for recalcitrant bursitis of the knee: case report and literature review. Case Rep Orthop 2012;2012: 593193.

29. Pelletier LL. Microbiology of the circulatory system. In: Baron S, editor. Medical microbiology. 4th edition. Galveston (TX): University of Texas Medical Branch at Galveston; 1996. Chapter 94.

30. Routt ML Jr, Simonian PT, Ballmer F. A rational approach to pelvic trauma. Resuscitation and early definitive stabilization. Clin Orthop Relat Res 1995;(318):61–74.

31. Harma A, Inan M, Ertem K. The Morel-Lavallee lesion: a conservative approach to closed degloving injuries. Acta Orthop Traumatol Turc 2004;38(4): 270–3 [in Turkish].

32. Penaud A, Quignon R, Danin A, et al. Alcohol sclerodhesis: an innovative treatment for chronic Morel-Lavallée lesions. J Plast Reconstr Aesthet Surg 2011;64(10):e262–4.

33. Bansal A, Bhatia N, Singh A, et al. Doxycycline sclerodesis as a treatment option for persistent Morel-Lavallee lesions. Injury 2013;44(1):66–9.

34. Lin HL, Lee WC, Kuo LC, et al. Closed internal de-gloving injury with conservative treatment. Am J Emerg Med 2008;26(2):254.e5–6.

35. Coulibaly NF, Sankale AA, Sy MH, et al. Morel-Lavallée lesion in orthopaedic surgery (nineteen cases). Ann Chir Plast Esthet 2011;56:27–32.

36. Seo BF, Kang IS, Jeong YJ, et al. A huge Morel-Lavallée lesion treated using a quilting suture method: a case report and review of the literature. Int J Low Extrem Wounds 2014;13(2):147–51.

37. Matava MJ, Ellis E, Shah NR, et al. Morel-Lavallée lesion in a professional American football player. Am J Orthop 2010;39(3):144–7.

38. Kilic D, Akay H, Kavukçu S, et al. Management of recurrent malignant pleural effusion with chemical pleurodesis. Surg Today 2005;35(8):634–8.

39. Zimmer PW, Hill M, Casey K, et al. Prospective randomized trial of talc slurry vs bleomycin in pleurodesis for symptomatic malignant pleural effusions. Chest 1997;112(2):430–4.

40. Suzuki T, Hak DJ, Ziran BH, et al. Outcome and complications of posterior transiliac plating for vertically unstable sacral fractures. Injury 2009;40(4):405–9.

41. Dodwad SN, Niedermeier SR, Yu E, et al. The Morel-Lavallée lesion revisited: management in spinopelvic dissociation. Spine J 2013;15(6):e1–7.

Management of Major Traumatic Upper Extremity Amputations

Mark K. Solarz, MD*, Joseph J. Thoder, MD,
Saqib Rehman, MD

KEYWORDS

• Trauma • Amputation • Upper extremity • Revision amputation • Management

KEY POINTS

- Initial management of the acute traumatic upper extremity amputation begins with the principles of advanced trauma life support including achievement of hemostasis, a thorough neurovascular examination, imaging, appropriate care for the amputate, debridement of devitalized tissue, antibiosis and tetanus prophylaxis, and fracture stabilization.
- Care for the traumatic amputee should be multidisciplinary to provide medical, surgical, rehabilitative, social, and psychological support.
- Replantation, when indicated, should be performed by a replantation specialist at a replantation center.
- Revision amputation should aim to preserve the maximum length of the limb and motion in the major joints, allowing for maximal function.
- Initial postoperative care should focus on preparation of the stump for prosthesis wear and minimizing complications.

INTRODUCTION

A major traumatic amputation of the upper limb, which includes injuries proximal to the carpus, is a rare but significant life-altering event. According to the National Trauma Databank, 0.09% of persons hospitalized after trauma sustained a major upper limb amputation[1] and 34,000 people are living with a major amputation in the United States alone.[2] Most of these injuries occur as the result of blunt trauma, with motor vehicle collisions being the most common mechanism. However, penetrating and blast injuries that result in upper limb amputation are becoming more prevalent with the US military's involvement in Iraq and Afghanistan during the past 14 years.[3–5]

Appropriate management of traumatic upper limb amputation is imperative to reduce associated morbidity and mortality while allowing the amputee to reestablish meaningful function in the effected limb. This article reviews contemporary management of traumatic upper limb amputations, with specific focus on initial management, tissue debridement, revision amputation, and postoperative complications.

INITIAL MANAGEMENT

Upper extremity amputations are usually the result of high-energy mechanisms; as such the initial evaluation begins with the principles of advanced trauma life support. Securing the airway and

The authors have no disclosures pertaining to this topic.
Department of Orthopaedics and Sports Medicine, Temple University Hospital, 3401 North Broad Street, Zone B 5th Floor, Philadelphia, PA 19140, USA
* Corresponding author.
E-mail address: mark.solarz@tuhs.temple.edu

Orthop Clin N Am 47 (2016) 127–136
http://dx.doi.org/10.1016/j.ocl.2015.08.013

cervical spine are of utmost importance, followed by lung ventilation. An oft encountered component of advanced trauma life support primary survey with major amputations is control of hemorrhage, which results from laceration or rupture of the major vessels. A tourniquet is used if necessary to prevent lethal exsanguination; however, hemostasis is preferably achieved with elevation and application of a compression dressing. Blind clamping of vessels in the trauma bay is not recommended because collateral damage to intact vessels and nerves may occur. Resuscitation should begin with intravenous crystalloid fluids, but it may be necessary to infuse packed red blood cells if there is significant blood loss. Broad-spectrum antibiotics and tetanus prophylaxis are initiated in the trauma bay as soon as possible. Typically, at least a first-generation cephalosporin is used for infection prophylaxis, although an aminoglycoside should be added if there is significant contamination. Penicillin is added if there is concern for *Clostridium* infection from farm or vegetative contamination. If the patient's immunization status is unknown or overdue, tetanus prophylaxis is required.

Once the patient is acutely stabilized and resuscitation efforts initiated, care is directed toward a thorough history and physical examination. The history should focus on injury and patient factors that are helpful when formulating a treatment plan. Injury factors include the mechanism, timing, location, and additional injuries. Patient factors include hand dominance, prior occupation, baseline functional level, and medical history (especially diabetes mellitus, peripheral vascular disease, and prior injury to the affected extremity). Although not a contraindication to replantation, patients with diabetes, peripheral vascular disease, and smokers have lower success rates.[6] Physical examination should focus on the remaining portion of the affected extremity, taking note of the level of injury and the amount and type of contamination. Active and passive motion of the proximal joints should be noted to aid with preoperative planning for a future prosthesis. The remaining muscle groups should be palpated and evaluated for compartment syndrome. A local anesthetic is particularly useful before ranging the limb to reduce the effect pain inevitably has on the examination. The amputate should undergo a thorough examination for additional sites or injury distal to the amputation. Significant additional injuries can preclude a replantation attempt. A thorough secondary examination is essential to identify additional injuries to other extremities or the axial skeleton.

Orthogonal radiographs of the residual limb and amputate are obtained to further characterize the bony injury to each. In particular, segmental injuries to the amputate may prohibit successful replantation and favor revision amputation.

REPLANT OR REVISION AMPUTATION

When a traumatic upper extremity amputation occurs, definitive treatment should focus on ultimately providing the patient with the highest level of function possible. The initial decision making should differentiate an injury that can be successfully replanted from one that requires a revision amputation. One must keep in mind the complexity of motion in the human upper extremity; therefore, a replanted "bad hand" may provide more function than is possible with a prosthesis following revision amputation. When the expected function of a replanted extremity is less than that of an amputation with or without a prosthesis, or the patient is not a candidate for replantation, the decision should be made to perform a revision amputation.

Graham and colleagues[7] compared late functional outcomes between major upper extremity amputation and replantation at an average of 7.3 years postinjury. Functional outcomes were determined using the Carroll Standardized Evaluation and Integrated Limb Function, which assesses one's ability to perform simple and complex tasks. Twenty-two major upper extremity replantations were compared with 22 similar level amputees with prostheses, and the functional abilities of the replantation group were significantly better than the prosthesis group.

Proper care of the amputate precludes any discussion regarding the ability to perform a successful replantation. It should be wrapped with sterile saline-soaked gauze to prevent desiccation and then placed into a sealed, impermeable plastic bag. This bag should then be immersed into ice water to help preserve the tissues, which is particularly important if the amputate contains a large amount of muscle because of its high metabolic demand.

The decision to perform a major upper extremity replantation depends on patient factors and the injury pattern. If the amputation is one injury of a polytrauma situation, the patient may not be able to tolerate a lengthy replantation procedure or may not be able to effectively participate in postreplantation rehabilitation. If the patient is hemodynamically unstable, extremity injuries should be treated in a damage control manner and avoid attempted replantation. In general, a smaller zone of injury, such as that from a sharp amputation, results in a more successful replantation. The amount of soft tissue damage that occurs with a severe crush injury precludes replantation in most cases, because of the lack of healthy tissue throughout a large zone of injury. Cold ischemia time following the traumatic amputation should not exceed 6 to 8 hours before vascular reanastomosis. Although there are classic indications and contraindications for replantation, the final treatment decision should be made by the surgeon who is to perform the procedure in accordance with the patient's goals and wishes.

Key points
1. A revision amputation is performed if the patient is not a candidate for replantation or the resulting functional outcome is better than a successful replantation.
2. Contraindications for major upper extremity replantation are polytrauma, hemodynamic instability, greater than 6 to 8 hours cold ischemia time, or severe crush injury.
3. Proper care of the amputate: wrapping in saline-soaked gauze within a sealed impermeable bag, and immersing in ice water.

PROCEDURE: REVISION OF MAJOR UPPER EXTREMITY AMPUTATION
Preoperative Planning

As with most surgical procedures, preoperative planning is key for a successful outcome. Preservation of length and motion of the remaining joints are key components that ultimately determine functional ability. If active motion of the shoulder and elbow are maintained, the stump or prosthesis can be placed in space to assist with or perform many functions. Skin grafts, flaps, and free tissue transfer should be considered to preserve length in amputations where the soft tissues are not adequate for coverage. Although it is tempting to

simply shorten the bone to achieve coverage, a longer limb allows for a higher level of function and thus should be preserved when able. Baccarani and coworkers[8] described the successful use of free tissue transfer in 13 patients to preserve length of the residual limb and allow prosthetic fitting. Even if replantation cannot be performed, the amputate can be used for "spare parts," such as skin grafting to minimize donor site morbidity.[9]

General Procedure Details

The patient is placed supine on the operating room table with the affected upper extremity on a hand table. As with all surgical procedures, a formal timeout is performed to correctly identify the patient, operative site, and procedure to be performed. An antibiotic with gram-positive bacteria coverage is typically infused intravenously within an hour of the procedure, if the patient is not already on a standing antibiotic regimen. General anesthesia is preferred for revision amputations, and a well-padded pneumatic tourniquet is placed to aid in identification of neurovascular structures and hemorrhage control. Antimicrobial skin preparation and sterile draping is performed according to the surgeon preference and level of anticipated amputation.

In many cases of upper extremity revision amputation following a traumatic injury, skin flaps for distal coverage are irregular depending on the vital tissue remaining. If the level of amputation is proximal to the remaining tissue, a fish-mouth-type incision is typically used (**Fig. 1**). The exception is a wrist disarticulation, where a volar flap of thick palmar skin provides more durable coverage. Care should be taken to leave enough skin and

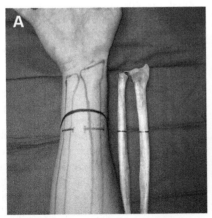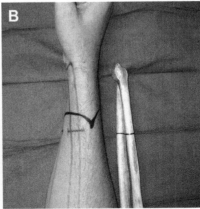

Fig. 1. (*A*, *B*) Clinical photographs and corresponding skeletal model demonstrating the planned fish-mouth surgical incision and osteotomy sites for a distal transradial amputation, seen in two planes.

soft tissue distal to the planned osteotomy level to provide adequate bone coverage for painless use with and without a prosthetic. Hemostasis of the superficial vessels is achieved using bipolar electrocautery. Blunt dissection is used to identify and isolate the major vessels and nerves at the proposed level of amputation. The tendons and muscle bellies are then sharply transected, taking care to preserve enough remaining tissue for stump coverage. If irregular skin and soft tissue flaps remain following the traumatic injury, it is best to preserve more than is necessary until closure. The excess can always be trimmed at that time once appropriate stump coverage is ensured.

The major vessels are ligated with a nylon suture or surgical clip, and subsequently sharply transected distal to this location. The proper handling of major nerves at the amputation level is important to prevent painful neuroma formation and preserve sensation to the stump. Nerves, including major sensory nerves, are isolated by blunt dissection, and gentle traction is applied before transection so that the nerve endings retract into the soft tissues. The goal is to provide abundant coverage of the nerve ending such that the inevitable neuroma formed is not superficial and, as such, easily irritated.

Once a tensionless distal skin closure is complete, a well-padded compressive stump dressing is applied for edema control. Early prosthesis fitting is recommended to facilitate stump maturation and start prosthesis training during the wound healing process. Wound healing issues from vascular insufficiency during early prosthesis use are less of a concern in a traumatic upper extremity amputation compared with most lower extremity amputations. Particularly in unilateral upper extremity amputations where delays in prosthesis fitting can allow the amputee to develop one-handed function, early prosthesis fitting is vital to provide an additional prehensile limb to assist the uninjured limb.

Early identification and treatment of psychological pathology is an important part of the postoperative rehabilitation period. Copuroglu and colleagues[10] followed 22 upper extremity amputees and found that whereas five required treatment of acute stress disorder, 17 required treatment of posttraumatic stress disorder 6 months after their injury. Grunert and co-workers[11] found that visualization and memory of the traumatic amputation is a risk factor for development of flashbacks and posttraumatic stress disorder. While postoperatively monitoring upper extremity amputees, it is important for the orthopedic surgeon to maintain a high level of suspicion for these psychological disorders and provide early referrals when necessary.

Targeted Muscle Reinnervation

Since the advent of myoelectric sensors, an equipped prosthesis can be cortically controlled by the patient through electromyography waves created by innervated muscles. For more proximal amputations, however, there are limited muscle groups remaining to control multiple functions simultaneously. Targeted muscle reinnervation solves this problem by transferring nerves that previously innervated distal muscle groups to motor nerves of remaining proximal muscle groups. The goal is to successfully reinnervate the new muscle, resulting in an amplified electromyography signal for myoelectric sensor detection.

Targeted muscle reinnervation has been used in the acute setting during revision amputation, particularly in proximal amputations, such as shoulder disarticulation or transhumeral amputations.[12] Mixed major nerve endings are transferred to nearby muscles to allow for future use with myoelectric prosthesis. An added benefit of targeted muscle reinnervation is reduction in symptomatic neuroma formation, because transfer of the nerve endings provides an end target for the transected nerve.[13,14]

Wrist Disarticulation

Irreparable injuries at the level of the carpus can be treated with wrist disarticulation (**Fig. 2**). Full pronation and supination of the remaining limb should be preserved at this level because of preservation of the distal radioulnar joint and triangular fibrocartilage complex. In comparison with a transradial amputation, painful impingement of the radius and ulna is not an issue. A historical disadvantage to wrist disarticulation was difficulty fitting a functional prosthesis at this length, leading many surgeons to prefer a transradial amputation. However, advances in modern prostheses allow satisfactory use of a functioning prosthesis at this level.

If the thick volar skin of the palm remains viable, it is best used as a flap for distal coverage. Any remaining carpal bones are excised, taking care to preserve the triangular fibrocartilage complex. The radial and ulnar styloids are maintained for later use in prosthesis fitting unless they prevent tensionless soft tissue coverage. Tenodesis of the flexor and extensor tendons should be performed to maintain appropriate resting tension of the muscles for later use with a myoelectric prosthesis. The median, superficial palmar cutaneous branch of the median, ulnar, dorsal ulnar cutaneous, and branches of the superficial radial

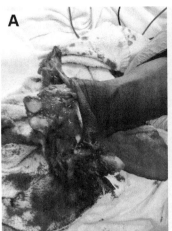
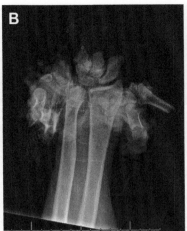
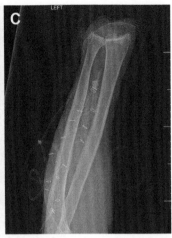

Fig. 2. (*A*, *B*) A 52-year-old man sustained an explosive injury to the left hand from a firework with extensive distal soft tissue and bone destruction. (*C*) Because of the significant damage from the carpus distally, a wrist disarticulation was performed, and a dorsal fasciotomy for compartment syndrome.

sensory nerve are encountered at this level and should be transected under traction so that the nerve endings retract into the proximal musculature. Failure to do so inevitably results in painful neuroma formation at the level of the amputation, limiting function with and without a prosthesis.

Transradial Amputation

Transradial amputations are the most common major upper extremity amputation and also have a high rate of prosthesis acceptance following surgery.[15] Amputation at this level can maintain some pronosupination depending on the relative location of the amputation. Although distal third transradial amputations retain much of their normal range of pronation and supination, proximal third transradial amputations retain little if any (**Fig. 3**). At least 6 to 8 cm of distal radius and ulna resection is recommended to provide adequate muscle coverage,[16] whereas a 10-cm resection may allow for easier prosthetic fitting.[17] If 5 cm of ulna distal to the elbow joint is salvaged, elbow flexion is preserved and a prosthesis can be fit.

A fish-mouth incision is typically used for transradial amputations, with the planned bone cuts 2 to 3 cm proximal to the skin incision. The radial and ulnar arteries are identified with blunt dissection and ligated. Depending on the level of amputation, the various nerves are encountered and must be treated properly with traction neurotomy to avoid painful neuroma formation. Along the with the median, ulnar, and superficial radial sensory nerves, one must keep in mind the anterior and posterior interosseous nerves and the medial, lateral, and posterior antebrachial cutaneous nerves. Once the radial and ulnar osteotomies

are performed, myodesis of the deep forearm muscles to the distal ends of the remaining bones is performed using suture passed through unicortical drill holes. This reduces or prevents soft tissue motion over to the distal bone cuts, which ultimately reduces bursitis formation.[18] Myoplasty of the superficial flexor muscles to the extensor muscles should place the muscles on the appropriate tension to allow muscle contractions for later use of a myoelectric prosthesis. If the injury requires a proximal third transradial amputation, the biceps tendon should be transferred to the proximal ulna to reduce the risk of flexion contracture formation.[19]

Elbow Disarticulation

If the radius and ulna cannot be salvaged, disarticulation at the elbow is performed as long as the humeral condyles are intact. Elbow disarticulation can allow rotation of a prosthesis fit to the humeral condyles, making it preferable to a transhumeral amputation.

Skin flap coverage may be irregular depending on the remaining viable tissue after the traumatic injury, or fashioned as a fish-mouth-type incision to create equal anterior and posterior flaps. Blunt dissection is carried down through the subcutaneous tissues to identify important neurovascular structures. Anteriomedially, the brachial artery is identified and ligated, along with any accompanying veins. Working from medial to lateral, the medial brachial cutaneous and medial antebrachial cutaneous nerves are identified and transected under tension. The median nerve is then identified medial to the brachial artery and the ulnar nerve is identified in the cubital tunnel or

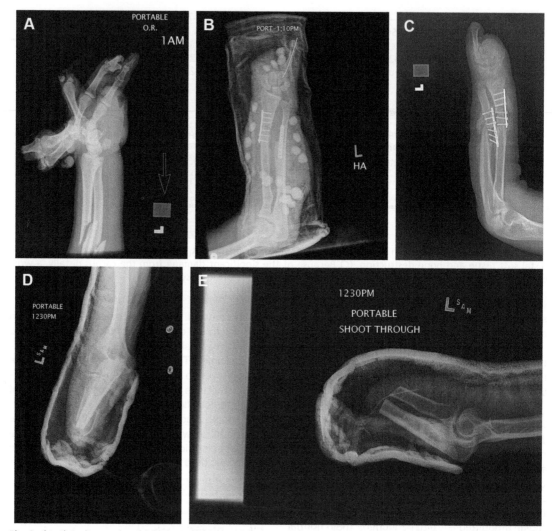

Fig. 3. (*A–E*) Radiographs of a 23-year-old man who sustained a partial left hand amputation and radial and ulnar diaphyseal fractures following a pipe bomb explosion (*A*). He was initially managed with revision amputation of the hand and segmental resection with open reduction internal fixation of the radius and ulna (*B*); however, he went on to infected nonunion of his radius and ulna with poor soft tissue healing (*C*). It should be noted that the implants used here are too small for fixation of a diaphyseal forearm fracture. He elected to undergo a proximal transradial amputation (*D, E*).

proximally. These are likewise transected under tension or inserted into local muscle by targeted muscle reinnervation. The brachialis tendon is freed from its insertion onto the coranoid and the distal biceps tendon is sharply transected from its radial insertion at the bicipital tuberosity. The lateral antebrachial cutaneous nerve is transected under tension such that it retracts beneath the biceps brachii muscle. The radial nerve is identified between the brachioradialis and brachialis muscles and transected under tension such that it retracts under cover of the triceps. The flexor-pronator and extensor common insertions are then freed from the medial and lateral condyles,

respectively. The elbow joint capsule is then divided in a circumferential manner to free the radius and ulna from the humerus. The subcutaneous and skin layers are then closed and the stump is dressed in the usual manner.

Transhumeral Amputation

As with a transradial amputation, the maximum length should be preserved when performing a transhumeral amputation (**Fig. 4**). Skin grafts and soft tissue transfers can be used if traumatic injury to the soft tissues cannot provide appropriate bony coverage. If the length of the amputation is

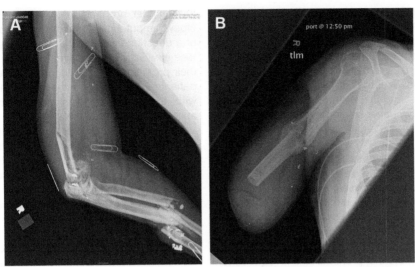

Fig. 4. (*A, B*) Preoperative and postoperative radiographs of a 31-year-old man who sustained multiple gunshot wounds to the right upper extremity, resulting in fractures at multiple levels and a brachial artery transaction (*A*). He underwent arterial repair acutely; however, his repair ultimately failed and he required a delayed transhumeral amputation (*B*).

at or proximal to the pectoralis major insertion, there is little functional benefit over a shoulder disarticulation because most shoulder motion at this level is lost. However, the stump does provide additional area for prosthesis fixation and should be preserved if possible.

A fish-mouth-type skin incision is made distal to the planned bone cut and dissection is carried down through the subcutaneous tissues to identify neurovascular structures. The brachial artery and its accompanying veins are ligated proximal to the humeral cut. The median and ulnar nerves are identified in the medial aspect of the arm and the location of the radial nerve depends on the level of the amputation. These are either divided under tension to allow for adequate soft tissue coverage or rerouted by targeted muscle reinnervation. The elbow flexors and extensors are transected circumferentially 1 to 2 cm distal to the proposed humeral cut and retracted proximally. The periosteum of the humerus is then incised at the planned level and the osteotomy is performed using an oscillating saw. Bone coverage is performed by suturing the fascia of the flexors and extensors, with or without myodesis of the muscles through bone tunnels. The subcutaneous and skin layers are then closed, and the usual stump dressing is applied.

Shoulder Disarticulation

If the proximal humerus cannot be salvaged following traumatic injury, shoulder disarticulation is indicated. Without the added contour of an upper extremity stump, fitting for a prosthesis becomes much more difficult at this level. Targeted muscle reinnervation should be considered at this level if the patient is a candidate for a myoelectric prosthesis, because there are few remaining muscles left to control motion for the entire prosthesis.

A fish-mouth-type incision is started at the coracoid and extended along the anterior border of the deltoid to its humeral insertion. This is extended posteriorly along the posterior deltoid, and an inferior flap is created in the axillary fold. Dissection is carried down through the subcutaneous tissues, and the cephalic vein is ligated proximally within the deltopectoral groove. The deltoid and pectoralis major tendons are divided at their humeral insertions and retracted proximally. The coracobrachialis and short head of the biceps brachii are then sharply transected at the insertion on the coracoids, taking care to leave the pectoralis minor insertion intact. The axillary artery and vein are identified below the conjoint tendon and ligated. The median, ulnar, radial, and musculocutaneous nerves are identified and transected either under tension such that they retract under the pectoralis minor or transferred to shoulder girdle muscles by targeted muscle reinnervation. The humerus is then externally rotated so the latissimus dorsi and teres major muscles are released at their humeral insertions. The biceps brachii and triceps are released proximally, allowing the rotator cuff muscles to be released from the lesser (subscapularis) and greater (supraspinatus, infraspinatus, and teres minor) tuberosities. The remaining glenohumeral joint capsule is then divided to complete the amputation. The pectoralis major and latissimus dorsi tendons are sutured to one another over the glenoid for further soft tissue coverage, and the fish-mouth flaps are closed in the usual two-layer fashion.

Key points
1. Wrist disarticulation allows for full forearm pronation-supination and modern techniques allow for prosthetic use at this level.
2. Maximum length should be preserved when performing a transradial or transhumeral amputation, even if additional measures are needed for distal soft tissue coverage.
3. Five centimeters of proximal ulna is required to preserve elbow flexion and allow for prosthetic fit in a transradial amputation.
4. Elbow disarticulation allows rotation of a prosthesis through its fit onto the humeral condyles.
5. Although shoulder function is lost with amputation at or proximal to the pectoralis major insertion, preserving the stump allows a better prosthetic fit.

UPPER LIMB AMPUTATION OUTCOMES

Traumatic amputation of the upper extremity is a life-altering event. The goal of revision amputation is a painless limb that maximizes function with and without a prosthesis. To objectively measure outcomes following traumatic upper extremity amputation, studies have looked at various postoperative factors, such as prosthetic use or rejection, return to work, or performance in various functional tests.

The regular use of a prosthesis is frequently as a marker of success following upper extremity amputation, because rejection of a prosthesis can be caused by discomfort or perceived lack of functional gain.[20] Raichle and colleagues[21] investigated patient-reported prosthetic use in the upper and lower extremities to determine which factors predict use or abandonment. Lower extremity amputees reported using their prosthesis more than upper extremity amputees at 84% to 56%, respectively. The only significant factor in predicting upper extremity prosthesis use was level of amputation, with below-elbow amputations predicting better prosthesis use. Wright and colleagues[15] found a 38% prosthesis rejection rate in major upper limp amputees at all levels, and percentage of use differed depending on level of amputation. Thirty-nine of 42 transradial amputees reported regularly using their prostheses, whereas

this number dropped to only 9 of 21 in above-elbow amputations. Davidson[22] reported results of a questionnaire sent to upper extremity amputees in which 56% reported rarely or never using their prosthesis. Interestingly, the amount of time patients wore their prostheses did not correlate with their level of satisfaction with functional abilities.

Although traumatic upper limb amputation results in a significant loss of upper extremity function, many amputees are able to return to work with the aid of a prosthesis. Pinzur and coworkers[23] found that 17 of 18 patients who underwent major upper limb amputation were able to recover enough function with their prosthesis to allow return to work. However, although most upper limb amputees are able to work in some fashion, a fewer number are able to reassume their preinjury occupation. Datta and colleagues[24] investigated upper limb amputees with elbow disarticulations and more proximal levels in the United Kingdom and found that although 73.2% were able to work following their injury, two-thirds had to change jobs. Likewise, Livingston and coworkers[25] investigated postoperative disability in 42 traumatic amputees and found that only one in five above-elbow and three of nine below-elbow amputees were able to return to their previous level of occupation.

Unfortunately, there is no accepted standardized test to evaluate function or quality of life following upper limb revision amputation and prosthesis use. Wright[26] performed a review of published outcome measures for upper limb amputees and found seven different methods used. These included amputee-specific outcome measures, such as the Assessment of Capacity for Myoelectric Control, and general upper limb functional assessments, such as the Disabilities of the Arm, Shoulder, and Hand. No test is universally used or accepted despite the multitude available, making objective assessment of postoperative function and comparison among tests difficult.

COMPLICATIONS

Neuroma formation after upper limb amputation is a significant source of stump pain and cause of prosthesis failure. Geraghty and Jones reported a 25% incidence of symptomatic neuroma formation in 32 upper extremity amputations,[27] although the exact percentage is likely underestimated. Incidence of painful neuroma formation is decreased by meticulous handling of nerves during revision amputation and performance of traction neurotomy to bury the severed nerve ending under soft tissue coverage. Targeted muscle reinnervation can also decrease painful neuroma formation when performed at the time of the amputation[12] or even as a treatment option after neuroma formation has already occurred.[13]

Phantom limb pain is one of the most common complications following any extremity amputation. Shukla and colleagues[28] reported 82% short-term incidence of phantom pain in 34 upper extremity amputees, compared with 54% in lower extremity amputees. Kooijman and coworkers[29] sent questionnaires to 124 upper limb amputees, and found that 51% experience phantom pain, of which 64% reported "moderate to very much suffering" as a result. Interestingly, only four patients received treatment of their phantom pain, making it a prevalent yet undertreated complication.

Heterotopic ossification has become an increasingly recognized complication following traumatic upper extremity amputation, particularly with combat-related injuries. Potter and coworkers[30] reviewed 213 amputations in 187 soldiers and found a 63% prevalence of heterotopic ossification formation. Risk factors for heterotopic ossification formation were a blast injury and performing the amputation in the zone of injury. Fortunately, most of these cases did not require surgical excision and those that did respond well to treatment. Although the prevalence of heterotopic ossification is higher in combat-related amputation, it should be a consideration with civilian amputations, particularly if from a blast injury.

SUMMARY

Traumatic upper extremity amputation is a life-altering event, and recovery of function depends on proper surgical management and postoperative rehabilitation. Replantation should be considered, when indicated, but many injuries require revision amputation and postoperative prosthesis fitting. The surgeon should be aware of current surgical techniques and advances in modern prostheses so that preoperative planning leads to maximal functional recovery while minimizing complications. Care should be taken to preserve maximal length of the limb and motion of the remaining joints. Skin grafting or free tissue transfer may be necessary for coverage in some cases to allow preservation of length. Early prosthetic fitting within 30 days of surgery should be performed so the amputee is able to start the rehabilitation process while the wound is healing and the stump is maturing. Multidisciplinary care, which includes the surgeon, therapist, prosthetist, and psychiatrist, is essential for the overall care of the patient following a traumatic amputation of the upper limb.

REFERENCES

1. Barmparas G, Inaba K, Teixeira PG, et al. Epidemiology of post-traumatic limb amputation: a national trauma databank analysis. Am Surg 2010;76(11):1214–22.

2. Ziegler-Graham K, MacKenzie EJ, Ephraim PL, et al. Estimating the prevalence of limb loss in the United States: 2005 to 2050. Arch Phys Med Rehabil 2008;89(3):422–9.

3. Clouse WD, Rasmussen TE, Perlstein J, et al. Upper extremity vascular injury: a current in-theater wartime report from Operation Iraqi Freedom. Ann Vasc Surg 2006;20(4):429–34.

4. Stansbury LG, Lalliss SJ, Branstetter JG, et al. Amputations in U.S. military personnel in the current conflicts in Afghanistan and Iraq. J Orthop Trauma 2008;22(1):43–6. ·

5. Fischer H. A guide to U.S. military casualty statistics: Operation Inherent Resolve, Operation New Dawn, Operation Iraqi Freedom and Operation Enduring Freedom. 2014. Available at: http://www.fas.org/sgp/crs/natsec/RS22452.pdf. Accessed May 12, 2015.

6. Beris AE, Lykissas MG, Korompilias AV, et al. Digit and hand replantation. Arch Orthop Trauma Surg 2010;130(9):1141–7.

7. Graham B, Adkins P, Tsai TM, et al. Major replantation versus revision amputation and prosthetic fitting in the upper extremity: a late functional outcomes study. J Hand Surg 1998;23(5):783–91.

8. Baccarani A, Follmar KE, De Santis G, et al. Free vascularized tissue transfer to preserve upper extremity amputation levels. Plast Reconstr Surg 2007;120(4):971–81.

9. Lin CH, Webb K, Neumeister MW. Immediate tissue transplantation in upper limb trauma: spare parts reconstruction. Clin Plast Surg 2014;41(3):397–406.

10. Copuroglu C, Ozcan M, Yilmaz B, et al. Acute stress disorder and post-traumatic stress disorder following traumatic amputation. Acta Orthop Belg 2010;76(1):90–3.

11. Grunert BK, Matloub HS, Sanger JR, et al. Treatment of posttraumatic stress disorder after work-related hand trauma. J Hand Surg 1990;15(3):511–5.

12. Cheesborough JE, Souza JM, Dumanian GA, et al. Targeted muscle reinnervation in the initial management of traumatic upper extremity amputation injury. Hand (N Y) 2014;9(2):253–7.

13. Pet MA, Ko JH, Friedly JL, et al. Does targeted nerve implantation reduce neuroma pain in amputees? Clin Orthop Relat Res 2014;472(10):2991–3001.

14. Souza JM, Cheesborough JE, Ko JH, et al. Targeted muscle reinnervation: a novel approach to postamputation neuroma pain. Clin Orthopaedics Relat Res 2014;472(10):2984–90.

15. Wright TW, Hagen AD, Wood MB. Prosthetic usage in major upper extremity amputations. J Hand Surg 1995;20(4):619–22.
16. Tintle SM, Baechler MF, Nanos GP III, et al. Traumatic and trauma-related amputations: Part II: upper extremity and future directions. J Bone Joint Surg Am 2010;92(18):2934–45.
17. Lake C, Dodson R. Progressive upper limb prosthetics. Phys Med Rehabil Clin N Am 2006;17(1): 49–72.
18. Singh R, Hunter J, Philip A. Fluid collections in amputee stumps: a common phenomenon. Arch Phys Med Rehabil 2007;88(5):661–3.
19. Jebson PJ, Louis DS, Bagg M. Amputations. In: Green DP, Wolfe SW, editors. Green's operative hand surgery. 6th edition. Philadelphia: Elsevier/ Churchill Livingstone; 2011. p. 1885–927.
20. Biddiss E, Chau T. Upper-limb prosthetics: critical factors in device abandonment. Am J Phys Med Rehabil 2007;86(12):977–87.
21. Raichle KA, Hanley MA, Molton I, et al. Prosthesis use in persons with lower- and upper-limb amputation. J Rehabil Res Dev 2008;45(7):961–72.
22. Davidson J. A survey of the satisfaction of upper limb amputees with their prostheses, their lifestyles, and their abilities. J Hand Ther 2002;15(1):62–70.
23. Pinzur MS, Angelats J, Light TR, et al. Functional outcome following traumatic upper limb amputation and prosthetic limb fitting. J Hand Surg 1994; 19(5):836–9.
24. Datta D, Selvarajah K, Davey N. Functional outcome of patients with proximal upper limb deficiency– acquired and congenital. Clin Rehabil 2004;18(2): 172–7.
25. Livingston DH, Keenan D, Kim D, et al. Extent of disability following traumatic extremity amputation. J Trauma 1994;37(3):495–9.
26. Wright V. Prosthetic outcome measures for use with upper limb amputees: a systematic review of the peer-reviewed literature, 1970 to 2009. J Prosthet Orthot 2009;21(9):1–63.
27. Geraghty TJ, Jones LE. Painful neuromata following upper limb amputation. Prosthet Orthot Int 1996; 20(3):176–81.
28. Shukla GD, Sahu SC, Tripathi RP, et al. A psychiatric study of amputees. Br J Psychiatry 1982;141:50–3.
29. Kooijman CM, Dijkstra PU, Geertzen JH, et al. Phantom pain and phantom sensations in upper limb amputees: an epidemiological study. Pain 2000;87(1): 33–41.
30. Potter BK, Burns TC, Lacap AP, et al. Heterotopic ossification following traumatic and combat-related amputations. prevalence, risk factors, and preliminary results of excision. J Bone Joint Surg Am 2007;89(3):476–86.

Application of Tranexamic Acid in Trauma and Orthopedic Surgery

John D. Jennings, MD*, Mark K. Solarz, MD[1],
Christopher Haydel, MD[1]

KEYWORDS

- Tranexamic acid • Orthopedics • Trauma • Transfusion • Hemorrhage • Antifibrinolytics

KEY POINTS

- Tranexamic acid has been approved by the Food and Drug Administration for the past 30 years as an antifibrinolytic and has recently been added to the World Health Organization's list of essential medications.
- Tranexamic acid is not only effective, but safe in trauma and orthopedics with no increased morbidity including deep venous thrombosis or pulmonary embolism. Furthermore, it is inexpensive and the cost-savings with its use have been confirmed.
- Tranexamic acid has become readily integrated into joint replacement and spine surgeries, although the optimal timing and dosing have not been established. Significant reduction in blood loss and transfusion requirements in this setting was again demonstrated.
- The role of tranexamic acid in orthopedic trauma is emerging, and to date there have only been a small number of heterogeneous studies, which mostly pertained to hip fractures. Results in this cohort are promising, however.
- Significant future investigation, particularly with regards to orthopedic trauma, is needed to maximize the benefit from this drug. Furthermore, optimal timing and dosing should be confirmed.

INTRODUCTION

The use of tranexamic acid (TXA) as an antifibrinolytic agent was initially approved by the Food and Drug Administration to reduce bleeding in hemophiliacs undergoing tooth extraction.[1] Over the ensuing 30 years its use has extended to virtually every aspect of medicine from acute trauma to elective surgeries and extensive investigation for its myriad applications continues. The use of TXA in traumatically injured patients has gained international recognition, because hemorrhage is the number one preventable cause of death in this population.[2] The World Health Organization added the drug to its list of essential medications in 2011 after several investigations suggested it may significantly reduce death caused by hemorrhage.[1]

As a synthetic derivative of lysine, TXA competitively inhibits the conversion of plasminogen to plasmin, effectively prohibiting fibrin degradation

J.D. Jennings and M.K. Solarz have no disclosures pertaining to this topic. C. Haydel receives speaking fees from Depuy Synthes.

Department of Orthopaedics and Sports Medicine, Temple University Hospital, 3401 North Broad Street, Zone B 5th Floor, Philadelphia, PA 19140, USA

[1] Present address: 3501 North Broad Street, Philadelphia, PA 19140, USA.

* Corresponding author. 3501 North Broad Street, Philadelphia, PA 19140.

E-mail address: john.jennings2@tuhs.temple.edu

Orthop Clin N Am 47 (2016) 137–143
http://dx.doi.org/10.1016/j.ocl.2015.08.014

and dissolution of formed clot.[3] In addition, its theorized anti-inflammatory properties have been proposed as a secondary mechanism for reducing mortality in hemorrhaging patients.[4] It may be administered intravenously, intra-articularly, topically into the surgical field, or even orally.[5] Dose of the drug and timing of administration have also been examined and recommendations vary based on the circumstances of its use.

Orthopedic surgeons have incorporated TXA into multiple elective surgeries as a means of reducing blood loss and transfusion requirements.[6] The safety and efficacy of TXA for total hip and total knee arthroplasty have been demonstrated, although debate continues regarding the most appropriate route for administration.[7,8] Multiple studies have also demonstrated the safety and use of TXA in reducing blood loss during elective spine surgery.[9,10] Unfortunately, the role for TXA in orthopedic trauma has yet to be elucidated, although the limited results from its use in hip and femur fractures to date are encouraging.[11,12]

TRANEXAMIC ACID

TXA (trans-4-[aminomethyl] cyclohexane carboxylic acid) (**Fig. 1**) was first developed in Japan in 1962 in an attempt to synthetically capture the plasminogen-inhibiting capabilities of lysine more effectively.[13,14] The initial goal of this research

was to reduce postpartum deaths caused by hemorrhage, yet its use in medicine and surgery has continued to expand.

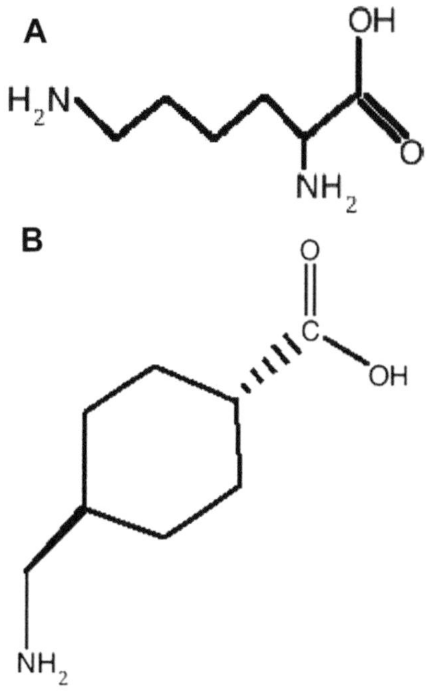

Mechanism and Pharmacokinetics

The interaction of plasminogen and the plasmin heavy chain is reversibly inhibited by TXA blockade of lysine-binding sites on plasminogen (**Fig. 2**).[15] Failure of fibrinolysis results as plasminogen is unable to bind to the fibrin molecules. At higher doses, TXA is secondarily able to directly inhibit plasmin activity and formation.[13] The plasma concentration needed to achieve approximately 80% inhibition of fibrinolysis is 10 µg/mL and maximum concentration is achieved approximately 1 hour after intravenous (IV) dosing.[14,16,17] The antifibrinolytic effects of TXA last from 8 to 17 hours after administration.[17–19]

Dosing and Timing of Administration

Orthopedic applications of TXA have effectively used IV, intra-articular, topical, and oral dosing

Fig. 1. Structure of lysine (A) and its synthetic derivative tranexamic acid (B).

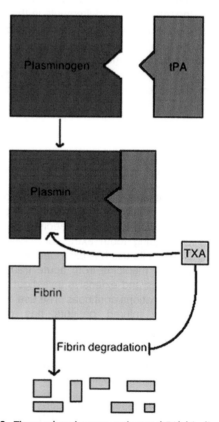

Fig. 2. Tissue plasminogen activator (tPA) binding to and activating plasminogen to plasmin. The lysine binding site for fibrin is blocked by tranexamic acid (TXA) thus inhibiting fibrin degradation and promoting clot stabilization.

(**Fig. 3**). The optimal dosing and timing have yet to be elucidated and is currently not standardized; however, the most common dosing by IV is 10 to 15 mg/kg before incision or inflation of the tourniquet if one is used and again before wound closure or tourniquet deflation.[17,20] Intra-articular dose of 250 mg to 2 g was most common and topical administration of 1 to 3 g mixed in normal saline is also reportedly effective for joint arthroplasty.[21] For trauma patients typical IV dosage is 1 g over 10 minutes followed by infusion of 1 g over the ensuing 8 hours.[22]

Cost

The cost for 1 g of TXA varies, with average estimates between $45 and $55. Multiple studies note the cost benefit of the drug because the implicit savings in units of blood may be extraordinary.[22,23] The estimated cost per life-year gained from administering TXA, according to the Clinical Randomization of an Antifibrinolytic in Significant Hemorrhage 2 (CRASH-2) study data, was $64.[22]

Safety

As an antifibrinolytic, the theoretic risk of using TXA is the formation of unwanted and harmful vascular thromboses. To date, the CRASH-2 trial

is the largest prospective, randomized, placebo-controlled study to evaluate the safety of TXA. More than 20,000 trauma patients were enrolled across 274 hospitals in 40 countries and there was no difference in the rate of thrombus or embolus formation between the TXA and placebo groups. The authors concluded TXA is safe and effective at reducing blood loss and transfusion requirements.

In orthopedics, Poeran and colleagues[7] retrospectively reviewed almost 900,000 elective joint replacement surgeries that used perioperative TXA and found no increased risk for thromboembolic events, acute renal failure, cardiac or cerebrovascular events, or in-hospital mortality.[24] Several meta-analyses have reiterated the safety profile of TXA, demonstrating no increased rates of deep vein thrombosis, pulmonary embolism, activated partial thromboplastin time, or prothrombin time.[5,7,25–27]

USE IN TRAUMA

Much has been published within the past decade regarding the use of TXA in the treatment of traumatic hemorrhage. Encouraging results of TXA use during elective surgery prompted the investigation of its use in trauma with the goal of reducing transfusion requirements and mortality from blood loss. Although these studies have shed light on the potential for TXA use in trauma, there remains no consensus for its use in trauma centers throughout the United States.

One of the most referenced trials regarding the use of TXA in trauma patients is the CRASH-2.[28] This international, randomized controlled study evaluated the effect of TXA following blunt or penetrating trauma. More than 20,000 trauma patients from 274 hospitals in 40 countries were randomized to either a standardized treatment with TXA or placebo; the primary outcome was death within 4 weeks of injury. The group that received TXA had significantly fewer deaths from hemorrhage despite no difference in vascular clot formation. The authors concluded that TXA is safe for use when trauma results in significant hemorrhage and should be administered as soon as possible. The results of this study led to the World Health Organization's addition of TXA to their list of essential mediations.[1]

A subgroup analysis of the CRASH-2 data has provided further details of the best use for TXA in trauma. Roberts and colleagues[22] demonstrated that TXA use provided the most survival benefit in patients who presented with systolic blood pressure below 75 mm Hg and those treated soon after their injury. The most benefit was seen

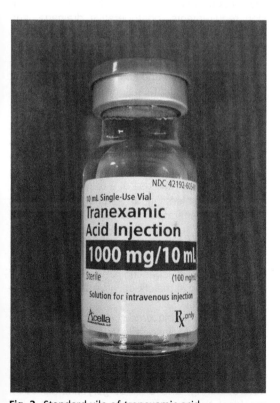

Fig. 3. Standard vile of tranexamic acid.

in those receiving TXA within 1 hour, followed by those receiving treatment within 3 hours. Interestingly, those receiving TXA after 3 hours had an overall increase in mortality.

To build on the civilian data of TXA use in trauma, Morrison and colleagues[27] demonstrated the benefit of TXA use with military injuries. The Military Application of TXA in Trauma Emergency Resuscitation study (MATTERs) was a retrospective study of 896 soldiers in southern Afghanistan who required a blood transfusion during treatment of a traumatic injury. Despite having higher Injury Severity Scores among those who received TXA, there was overall reduction in mortality with TXA use, particularly in those who required massive transfusions. There was no difference in thrombotic events between groups when their data were corrected for Injury Severity Scores. They expanded on their data with the MATTERs II study, which demonstrated that the addition of cryoprecipitate to TXA reduced mortality when compared with administration of TXA or cryoprecipitate alone.[29]

Although data from CRASH-2 and MATTERs have demonstrated improved survival with TXA use and an economic analysis has shown it to be cost effective and to reduce hospital stays, there has not been widespread adoption of standard TXA protocols at trauma centers in the United States.[30] In a national survey of trauma surgeons in 2014, only 38% reported regularly using TXA and less than 25% use it one to two times per year. The main reasons for not using TXA were uncertainty of clinical benefit and unfamiliarity with the drug.[31] Because some recent data suggest that TXA may increase mortality for a subset of patients in severe hemorrhagic shock, more randomized studies are needed to delineate which patients benefit most from TXA use and allow for its potential incorporation into widespread use.[32]

USE IN ORTHOPEDICS

The use of TXA in orthopedics has primarily been described in the context of total hip arthroplasty and total knee arthroplasty, which may be associated with significant bleeding and related complications.[5,19,33] Patients with acute blood loss anemia from significant intraoperative or postoperative bleeding may require transfusion of blood products, which is an independent predictor of morbidity.[34] Furthermore, allogenic blood transfusion is not only expensive, but carries a risk of hemolytic or anaphylactic transfusion reactions, transmission of infection (hepatitis, human immunodeficiency virus, cytomegalovirus, and so forth),

increased length of hospital stay, and is a scarce resource.[5,19] For this reason, a plethora of studies have emerged examining the use of TXA in reducing blood loss and blood transfusion requirements in multiple elective orthopedic surgical procedures.

Total Hip Arthroplasty

The use of IV and topical TXA has been well described in total hip arthroplasty, because the procedure is regularly associated with significant blood loss. With the exception of a few studies, most investigations found TXA to consistently reduce blood transfusion requirements in patients undergoing total hip arthroplasty.[16,33,35] This finding was independent of dose, timing, type of anesthesia, or whether a press-fit or cemented prosthesis was used.[33] Moreover, a significant reduction in intraoperative and postoperative blood loss, postoperative drainage, and cost was consistently demonstrated.[23,33] TXA significantly reduces transfusion rates for patients regardless of preoperative hemoglobin levels.[36]

When comparing route of administration, topically applied TXA was initially investigated to circumvent the theoretically increased risk of thromboembolic events with IV systemic delivery. In large prospective studies and meta-analyses, topical application decreases blood loss, transfusion requirements, postoperative drainage, and decline in hemoglobin without increasing the risk for deep venous thrombosis or pulmonary embolism.[37] Another study safely added dilute epinephrine to topical TXA and found an additive effect that was superior to TXA alone.[19]

Total Knee Arthroplasty

The use of TXA in knee replacement surgery has likewise been extensively studied and has the added variable of routine tourniquet use during surgery. Although the use of a tourniquet reduces intraoperative bleeding, an augmented fibrinolytic response is generated that may lead to increased postoperative bleeding and drainage.[17,21] As such, Benoni and coworkers[38] and Hippala and coworkers[39] investigated the use of TXA with promising results, sparking an ensuing cohort of studies looking at the effectiveness of this prophylactic treatment.[24]

As with hip replacement, the use of TXA in total knee arthroplasty effectively reduces blood loss, need for transfusions, and postoperative drainage.[21] These positive effects were demonstrated at multiple doses given at various points before, during, and after surgery and as such, the ideal timing and dosage has not yet been established.[40,41] Furthermore, topical application is at least as effective as IV administration and results in negligible systemic absorption.[8,18,24,42]

In a multicenter, randomized clinical trial, topical and IV TXA were each deemed safe and superior to routine hemostasis in reducing blood loss and transfusion requirements, yet no difference was elucidated between the two routes of administration.[21] As such, topical TXA is an attractive option, particularly for patients with increased risk for thromboembolic events or with renal failure.

Spine Surgery

Significant bleeding in spine surgery is often attributed to long procedures, large surgical wounds, and the vascular cancellous bone of the spine.[9] As such, marked interest in strategies to conserve blood has been undertaken, and recent investigation has demonstrated an important place for TXA in this domain.

Clinical trials have proved that TXA is an effective tool in reducing blood loss in spine surgery with no incremental risk or complications.[43,44] In a recent meta-analysis, Cheriyan and coworkers[9] demonstrated a 33% reduction in transfusion rates with the administration of TXA and concomitantly found reduced intraoperative, postoperative, and total blood loss. The safety and efficacy of TXA in spine surgery has been confirmed in multiple other studies; however, as with total joint surgeries, no unified recommendation for timing or dose exists to date.[44–46]

Orthopedic Trauma

Although the use of TXA in joint replacement and spine surgery has been verified and extensively studied, its place in orthopedic trauma is still under early investigation. For this patient population, perioperative blood loss attributed to the fracture and subsequent surgery may be significant and lead to significant morbidity.[47,48]

For patients with hip fractures undergoing hemiarthroplasty, TXA is a safe, effective, and cost-efficient adjunct in reducing blood loss.[47,49] Recently, Lee and colleagues[47] reviewed 271 patients with hip fractures managed with hemiarthroplasty and found that when compared with standard treatment, patients who received a 1-g TXA bolus preoperatively had less blood loss and a lower transfusion rate with no increase in 30- or 90-day mortality. They noted the importance of blood conservation in this patient population in particular, because they are more susceptible to anemia and required transfusions postoperatively.

Similarly, in a randomized, double-blind, controlled trial conducted by Zufferey and colleagues,[12] 15 mg/kg at skin incision and 3 hours later was found to reduce transfusion rates by 30% compared with placebo. These authors did note that roughly one-third of the blood loss in these patients occurred before surgery and was thus an added variable when compared with elective surgeries.

The positive effects of TXA in patients with hip fracture have been confirmed in several other studies, although heterogeneity makes comparisons difficult.[11,49,50] For instance, no studies to date stratify these patients by intracapsular versus extracapsular fractures, which has a significant contribution to overall blood loss.

Benefits have been demonstrated with variable doses and, as with its use in general trauma, early administration may be advantageous. However, optimal timing for the initial or subsequent doses has not been established. The value of TXA has been replicated in multiple prospective trials for patients with hip and femur fractures when compared with placebo; however, its use in this setting remains off-label.[11,12]

FUTURE INVESTIGATION

Although TXA has been extensively studied and is certainly an excellent addition to the armamentarium of orthopedic and trauma surgeons alike, knowledge of its full benefits and limitations continues to grow. Dosing and timing of administration, for example, is highly variable between centers and therefore prompts future exploration to find the highest benefit at the lowest cost.

Furthermore, the presence of TXA in several elective orthopedic surgical practices has been established, yet knowledge of its potential benefits and limitations in other realms of orthopedics has yet to be elucidated. In trauma, for example, most research to date has understandably focused on hip fracture surgery. However, pelvic and other long bone fracture surgery can likewise be associated with significant blood loss and may stand to benefit from TXA.

Lastly, the route of administration and limitations in patients with other comorbidities are not yet fully understood. Multiple studies have demonstrated the effectiveness of TXA applied topically to the surgical field when compared with IV dosing; whether this holds true outside of joint replacement is still unknown. The efficacy of topical application was predicated on a concern for using TXA in patients with renal failure or a predisposition to thromboembolic events. The systemic effects from topical application are still under investigation and appropriate IV dosing is likewise yet to be established.

SUMMARY

Over the past 30 years, TXA has become a significant tool in reducing perioperative blood loss, transfusion requirements, and morbidity in patients across multiple specialties. Its indications have continued to expand as its effectiveness and safety endure the growing list of applications, particularly in orthopedic surgery. Although questions remain about optimal timing, dosing, patient limitations, and route of administration, overwhelming evidence supports its use as a cost-effective measure in blood management and routine use is likely in the future.

REFERENCES

1. Napolitano LM, Cohen MJ, Cotton BA, et al. Tranexamic acid in trauma: how should we use it? J Trauma Acute Care Surg 2013;74(6):1575–86.
2. Perel P, Clayton T, Altman DG, et al. Red blood cell transfusion and mortality in trauma patients: risk-stratified analysis of an observational study. PLoS Med 2014;11(6):e1001664.
3. McCormack PL. Tranexamic acid: a review of its use in the treatment of hyperfibrinolysis. Drugs 2012; 72(5):585–617.
4. Jimenez JJ, Iribarren JL, Lorente L, et al. Tranexamic acid attenuates inflammatory response in cardiopulmonary bypass surgery through blockade of fibrinolysis: a case control study followed by a randomized double-blind controlled trial. Crit Care 2007;11(6): R117.
5. Wei Z, Liu M. The effectiveness and safety of tranexamic acid in total hip or knee arthroplasty: a meta-analysis of 2720 cases. Transfus Med 2015; 25(3):151–62.
6. Danninger T, Memtsoudis SG. Tranexamic acid and orthopedic surgery-the search for the holy grail of blood conservation. Ann Transl Med 2015;3(6):77.
7. Poeran J, Rasul R, Suzuki S, et al. Tranexamic acid use and postoperative outcomes in patients undergoing total hip or knee arthroplasty in the United States: retrospective analysis of effectiveness and safety. BMJ 2014;349:g4829.
8. Digas G, Koutsogiannis I, Meletiadis G, et al. Intra-articular injection of tranexamic acid reduce blood loss in cemented total knee arthroplasty. Eur J Orthop Surg Traumatol 2015;25(5):1–8.
9. Cheriyan T, Maier SP, Bianco K, et al. Efficacy of tranexamic acid on surgical bleeding in spine surgery: a meta-analysis. Spine J 2015;15(4):752–61.
10. Li ZJ, Fu X, Xing D, et al. Is tranexamic acid effective and safe in spinal surgery? A meta-analysis of randomized controlled trials. Eur Spine J 2013;22(9):1950–7.
11. Vijay BS, Bedi V, Mitra S, et al. Role of tranexamic acid in reducing postoperative blood loss and transfusion requirement in patients undergoing hip and femoral surgeries. Saudi J Anaesth 2013;7(1): 29–32.
12. Zufferey PJ, Miquet M, Quenet S, et al. Tranexamic acid in hip fracture surgery: a randomized controlled trial. Br J Anaesth 2010;104(1):23–30.
13. Hunt BJ. The current place of tranexamic acid in the management of bleeding. Anaesthesia 2015; 70(Suppl 1):50–3. e18.
14. Tengborn L, Blombäck M, Berntorp E. Tranexamic acid: an old drug still going strong and making a revival. Thromb Res 2015;135(2):231–42.
15. Dunn CJ, Goa KL. Tranexamic acid: a review of its use in surgery and other indications. Drugs 1999; 57(6):1005–32.
16. Benoni G, Lethagen S, Fredin H. The effect of tranexamic acid on local and plasma fibrinolysis during total knee arthroplasty. Thromb Res 1997;85(3): 195–206.
17. Dahuja A, Dahuja G, Jaswal V, et al. A prospective study on role of tranexamic acid in reducing postoperative blood loss in total knee arthroplasty and its effect on coagulation profile. J Arthroplasty 2014; 29(4):733–5.
18. Wang CG, Sun ZH, Liu J, et al. Safety and efficacy of intra-articular tranexamic acid injection without drainage on blood loss in total knee arthroplasty: a randomized clinical trial. Int J Surg 2015;20:1–7.
19. Gao F, Sun W, Guo W, et al. Topical application of tranexamic acid plus diluted epinephrine reduces postoperative hidden blood loss in total hip arthroplasty. J Arthroplasty 2015. [Epub ahead of print].
20. Panteli M, Papakostidis C, Dahabreh Z, et al. Topical tranexamic acid in total knee replacement: a systematic review and meta-analysis. Knee 2013;20(5): 300–9.
21. Aguilera X, Martínez-Zapata MJ, Hinarejos P, et al. Topical and intravenous tranexamic acid reduce blood loss compared to routine hemostasis in total knee arthroplasty: a multicenter, randomized, controlled trial. Arch Orthop Trauma Surg 2015; 135(7):1017–25.
22. Roberts I, Shakur H, Coats T, et al. The CRASH-2 trial: a randomised controlled trial and economic evaluation of the effects of tranexamic acid on death, vascular occlusive events and transfusion requirement in bleeding trauma patients. Health Technol Assess 2013;17(10):1–79.
23. Johansson T, Pettersson LG, Lisander B. Tranexamic acid in total hip arthroplasty saves blood and money: a randomized, double-blind study in 100 patients. Acta Orthop 2005;76(3):314–9.
24. Oremus K. Tranexamic acid for the reduction of blood loss in total knee arthroplasty. Ann Transl Med 2015;3(Suppl 1):S40.
25. Yang ZG, Chen WP, Wu LD. Effectiveness and safety of tranexamic acid in reducing blood loss in total

knee arthroplasty: a meta-analysis. J Bone Joint Surg Am 2012;94(13):1153–9.

26. Tan J, Chen H, Liu Q, et al. A meta-analysis of the effectiveness and safety of using tranexamic acid in primary unilateral total knee arthroplasty. J Surg Res 2013;184(2):880–7.

27. Morrison JJ, Dubose JJ, Rasmussen TE, et al. Military Application of Tranexamic Acid in Trauma Emergency Resuscitation (MATTERs) Study. Arch Surg 2012;147(2):113–9.

28. Shakur H, Roberts I, Bautista R, et al. Effects of tranexamic acid on death, vascular occlusive events, and blood transfusion in trauma patients with significant haemorrhage (CRASH-2): a randomised, placebo-controlled trial. Lancet 2010;376(9734): 23–32.

29. Morrison JJ, Ross JD, Dubose JJ, et al. Association of cryoprecipitate and tranexamic acid with improved survival following wartime injury: findings from the MATTERs II study. JAMA Surg 2013; 148(3):218–25.

30. Guerriero C, Cairns J, Perel P, et al, CRASH 2 Trial Collaborators. Cost-effectiveness analysis of administering tranexamic acid to bleeding trauma patients using evidence from the CRASH-2 trial. PLoS One 2011;6(5):e18987.

31. Jawa R, Singer A, McCormack J, et al. Use of tranexamic acid in civilian US trauma centers: results of a national survey. Las Vegas (Nevada): Academic Surgical Congress; 2015.

32. Valle EJ, Allen CJ, Van Haren RM, et al. Do all trauma patients benefit from tranexamic acid? J Trauma Acute Care Surg 2014;76(6):1373–8.

33. Sukeik M, Alshryda S, Haddad FS, et al. Systematic review and meta-analysis of the use of tranexamic acid in total hip replacement. J Bone Joint Surg Br 2011;93(1):39–46.

34. Lemaire R. Strategies for blood management in orthopaedic and trauma surgery. J Bone Joint Surg Br 2008;90(9):1128–36.

35. Garneti N, Field J. Bone bleeding during total hip arthroplasty after administration of tranexamic acid. J Arthroplasty 2004;19(4):488–92.

36. Whiting DR, Duncan CM, Sierra RJ, et al. Tranexamic acid benefits total joint arthroplasty patients regardless of preoperative hemoglobin value. J Arthroplasty 2015. [Epub ahead of print].

37. Wang C, Xu GJ, Han Z, et al. Topical application of tranexamic acid in primary total hip arthroplasty: a systemic review and meta-analysis. Int J Surg 2015;15:134–9.

38. Benoni G, Carlsson A, Petersson C, et al. Does tranexamic acid reduce blood loss in knee arthroplasty? Am J Knee Surg 1995;8(3):88–92.

39. Hiippala S, Strid L, Wennerstrand M, et al. Tranexamic acid (Cyklokapron) reduces perioperative blood loss associated with total knee arthroplasty. Br J Anaesth 1995;74(5):534–7.

40. Kundu R, Das A, Basunia SR, et al. Does a single loading dose of tranexamic acid reduce perioperative blood loss and transfusion requirements after total knee replacement surgery? A randomized, controlled trial. J Nat Sci Biol Med 2015;6(1):94–9.

41. Ishii Y, Noguchi H, Sato J, et al. Effect of a single injection of tranexamic acid on blood loss after primary hybrid TKA. Knee 2015;22(3):197–200.

42. Sabatini L, Atzori F. Topical intra-articular and intravenous tranexamic acid to reduce blood loss in total knee arthroplasty. Ann Transl Med 2015; 3(Suppl 1):S18.

43. Farrokhi MR, Kazemi AP, Eftekharian HR, et al. Efficacy of prophylactic low dose of tranexamic acid in spinal fixation surgery: a randomized clinical trial. J Neurosurg Anesthesiol 2011;23(4):290–6.

44. Raksakietisak M, Sathitkarnmanee B, Srisaen P, et al. Two doses of tranexamic acid reduce blood transfusion in complex spine surgery: a prospective randomized study. Spine (Phila Pa 1976) 2015. [Epub ahead of print].

45. Yang B, Li H, Wang D, et al. Systematic review and meta-analysis of perioperative intravenous tranexamic acid use in spinal surgery. PLoS One 2013; 8(2):e55436.

46. Xie J, Lenke LG, Li T, et al. Preliminary investigation of high-dose tranexamic acid for controlling intraoperative blood loss in patients undergoing spine correction surgery. Spine J 2015;15(4):647–54.

47. Lee C, Freeman R, Edmondson M, et al. The efficacy of tranexamic acid in hip hemiarthroplasty surgery: an observational cohort study. Injury 2015. [Epub ahead of print].

48. Kadar A, Chechik O, Steinberg E, et al. Predicting the need for blood transfusion in patients with hip fractures. Int Orthop 2013;37(4):693–700.

49. Sadeghi M, Mehr-Aein A. Does a single bolus dose of tranexamic acid reduce blood loss and transfusion requirements during hip fracture surgery? A prospective randomized double blind study in 67 patients. Acta Med Iran 2007;45(6):437–42.

50. Emara WM, Moez KK, Elkholy AH. Topical versus intravenous tranexamic acid as a blood conservation intervention for reduction of post-operative bleeding in hemiarthroplasty. Anesth Essays Res 2014;8(1):48–53.

Pediatrics

Preface
Patellar Instability

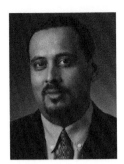

Shital N. Parikh, MD, FACS
Editor

From an evolutionary standpoint, the patella appeared much later than the condyles, meniscus, and cruciate ligaments of the knee. Compared with lower animals, the patella gradually increased in size and function and gained more importance as a facilitator for the extensor mechanism in erect humans. Being low in the evolutionary chain and high in functional demand, the patellofemoral joint is indeed unique. In past decades, various patellar instability patterns have been described in the literature and so has the various surgical options to treat it, ranging from patellectomy to patellofemoral replacement. Recently, the medial patellofemoral ligament has been recognized as the most important contributor to patellar stability, and its reconstruction as the ultimate treatment. However, all patellar instability patterns are not the same, and all instability patterns cannot be managed by the same ligament reconstruction. In the article "Classification of Lateral Patellar Instability in Children and Adolescents," the authors have first tried to define the common nomenclature related to lateral patellar instability. This is followed by a classification system to differentiate the four recognizable patterns of instability (types I–IV) with each higher type representing increasing severity and requiring more complex surgery. The classification system would help guide the medical decision-making process and decrease heterogeneity in the literature for research and communication purposes.

The second article in this series is on congenital anomalies of the hand and its management principles. The authors briefly describe the epidemiology, classification, and embryology of congenital hand anomalies and focus on three common anomalies (syndactyly, polydactyly, and hypoplastic thumb). Since several congenital hand anomalies are associated with systemic malformations, sometimes fatal, it is important to identify such associations. Each anomaly is discussed in detail, including its types, principles of management, technical considerations during surgery, postoperative course, and outcomes. The authors stress the importance of getting the family involved in treatment discussions because distinction needs to be made between the expected cosmetic and functional outcomes related to the anomaly. Also, there are various cultural and social differences between patients; hence, preoperative counseling and patient and family expectations play a big role in decision-making.

I am sure the readers would enjoy these informative articles. As a medical student and resident, I remember the *Orthopedic Clinics of North America* as the go-to reference for up-to-date information. It continues to be so. It has been an honor and pleasure serving on the editorial board of this prestigious series. Besides the authors, I would like to thank the office and support staff who worked tirelessly to get timely information to the readers. Best wishes to the new editorial board and to the future of this series.

Shital N. Parikh, MD, FACS
Cincinnati Children's Hospital Medical Center
3333 Burnet Avenue
Cincinnati, OH 45229, USA

E-mail address:
Shital.Parikh@cchmc.org

orthopedic.theclinics.com

Classification of Lateral Patellar Instability in Children and Adolescents

Shital N. Parikh, MD[a],*, Marios G. Lykissas, MD[b]

KEYWORDS

- Patella • Patellofemoral • Instability • Subluxation • Dislocation • Nomenclature • Classification
- Habitual

KEY POINTS

- Standardized nomenclature should be used when describing patellar instability patterns to avoid heterogeneity related to the causes and treatment of varied instability patterns.
- Type I (first-time patellar dislocation) and type II (recurrent patellar instability) represent the most common patterns of patellar instability seen in adolescent and young adult patients.
- Medial patellofemoral ligament (MFPL) reconstruction may suffice for most type II patellar instability patients, although all contributing factors should be analyzed.
- Type III (dislocatable) and type IV (dislocated) instability patterns are typically seen in children, although if ignored or in asymptomatic patients, presentation may be delayed.
- MPFL reconstruction would not suffice as an adequate treatment option for type III and type IV instability patterns. Quadricepsplasty is frequently required to realign or lengthen the quadriceps mechanism to stabilize the patella.

INTRODUCTION

Instability of the patellofemoral joint is a common, often challenging, problem that affects between 7 and 49 people per 100,000.[1,2] The highest risk is noted for young individuals in the second decade of life with a prevalence of first-time patellar dislocation of 31 per 100,000.[2] The annual prevalence drops to 11 per 100,000 in the third decade and to 1.5 to 2 per 100,000 for patients between 30 and 59 years of age.[2] Because of the varied cause, varied time of presentation, and its multifactorial nature, treatment of patellar instability is varied as well. Historically, more than 100 different surgical procedures have been described in the literature to address patellar instability, although in the last 2 decades, the role of medial patellofemoral ligament (MPFL) reconstruction has received the most attention.[3]

Patellar instability is predominantly in a lateral direction due to the obliquity of the femur in humans as compared with other primates.[4] Although medial, superior, inferior, rotational, intra-articular, and multidirectional instability patterns have been described, these are rare. For the current article, patellar instability would imply lateral patellar instability. Patellar instability encompasses patellar subluxation and dislocation.

There is significant heterogeneity in the literature related to the causes, contributing factors, and treatment of lateral patellar instability. To address

The authors have nothing to disclose.
[a] Division of Pediatric Orthopaedics, Cincinnati Children's Hospital Medical Center, 3333 Burnet Avenue, Cincinnati, OH 45229, USA; [b] Department of Orthopaedic Surgery, University of Ioannina School of Medicine, Dompoli 30, Ioannina, PC 45110, Greece
* Corresponding author.
E-mail address: shital.parikh@cchmc.org

orthopedic.theclinics.com

such a multifactorial issue of patellar instability, the first task is to classify the instability pattern. Ideally, classification systems are used to assess a clinical entity, to enable surgeons to recommend specific treatment options, and to allow comparison of different treatment methods. It should be objective, easy to understand, and of practical value in a clinical setting. The aim of this article is to review the nomenclature and existing patellar instability classification systems and analyze the different instability patterns into a comprehensive system.

EXISTING CLASSIFICATION

The classification systems that are most often used to describe patellar instability are based on either the clinical symptoms or the pattern/cause of the patellar dislocation. Dejour and colleagues[5] classified patellar instability into 3 types based on the presence of patellofemoral anatomic abnormalities or patellar pain:

1. In major patellar instability, there are more than one documented dislocations.
2. In objective patellar instability, there is one documented dislocation and associated anatomic abnormality.
3. In potential patellar instability, the patient has patellar pain with associated radiographic abnormalities.

The classification system as described by Garin and colleagues[6] includes major dislocation (permanent or habitual) and recurrent dislocation (potential or objective). Chotel and colleagues,[7] however, did not recognize potential patellar instability as described by Dejour and Garin and considered it a vague and controversial condition. The authors proposed a more detailed classification system that distinguished 5 clinical patterns, more commonly seen in children. Their classification system did not include traumatic dislocation. The clinical patterns of the Chotel classification system, based on the age of presentation, were as follows:

1. Congenital dislocation: present at birth
2. Permanent dislocation: appeared before the age of 5 years
3. Habitual dislocation during knee flexion: appeared between 5 to 8 years
4. Habitual dislocation during knee extension
5. Recurrent dislocation: in adolescents

Although age may help to diagnose the instability pattern, it cannot be relied on much because patients and families may ignore the instability;

they may be misdiagnosed, or they may present late if the instability was asymptomatic. Sillanpaa[8] preferred to use the term primary patellar dislocation when patellar dislocation occurred for the first time and secondary patellar dislocation when a dislocation had occurred once previously and occurred again.[8] The use of the term acute patellar dislocation was discouraged, because it did not differentiate between a first-time dislocation and recurrent dislocation. Hiemstra and colleagues[9] classified patellar instability as WARPS (weak, atraumatic, risky anatomy, pain, and subluxation) or STAID (strong, traumatic, anatomy normal, instability, and dislocation) with some patients having mixed characteristics. Their classification system was based on the shoulder instability classification system of TUBS (traumatic, unilateral, Bankart lesion, surgery) and AMBRI (atraumatic, multidirectional, bilateral, rehabilitation, inferior shift). Although the existing classification systems are useful, they are not comprehensive.

Before the discussion of the comprehensive classification system, a standardized nomenclature would help in communication and understanding of various terminology used to describe patterns of patellar instability.

NOMENCLATURE

Grelsamer[10] recognized that the study of the patellofemoral joint is complicated by the use of expressions and terms that lack proper definition. Several of these terms, including chondromalacia, subluxation, maltracking, patellofemoral syndrome, and anterior knee pain, may mean different things to different physicians. Similarly, the literature related to patellar instability is confusing because of the lack of standard terminology to describe various patterns of instability.[11] For example, the term mild patellofemoral instability has been used in the literature, although no formal definition or grade of severity of instability has been previously defined.[12] Similarly, the term chronic patellar instability may mean recurrent patellar dislocations or persistent symptoms after first-time patellar dislocation. A recent study on the treatment of habitual patellar dislocation in adolescents included patients with recurrent patellar dislocation creating controversial recommendations requiring clarification by the authors.[13,14] Thus, any discussion related to patellar instability should include precise terms and definitions. **Table 1** includes the definition of terms used to describe various forms of instability in the classification system. The term subluxation merits special description, because it has more ambiguity associated with it.

Table 1
Nomenclature for lateral patellar instability

Terminology	Description
Patellar subluxation	Partial lateral movement of patella out of trochlea but presence of articular contact between the patella and the trochlea (based on symptoms, signs, or radiographs)
Patellar dislocation	Complete lateral movement of patella out of trochlea with no articular contact between them
Patellar instability	Patellar subluxation or patellar dislocation
First-time patellar dislocation	The first true episode of patellar dislocation wherein the deformity had to be reduced or self-reduced
Recurrent patellar dislocation	Second or subsequent episode of patellar dislocation wherein deformity had to be reduced or self-reduced
Passive patellar dislocation	Dislocatable patella with an apprehension maneuver or in certain knee position
Habitual patellar dislocation	Involuntary patellar dislocation and relocation with every cycle of knee flexion and extension
Congenital patellar dislocation	Intrauterine patellar dislocation with associated characteristic limb deformities
Developmental patellar dislocation	Patellar instability not present at birth but develops after walking age
Voluntary patellar dislocation	Patellar dislocation and relocation that can be demonstrated by selective muscle contraction without significant movement of the knee joint
Syndromic patellar dislocation	Patellar dislocation associated with a neuromuscular disorder, connective tissue disorder, or syndrome

Patellar subluxation could be a clinical symptom, clinical sign, or radiographic diagnosis.[10] It is defined as a partial loss of contact between the articular surface of patella and the trochlea. As a clinical symptom, Hughston[15] first described patellar subluxation as a frequently missed diagnosis in athletes. Patients present with frequent giving-way episodes with activities. The other presenting symptoms may include pain, swelling, or locking. These symptoms could be quite disabling. They frequently start after an initial patellar dislocation episode, but at times, could be present without a definite or known dislocation history. As a clinical sign, a hypermobile patella or positive apprehension sign could be regarded as patellar subluxation. As a radiologic diagnosis of subluxation, lateral displacement of the patella could be seen on axial imaging.

COMPREHENSIVE CLASSIFICATION

The proposed classification system was developed based on review of literature and more than 300 cases of patellar instability treated at the authors' institution from 2008 to 2015. It is comprehensive because all forms of patellar instability encountered in children and adolescents are included (**Table 2**). It is easy to understand and memorize, as type I dislocation means first-time patellar dislocation, and type II means second or subsequent patellar dislocation or continued symptoms after an initial instability episode. These patterns are commonly seen in adolescent and

Table 2
Classification of patellar instability

Type I	First patellar dislocation
A	With osteochondral fracture
B	Without osteochondral fracture
Type II	Recurrent patellar instability (most common pattern)
A	Recurrent patellar subluxation
B	Recurrent ($\geq$2) patellar dislocation
Type III	Dislocatable patella
A	Passive patellar dislocation
B	Habitual patellar dislocation—in flexion or extension
Type IV	Dislocated patella
A	Reducible
B	Irreducible

young adult patients. Type III (dislocatable patella) and type IV (dislocated patella) represent instability patterns typically seen in children. The classification pattern would help in identification of the common pathologic factors and aid in the decision-making process during its management. The complexity of treatment increases with the type of instability, in that most type I instability patients could be managed nonoperatively, whereas most type IV instability patients would need a complex realignment procedure. Any instability pattern could be associated with patellofemoral arthritis, which then would change the treatment options and eventual outcomes. Thus patellofemoral instability with arthritis is excluded from the classification system.

TYPE I: FIRST TIME PATELLAR DISLOCATION

The first episode of patellar dislocation may be traumatic and could lead to knee effusion. It is associated with an osteochondral fracture or chondral injury in 30% of the patients (type IA).[16] The osteochondral fracture or chondral injury usually involves the medial aspect of the patella, and less frequently, the middle third of the lateral femoral condyle.[1] In the presence of a knee effusion after patellar dislocation, an MRI can help identify the presence of an osteochondral fracture or other associated intra-articular injuries.[17] The osteochondral fracture of the patella needs to be differentiated from the medial rim avulsion fracture of the patella, which seldom needs to be addressed.[18] The presence of an osteochondral fracture or chondral fragment may necessitate surgical intervention to either excise or fix the fragment depending on its size (10–15 mm) and status of the cartilage within the piece. If surgery is required to address the osteochondral fracture or chondral fragment, then a concomitant or staged patellar stabilization procedure could be performed to prevent subsequent instability episodes. Most patients with traumatic patellar dislocation have normal underlying bony anatomy.

In contrast, atraumatic first-time patellar dislocation or dislocation after trivial trauma (eg, walking down steps, turning or pivoting maneuver during a routine activity) is frequently associated with underlying anatomic abnormalities and is seldom accompanied by an osteochondral fracture (type 1B).

In clinical studies comparing the nonoperative and operative treatment of acute patellar dislocations, medial-sided primary repair has not shown improvement in long-term subjective or functional outcomes.[19–23] The operative repair consisted of primary repair of the MPFL and medial retinacular

structures in these studies. These studies favored conservative treatment, which includes casting or splinting for 3 to 4 weeks, followed by rehabilitation, activity modification, and gradual return to full activities. A recent randomized controlled study, however, has shown favorable results of MPFL reconstruction for first-time patellar dislocation, when compared with nonoperative treatment.[24] Some investigators have recommended patellar stabilization after first-time patellar dislocation based on femoral-sided MPFL tear or significant medial tissue disruption, although systematic review supports nonoperative treatment of first-time patellar dislocation.[16,25]

TYPE II: RECURRENT PATELLAR INSTABILITY

Type II or recurrent patellar instability is the most common type of patellar instability seen in clinical practice, typically in female adolescents. After first-time dislocation, patients may continue to have pain, episodic feeling of their patella slipping out, locking, or other disabling symptoms suggestive of recurrent patellar subluxation (type IIA), or patients may have frank recurrent dislocations (type IIB).[15] Natural history studies of nonoperative treatment after first-time dislocation have shown 15% to 44% recurrent dislocation rates and up to 50% of patients could continue to have either subluxation or pain without frank dislocations.[11,16,26,27] Previous history of patellar instability, family history of patellar instability, and female gender have been associated with increased risk of re-dislocation.[28]

Patients with recurrent patellar subluxation (type IIA) typically have a positive apprehension sign. A structured rehabilitation program would be the first choice of treatment. A patellar stabilizing brace may be of benefit. Once conservative treatment is exhausted and for patients with recurrent patellar dislocation (type IIB), surgical intervention is recommended. Dysplastic features of patellofemoral joint and lower extremity, contributing to the development of patellofemoral instability, should be evaluated. These instabilities include patella alta, trochlear dysplasia, vastus medialis obliqus insufficiency, lateral patellar tilt and tight lateral structures, quadriceps malalignment or shortening, joint hyperlaxity, lower limb malalignment, and excessive lateralization of tibial tubercle.[5] Although some surgeons deem it necessary to address several or all risk factors during surgery for patellar stabilization, others perform an isolated MPFL reconstruction knowingly ignoring some or most of the risk factors. There is low-level evidence to support each treatment philosophy. For example, MPFL reconstruction and trochleoplasty are recommended in patients with patellar instability and trochlear dysplasia; however, isolated MPFL reconstruction has shown promising results even in the presence of trochlear dysplasia.[29,30] Similarly, some authors have recommended patellar distalization for patella alta, although isolated MPFL reconstruction has been shown to decrease patellar height at short-term follow-up.[31] It is possible that isolated MPFL reconstruction can compensate for lower degrees or lower number of risk factors, and it might fail beyond a certain threshold. Although attempts have been made to quantify such thresholds for each individual risk factor, a composite scoring system that would consider all established risk factors to help guide comprehensive management for patellar instability has not been validated.

TYPE III: DISLOCATABLE PATELLA

A dislocatable patella would have trochlear articulation to begin with, then would dislocate laterally with a maneuver, and then relocate itself in the trochlear groove once the dislocating force is discontinued. The maneuver required to dislocate the patella could be an apprehension sign maneuver, static position of the knee, or dynamic motion of the knee. Passive patellar dislocation (type IIIA) is when the patella can be dislocated either with an apprehension maneuver, that is, pushing the patella laterally, or by placing the knee in certain position. It is differentiated from habitual patellar dislocation (type IIIB) in that type A is episodic. It is seen in patients with significantly incompetent or lax medial structures, as seen in patients with joint hypermobility syndromes. It could also be seen in patients with hypotonia or poorly developed muscle restraints (eg, Down syndrome). A referral to a geneticist may help to diagnose an underlying syndrome, especially in patients with bilateral dislocatable patellae. Surgical treatment should be considered if the patient remains symptomatic after initial conservative treatment. The rotational and coronal plane alignment should be assessed because genu valgum or femoral anteversion may be contributing factors that may have to be considered during the surgical decision-making process. An MPFL reconstruction would help with patellar stabilization, although a stiffer graft (quadriceps tendon autograft or soft tissue allograft) may prevent stretching and failure over time in patients with hypermobility syndromes. A lateral retinacular release in the setting of hyperlaxity may lead to iatrogenic medial instability and should be avoided.[32]

Habitual dislocation of the patella (type IIIB) is defined as dislocation of patella with every cycle of flexion and extension motion of the knee. This pattern of instability is frequently seen in children, although, if ignored or asymptomatic during the first decade of life, they may present at a later age. A referral to the geneticist may help to diagnose any underlying syndrome. Habitual dislocation in flexion is more common than habitual dislocation in extension. Habitual dislocation of the patella is a function of knee motion and is involuntary. The other terms used in the literature to describe this entity are obligatory or mandatory dislocation of patella, which reiterates that the dislocation event is not under the patient's control.

Habitual dislocation in flexion means that the patella would dislocate spontaneously when the knee is flexed and reduce spontaneously when the knee is extended.[33,34] The degree of knee flexion when the patella would dislocate is inversely proportional to the severity of the condition, that is, in severe forms, the patella would dislocate in early flexion and would remain dislocated with further flexion. There is usually a tether between the patella and the lateral structures (vastus lateralis, iliotibial band, lateral retinaculum), and the quadriceps mechanism is shortened and externally rotated. The lateral tether with accompanied short quadriceps tendon and trochlear dysplasia will pull the patella laterally in order to allow the knee to flex. Once dislocated, the extensor mechanism functions as a knee flexor, and hence, it may be difficult or impossible for the patient to extend the knee actively once the patella is dislocated. If the patella is not allowed to dislocate laterally by manual force, then knee flexion would be restricted, because of the short extensor mechanism coursing the anterior aspect of knee. The rationale for early treatment (before the age of 10 years) for these conditions is that repositioning of the patella and the extensor mechanism can help remodel the trochlea and prevent worsening symptoms.[33] The mainstay of surgical treatment is the release of the lateral tether and a quadricepsplasty to de-rotate or lengthen the extensor mechanism. An MPFL reconstruction may or may not be required. Because a tibial tubercle osteotomy is contraindicated in skeletally immature patient, medial transposition of the lateral half of patellar tendon or similar patellar tendon distal realignment procedure may be required, if there is a significant lateral position of the tibial tubercle.[35]

Habitual dislocation in extension means that the patella would dislocate when the knee is extended and would relocate with knee flexion.[7] It is usually associated with patella alta or a short trochlea. As the patient attempts to extend the knee from a flexed position, the patella would dislocate laterally by jumping over a dysplastic lateral trochlea. The degree of knee flexion at which the patella would dislocate is directly proportional to the severity of the condition, that is, in severe forms, the patella would dislocate near full flexion and would remain dislocated as the knee moves from flexion to extension. The severity of the condition would also be based on underlying dysplasia, as milder forms may have normal trochlear morphology and would present as a positive J sign at near full knee extension. Isolated MPFL reconstruction usually cannot restore patellofemoral stability in such cases. Lateral retinacular lengthening or release, quadricepsplasty, or distal realignment may have to be combined with MPFL reconstruction to help restore stability.[36] Stabilization of the patella at an early age could allow the trochlea to remodel with growth.

TYPE IV: DISLOCATED PATELLA

A dislocated patella is defined as a permanent dislocation of the patella on the lateral side of the knee with no articulation with the trochlea. It could be reducible (type IVA) or irreducible (type IVB). Patellar dislocation could be present at birth (congenital patellar dislocation) or it may present during early childhood (developmental patellar dislocation). The literature is confusing because of the lack of a clear distinction and frequent overlapping between these 2 categories. Many developmental patellar dislocations in children have been inappropriately referred to as congenital patellar dislocations. True congenital patellar dislocation is rare and is due to intrauterine failure of the internal rotation of the lower limb leading to an irreducible dislocated patella with knee flexion contracture, external rotation of the lower limb, and genu valgum.[37] Some patients with congenital patellar dislocation may not be diagnosed at birth and present later in life. The diagnosis could be missed early on, because the patella is small and difficult to palpate. As the patella is unossified, radiographs are normal, and thus, an ultrasound or MRI can help with the diagnosis. In contrast, developmental dislocation of the patella is seen after walking age and is not accompanied by the typical limb deformities that are seen with congenital patellar dislocation. The patient is brought by the family because of frequent falls, gait abnormalities, developing deformity, and differential development of the limb in unilateral cases. Initially, the patella may be reducible, but with time becomes irreducible. Rarely, permanent dislocation can be posttraumatic. A femur fracture, knee dislocation, or missed traumatic patellar dislocation treated with cast immobilization can develop permanent dislocation.

Children with dislocated patella should be screened for genetic conditions or syndrome.[7] They should be offered surgical treatment at the time of diagnosis: the rationale being that earlier surgery would prevent further contractures and deformity and could potentially help remodel the trochlea.[32] Surgical treatment would include extended lateral release or lengthening, quadricepsplasty, patellar tendon transposition, medial-sided reconstruction, or a combination of these procedures. Quadricepsplasty is the key to the success of surgery because the extensor mechanism has to be de-rotated to counter its external rotation and flexion force and may have to be lengthened. Several types of quadricepsplasty have been described in the literature, including Thompson, Judet, Stanisavljevic, and V-Y quadricepsplasty.[38–40] After relocation of the patella, a large lateral defect would be left in the area where the patella was dislocated. This defect can be left alone or can be closed with lengthened lateral retinaculum, fascia lata, acellular dermis or similar synthetic, or allograft patch.

Besides the previously described instability patterns, voluntary instability and syndromic patellar instability merit separate discussion because of their unique characteristics and considerations.

VOLUNTARY PATELLAR INSTABILITY

Rarely, patients can voluntarily sublux or dislocate their patella by selective contraction of parts of quadriceps muscles. It has been observed in female adolescents and may present with anterior knee pain. They can demonstrate the voluntary instability without significant pain or anxiety. They flex their knees to tighten the quadriceps muscle and then can dislocate the patella by selective contraction of the vastus lateralis muscle. It could be unilateral or bilateral. The apprehension sign is typically negative. Voluntary patellar instability is different from habitual dislocation of patella, wherein the dislocation is involuntary and is a function of knee motion. Voluntary patellar instability is somewhat similar to voluntary posterior dislocation of the shoulder. Treatment is mainly nonoperative and includes observation, physical therapy, and reassurance.

SYNDROMIC PATELLAR INSTABILITY

Syndromic patellar instability encompasses patients with neuromuscular disorders (eg, cerebral palsy), connective tissue disorder (eg, Ehlers-Danlos syndrome), or other syndromes (eg, nail-patella syndrome).[41] It is important to recognize that patellar instability may be the first presenting symptom in a patient with syndromic patellar instability. Depending on each patient, the role of the orthopedic surgeon would be to make appropriate referrals, like referral to geneticist for syndrome identification or referral to other subspecialists for cardiac, ophthalmic, or urology screening. These patients can present with any type of patellar instability (type I to IV), although most patients have complex (type III and IV) instability patterns. Female adolescents with joint hypermobility disorders like Ehlers-Danlos syndrome may present with first-time (type I) or recurrent (type II) patellar dislocation, and if not recognized, may pose a challenge to management of their patellar instability due to higher rates of failure of surgery, pain management issues, and medical comorbidities. Similarly, patients with Down syndrome or Ellis-van Creveld syndrome may have genu valgum along with patellar instability, which might have to be addressed to correct the underlying deformity.[42] Other well-known syndromes that have patellar instability as one of their features include nail-patella syndrome, Rubenstein-Taybi syndrome, Kabuki syndrome, and absent/small patella syndromes.[7]

SUMMARY

Several types of patellar instability patterns have been recognized. Type I and II are more common, seen in adolescent or young adult patients, and frequently treated by an adult orthopedic surgeon. Type III and IV are less common, typically seen in children, and frequently treated by a pediatric orthopedic surgeon. However, there may be overlap, and it is imperative for an orthopedic surgeon to be familiar with all types of patellar instability patterns because surgical treatment is more complex with type III and IV instability. Although MPFL reconstruction has gained increasing popularity in the last 2 decades, it alone would not suffice for all instability patterns. The surgeon needs to be familiar with a wide range of surgical treatment options to individualize the treatment to each patient.

REFERENCES

1. Nietosvaara Y, Aalto K, Kallio PE. Acute patellar dislocation in children: incidence and associated osteochondral fractures. J Pediatr Orthop 1994;14: 513–5.
2. Atkin DM, Fithian DC, Maranji KS, et al. Characteristics of patients with primary acute lateral patellar dislocation and their recovery within the first six months of injury. Am J Sports Med 2000;4:472–9.
3. Ellera Gomes JL. Medial patellofemoral ligament reconstruction for recurrent dislocation of the patella: a preliminary report. Arthroscopy 1992;8:335–40.
4. Tardieu C, Glard Y, Garron E, et al. Relationship between formation of the femoral bicondylar angle and trochlear shape: independence of diaphyseal and epiphyseal growth. Am J Phys Anthropol 2006;130: 491–500.
5. Dejour H, Walch G, Nove-Josserand L, et al. Factors of patellar instability: an anatomic radiographic study. Knee Surg Sports Traumatol Arthrosc 1994; 2:19–26.
6. Garin C, Chaker M, Dohin B, et al. Permanent, habitual dislocation and recurrent dislocation of the patella in children: surgical management by patellar ligamentous transfer in 50 knees. Rev Chir Orthop 2007;93:690–700.
7. Chotel F, Bérard J, Raux S. Patellar instability in children and adolescents. Orthop Traumatol Surg Res 2014;100(1 Suppl):S125–37.
8. Sillanpaa P. Terminology of patellar dislocation. In: Sillanpaa P, editor. Traumatic patellar dislocation. Saarbrucken (Germany): Lambert Academic Publishing; 2010. p. 16–8.
9. Hiemstra LA, Kerslake S, Lafave M, et al. Introduction of a classification system for patients with patellofemoral instability (WARPS and STAID). Knee Surg Sports Traumatol Arthrosc 2014;22:2776–82.
10. Grelsamer RP. Patellar nomenclature: the Tower of Babel revisited. Clin Orthop Relat Res 2005;436: 60–5.
11. Arendt EA, Fithian DC, Cohen E. Current concepts of lateral patella dislocation. Clin Sports Med 2002; 21:499–519.
12. Halbrecht JL. Mild patellar instability: arthroscopic reconstruction. In: Fulkerson JP, editor. Common patellofemoral problems. Rosemont (IL): American Academy of Orthopaedic Surgeons; 2005. p. 29.
13. Ji G, Wang F, Zhang Y, et al. Medial patella retinaculum plasty for treatment of habitual patellar dislocation in adolescents. Int Orthop 2012;36:1819–25.
14. Batra S. Recurrent dislocation is different from habitual dislocation of patella. Int Orthop 2014;38:2223.
15. Hughston JC. Subluxation of the patella. J Bone Joint Surg Am 1968;50:1003–26.
16. Stefancin JJ, Parker RD. First-time traumatic patellar dislocation: a systematic review. Clin Orthop Relat Res 2007;455:93–101.
17. Abbasi D, May MM, Wall EJ, et al. MRI findings in adolescent patients with acute traumatic knee hemarthrosis. J Pediatr Orthop 2012;32:760–4.
18. Sillanpää PJ, Salonen E, Pihlajamäki H, et al. Medial patellofemoral ligament avulsion injury at the patella: classification and clinical outcome. Knee Surg Sports Traumatol Arthrosc 2014;22:2414–8.
19. Apostolovic M, Vukomanovic B, Slavkovic N, et al. Acute patellar dislocation in adolescents: operative

versus nonoperative treatment. Int Orthop 2011;35: 1483–7.

20. Palmu S, Kallio PE, Donell ST, et al. Acute patellar dislocation in children and adolescents: a randomized clinical trial. J Bone Joint Surg Am 2008;90: 463–70.

21. Christiansen SE, Jakobsen BW, Lund B, et al. Isolated repair of the medial patellofemoral ligament in primary dislocation of the patella: a prospective randomized study. Arthroscopy 2008;24:881–7.

22. Nikku R, Nietosvaara Y, Kallio PE, et al. Operative versus closed treatment of primary dislocation of the patella. Similar 2-year results in 125 randomized patients. Acta Orthop Scand 1997;68:419–23.

23. Sillanpää PJ, Mäenpää HM, Mattila VM, et al. Arthroscopic surgery for primary traumatic patellar dislocation: a prospective, nonrandomized study comparing patients treated with and without acute arthroscopic stabilization with a median 7-year follow-up. Am J Sports Med 2008;36:2301–9.

24. Bitar AC, Demange MK, D'Elia CO, et al. Traumatic patellar dislocation: nonoperative treatment compared with MPFL reconstruction using patellar tendon. Am J Sports Med 2012;40:114–22.

25. Sillanpää PJ, Peltola E, Mattila VM, et al. Femoral avulsion of the medial patellofemoral ligament after primary traumatic patellar dislocation predicts subsequent instability in men: a mean 7-year nonoperative follow-up study. Am J Sports Med 2009;37: 1513–21.

26. Hawkins RJ, Bell RH, Anisette G. Acute patellar dislocations: the natural history. Am J Sports Med 1986; 14:117–20.

27. Cofield RH, Bryan RS. Acute dislocation of the patella: results of conservative treatment. J Trauma 1977;17:526–31.

28. Fithian DC, Paxton EW, Stone ML, et al. Epidemiology and natural history of acute patellar dislocation. Am J Sports Med 2004;32:1114–21.

29. Steiner TM, Torga-Spak R, Teitge RA. Medial patellofemoral ligament reconstruction in patients with lateral patellar instability and trochlear dysplasia. Am J Sports Med 2006;34:1254–61.

30. Bollier M, Fulkerson JP. The role of trochlear dysplasia in patellofemoral instability. J Am Acad Orthop Surg 2011;19:8–16.

31. Lykissas MG, Li T, Eismann EA, et al. Does medial patellofemoral ligament reconstruction decrease patellar height? A preliminary report. J Pediatr Orthop 2014;34:78–85.

32. Hughston JC, Deese M. Medial subluxation of the patella as a complication of lateral retinacular release. Am J Sports Med 1988;16:383–8.

33. Benoit B, Laflamme GY, Laflamme GH, et al. Long-term outcome of surgically-treated habitual patellar dislocation in children with coexistent patella alta. Minimum follow-up of 11 years. J Bone Joint Surg Br 2007;89:1172–7.

34. Bergman NR, Williams PF. Habitual dislocation of the patella in flexion. J Bone Joint Surg Br 1988;70:415–9.

35. Goldthwait JE. Slipping or recurrent dislocation of the patella. With the report of eleven cases. Boston Med Surg J 1904;150:169–74.

36. Lattermann C, Toth J, Bach BR Jr. The role of lateral retinacular release in the treatment of patellar instability. Sports Med Arthrosc 2007;15:57–60.

37. Ghanem I, Wattincourt L, Seringe R. Congenital dislocation of the patella. Part I: pathologic anatomy. J Pediatr Orthop 2000;20:812–6.

38. Thompson TC. Quadricepsplasty. Ann Surg 1945; 121:751–4.

39. Daoud H, O'Farrell T, Cruess RL. Quadricepsplasty. The Judet technique and results of six cases. J Bone Joint Surg Br 1982;64:194–7.

40. Stanisavljevic S, Zemenick G, Miller D. Congenital, irreducible, permanent lateral dislocation of the patella. Clin Orthop Relat Res 1976;(116):190–9.

41. Bongers EM, van Kampen A, van Bokhoven H, et al. Human syndromes with congenital patellar anomalies and the underlying gene defects. Clin Genet 2005;68:302–19.

42. Dugdale TW, Renshaw TS. Instability of the patellofemoral joint in Down syndrome. J Bone Joint Surg Am 1986;68:405–13.

Congenital Anomalies of the Hand—Principles of Management

Kevin J. Little, MD*, Roger Cornwall, MD

KEYWORDS

- Congenital hand • Syndactyly • Polydactyly • Thumb hypoplasia • Opponensplasty • Pollicization

KEY POINTS

- Although congenital hand anomalies are relatively rare, pediatric orthopedic surgeons and hand surgeons will frequently see them during the course of clinical practice.
- The clinician should be aware of the associated malformations and conditions that may, in some cases, be fatal if not recognized and treated appropriately.
- The goals of surgery are to improve hand function and cosmesis while limiting complications that could impair function long term.
- The surgeon must balance functional, cosmetic, and cultural goals and align those goals with the proper surgical techniques in order to maximize patient and parent satisfaction following surgical intervention.
- This article discusses syndactyly, preaxial polydactyly and postaxial polydactyly, and the hypoplastic thumb.

INTRODUCTION

Congenital anomalies of the upper extremity, although less common than congenital heart disease, are noted in approximately 2 per 1000 live births.[1,2] This incidence varies by country due to higher incidence of certain malformations in patients of certain ethnic backgrounds, such as polydactyly in those of African descent or amniotic bands in Japanese. Although many of these malformations lead to minor functional deficits, they can pose a concern for the parents and lead to psychological distress in children.[3] In addition, the 1-year mortality of patients with hand malformations is 14% to 16% due to associated malformations, often involving the heart, kidneys, or tracheoesophageal complex.[4] Boys are affected more commonly than girls by a 3:2 ratio, and mothers older than 40 years of age are twice as likely to have children with congenital hand differences as those only 10 years younger.[5,6]

Malformations of the hand and forearm were classified by Swanson[7] in 1964 and adopted by the International Federation of Societies for Surgery of the Hand (**Table 1**). Although this classification has its use, it is generally hard to use in clinical instances, because patients may be classified into several categories at once, and it does not guide treatment or prognosis. Oberg and colleagues[8] proposed a modified classification based on a more recent understanding of the embryology of congenital hand malformations. Using this classification, malformations are divided into malformations, deformations, and dysplasias, and then further subdivided (**Table 2**).

Division of Pediatric Orthopaedics, Department of Orthopaedic Surgery, Cincinnati Children's Hospital Medical Center, University of Cincinnati School of Medicine, 3333 Burnet Avenue, ML 2017, Cincinnati, OH 45229, USA
* Corresponding author.
E-mail address: kevin.little@cchmc.org

Orthop Clin N Am 47 (2016) 153–168
http://dx.doi.org/10.1016/j.ocl.2015.08.015
0030-5898/16/$ – see front matter © 2016 Elsevier Inc. All rights reserved.

Table 1
Swanson classification system for congenital hand differences

Type I	Failure of formation
	 • Transverse deficiency
	 • Longitudinal deficiency
	   ○ Preaxial: Hypoplasia of thumb and/or radius
	   ○ Central: Typical and atypical cleft hand
	   ○ Postaxial: Hypoplasia of ulna and/or hypothenar hand

Type II	Failure of differentiation • Soft tissue (syndactyly, Poland syndrome, camptodactyly) • Skeletal (synostosis, carpal coalition, complex syndactyly)
Type III	Duplication (polydactyly, mirror hand)
Type IV	Overgrowth (macrodactyly)
Type V	Undergrowth (radial hypoplasia, symbrachydactyly, brachydactyly)
Type VI	Congenital constriction ring syndrome (amniotic band syndrome)
Type VII	Generalized skeletal abnormalities

From Swanson AB. A classification for congenital malformations of the hand. N J Bull Acad Med 1964;10:166.

Embryology

Fetal limb development is initiated with the appearance of a limb bud, consisting of undifferentiated mesenchyme, at the lateral body wall 26 to 28 days after fertilization. Subsequently, the limb develops rapidly in a proximal-to-distal direction over the next 4 weeks. Complex interactions between signaling centers orchestrate this embryonic differentiation.[9–12] The first axis to form in the limb bud is the preaxial-postaxial (radial-ulnar) axis, which is defined by the zone of polarization activity. The next axis to form is the dorsal-volar axis defined by the apical ectodermal ridge (AER). Finally, the AER defines the limb proximal-distal axis and controls interdigital cellular apoptosis. Signaling pathways critical to limb formation include sonic hedgehog (Shh), wingless-type, and fibroblast growth factors. Ectopic Shh expression is a known source of polydactyly because of its role in digit number and identity.[9–17]

INDICATIONS/CONTRAINDICATIONS

For all congenital hand malformations, the primary surgical indication is to improve hand function and cosmesis. Contraindications include patients with surgical reconstruction that interferes with function, such as for a centralization procedure in a patient with poor elbow function or with a primary

Table 2
Oberg classification system for congenital hand differences

I: Malformations	A. Abnormal axis formation/differentiation: entire upper limb
	   i. Proximal-distal axis
	   ii. Radial-ulnar (anterior-posterior) axis
	   iii. Dorsal-ventral axis
	   iv. Unspecified axis
	 B. Abnormal axis formation/differentiation: Hand plate
	   i. Proximal-distal axis
	   ii. Radial-ulnar (anterior-posterior) axis
	   iii. Dorsal-ventral axis

II: Deformations	Constriction ring syndromes, trigger digits

III: Dysplasia	A. Hypertrophy
	   i. Whole limb
	   ii. Partial limb
	 B. Tumorous conditions
	   i. Vascular
	   ii. Neurologic
	   iii. Connective tissue
	   iv. Skeletal

IV: Syndromes	A. Specified B. Others

From Oberg KC, Feenstra JM, Manske PR, et al. Developmental biology and classification of congenital anomalies of the hand and upper extremity. J Hand Surg Am 2010;35(12):2073; with permission.

postaxial pinch. Relative contraindications include separating functionless or stiff digits, whereby reconstruction will only improve cosmesis and not alter function, or adult patients who function well with minor cosmetic deformity. In addition, the cultural aspects of congenital hand malformations should be considered before surgery is performed, because a malformation considered intolerable in one culture may be tolerable or even desirable in another.[18]

SYNDACTYLY

Syndactyly is a narrowed or fused web space between adjacent fingers. Syndactyly occurs in approximately 2 to 3 patients per 10,000 live births, affecting male patients more commonly than female patients.[19,20] Unilateral presentation is equally as common as bilateral presentation.[21] Heritable forms of syndactyly are transmitted in an autosomal-dominant pattern with variable penetrance and are often associated with syndactyly between the second and third toes.[19–21] Syndactyly is often classified by the length of the web, where complete syndactyly extends to the tips of the fingers; incomplete syndactyly does not include the fingertips. In addition, complex syndactyly describes bony fusions, which are typically identified with a single nail plate (synonychia), while simple syndactyly describes only soft tissue connections. Formal classification of syndactyly was originally proposed by Temtamy and McKusick,[22] breaking it down into 5 distinct subtypes based on phenotype and the underlying genetic abnormalities. This classification has been expanded many times and now includes 9 types and numerous subtypes.[23]

Syndactyly can be associated with other skeletal manifestations, including cleft hand, symbrachydactyly, and synpolydactyly, where extra digits are syndactylized in the central digits. Syndactyly is also associated with other genetic syndromes, including acrocephalosyndactyly (Apert, Pfeiffer, and Crouzon syndrome), characterized by craniosynostosis, midface hypoplasia, and complex syndactyly that can involve all 5 digits, as well as acrocephalopolysyndactyly (Noack and Carpenter syndrome), manifested by craniosynostosis, syndactyly, and preaxial polydactyly. Fourth web space syndactyly, between the ring and small fingers, is commonly associated with oculodentodigital dysplasia, where patients can have optic nerve hypoplasia, small teeth with numerous caries, and a narrow midface. Amniotic band syndrome or amniotic disruption sequence is often associated with multiple constriction bands, digital amputations, and acrosyndactyly, with digital fusion at the fingertips along with a variably patent web space proximally (**Fig. 1**).

Surgical Procedure

The treatment of syndactyly requires good preoperative planning and a thorough discussion of the risks and benefits with the family. Syndactyly release should be performed at 3 to 6 months of age only in patients with mismatched finger size where growth is leading to deviation of the fingers. Otherwise, it can be delayed until 1 to 2 years of age. Adjacent web spaces should not be released in the same setting to avoid vascular compromise. A simple, longitudinal separation creates significant scar tissue, which can impede growth and create deformity and joint contractures. Thus zigzag flaps have been advocated to break up longitudinal scar lines. The commissure should be created with supple dorsal skin flaps, and grafts should be avoided in this area to limit scarring and web creep. Furthermore, thumb-index syndactyly separation is more complicated than finger syndactyly and should be treated with a 2 or 4 flap z-plasty for mild narrowing, or with a dorsal rotational advancement flap for isolated complete syndactyly[24] (**Fig. 2**). It is essential to remember that the decision-making process needs to include input from families as well as the health care team (physician, therapist, and so on), and it often can be dominated by the families' perspective of the condition.

- A nonsterile brachial tourniquet inflated to no more than 100 mm Hg greater than systolic pressure and the use of a hand table and loupe magnification is recommended.

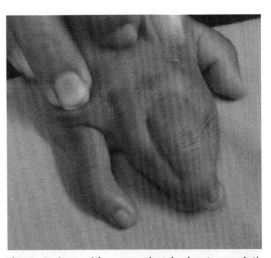

Fig. 1. Patient with acrosyndactyly due to amniotic band syndrome. Note the distal syndactyly with apparent digital separation proximally.

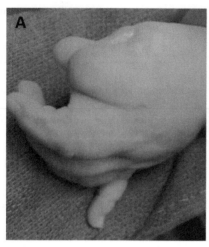
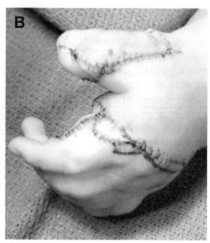

Fig. 2. (*A*) Patient with thumb-index syndactyly. (*B*) Same patient treated with a dorsal advancement flap.

- A dorsal rectangular or hourglass commissure flap is marked out two-thirds of the length of the proximal phalanx, the width equal to the center of each adjacent metacarpophalangeal joint (MCP) joint (**Fig. 3**).
- Zigzag flaps are marked out between the midsagittal axis of each digit dorsally and volarly such that the apex of each dorsal flap will interdigitate with the axilla of each volar flap and vice versa (**Fig. 4**).
- For complete syndactyly, double opposing fingertip skin flaps are created for the lateral nail folds via the Buck-Gramcko technique (**Fig. 5**).
- The distal bone connection is transected, and the neurovascular bundle is dissected proximally to its bifurcation. If a distal bifurcation of the artery is present, place a microvascular clamp on the artery branch to be ligated and

deflate the tourniquet to ensure immediate reperfusion to that digit.
- Distal nerve bifurcation can be addressed with intrafascicular dissection of the nerve branches until sufficiently proximal separation is achieved.
- The commissure flap is inset first, using a fast-absorbable 5-0 or 6-0 suture followed by closure of triangular flaps without tension.
- Areas that cannot be closed, typically along the lateral commissure, should be covered by defatted, full-thickness skin graft. The tourniquet should be deflated before placing dressings to ensure quick reperfusion to the digit.

Postoperative Care

Patients are typically discharged the day of surgery and return in 3 weeks for cast and dressing removal. The wounds are inspected for signs of infection, flap necrosis, or excessive scarring. Patients are encouraged to begin active range of motion (ROM) after cast removal and begin scar and web space massage once wounds have healed. The use of a silicone scar pad has been advocated to improve scar suppleness and appearance. Occupational therapy can be used to help with scar appearance, to help with ROM exercises in young patients, and to alleviate minor postoperative scar contracture.

Complications and Management

The most common immediate complication is vascular compromise to one of the digits. The best management is prevention, including avoiding operating on both sides of the digit in the same setting, and careful choice of digital

Fig. 3. Patient with syndactyly showing a standard rectangular dorsal flap.

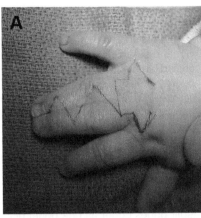
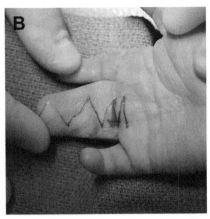

Fig. 4. Patient with syndactyly demonstrating the (*A*) dorsal and (*B*) volar alternating triangular flaps.

artery ligation for distal bifurcation. In cases of a white finger after skin closure, warm the finger with warm saline gauze and reassess after 5 to 10 minutes. If reperfusion is delayed, inspect the fingers for tight flaps and release tight sutures as needed. It is always better to add skin grafts to an open wound than to have too much tension on a skin flap. Infection can be seen, especially with loss of skin flaps or grafts, and should be treated appropriately with antibiotics and skin grafts should be repeated as needed. The most common late complication is web creep due to scar contracture at the commissure (**Fig. 6**). Occasionally this necessitates revision surgery. In addition, bony deformity and nail abnormalities are more common following complex syndactyly release and can be treated with digital osteotomy or lateral nail fold reconstruction.

Outcomes

There are more than 40 different descriptions of flaps used to release digital syndactyly, and most have reported good outcomes in the most patients. Barabás and Pickford[25] recently reported on 144 patients with an average of 5 years of follow-up following syndactyly release via a traditional Flatt technique. They reported 7 cases of graft failure and a 4.2% rate of web creep requiring revision surgery, although they noted that most of the cases with graft failure did not result in significant web creep. Vekris and colleagues[26] reported on the follow-up of 131 patients with an average of 11.5 years of follow-up. They noted worse results in complex syndactyly, in adjacent digits of dissimilar length, in cases of delayed presentation, and with the use of dorsal and palmar triangular flaps rather than a large

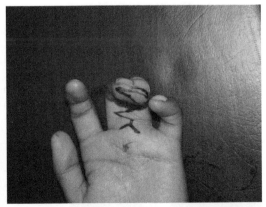

Fig. 5. Patient with syndactyly demonstrating the Buck-Gramcko Flaps used to restore the lateral nail folds.

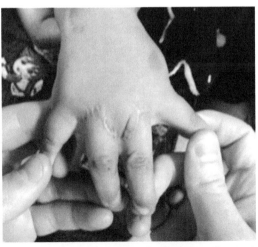

Fig. 6. Patient with syndactyly demonstrating web creep 2 years following syndactyly release.

dorsal rectangular flap. In addition, Lumenta and colleagues[27] reported on 26 patients with average 11.5-year follow-up and noted 7.7% web creep with an additional 42% showing signs of web thickening without creep. An additional 7.7% demonstrated loss of the lateral nail fold without nail abnormality, and 70% demonstrated hair growth from the groin full-thickness skin graft. Short-term follow-up studies are available for several graftless syndactyly releases with similar results in terms of web creep and revision surgery,[28–30] but long-term results greater than 5 years have not yet been published.

POLYDACTYLY

Polydactyly is categorized into preaxial (radial), central, and postaxial (ulnar) types. In addition, rare variants, including ulnar dimelia and mirror hand, may allow for up to 9-digit duplication. Preaxial polydactyly incidence varies greatly and is most commonly reported as 1 per 3000 live births.[31–34] Overall, preaxial polydactyly affects male patients more commonly than female patients, and whites are more commonly affected than blacks. Postaxial polydactyly has a racial predilection that is opposite from preaxial polydactyly, affecting blacks more commonly than whites at a ratio of 10:1. Overall, the incidence in blacks is estimated to be as high as 1 in 300 live births, whereas whites are estimated to be affected every 1 in 3000 live births.[31–34] With further subclassification of postaxial polydactyly, this racial disparity has been isolated to type B postaxial polydactyly, or the rudimentary digit. Postaxial type A has been reported to have similar racial characteristics.[35] However, Watson and Hennrikus[36] reported an incidence of postaxial polydactyly type B as high

as 1 in 143 black infants and 1 in 1334 white infants.

Preaxial and postaxial polydactyly possess individual classification systems aimed to provide a unified language between surgeons. Preaxial polydactyly is described using the Wassel-Flatt classification, which defines the anatomic level of duplication from distal to proximal.[37] The Wassel-Flatt classification consists of 7 categories and uses even numbers to represent complete duplications and odd numbers to represent incomplete duplications. An easy way to remember this classification is to start at the most distal normal bone and count the number of separate bones (split bones count as one bone) distal to that. An exception is the final category, type VII, which is the triphalangeal thumb[9] (**Fig. 7**).

Another difficulty with preaxial polydactyly nomenclature is that neither of the duplicated thumbs is normal. A better term for this condition would be a split thumb, implying that a normal thumb was split into 2 or more parts, where the polydactylous digits are typically asymmetrically split. This nomenclature has more implications for treatment, suggesting that treatment to restore normal anatomy is not possible, because normal anatomy does not exist in either duplicated digit.

Temtamy and McKusik[33] classified postaxial polydactyl into a simple 2-part scheme of phenotypic expression. Type A postaxial polydactyly (**Fig. 8**) is defined as a fully developed extra digit, whereas type B is a rudimentary digit. In whites, the occurrence of type A and type B are equivalent; however, in blacks, type B is more common.[31]

Despite several classification systems in the current literature, many surgeons prefer to use a focused descriptive approach to the duplicated

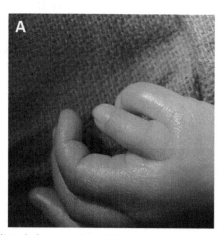
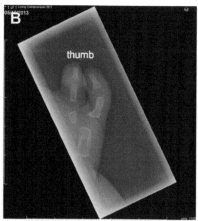

Fig. 7. (*A*) Clinical photograph and (*B*) posteroanterior radiograph of a patient with a triphalangeal thumb duplication (Wassel-Flatt VII).

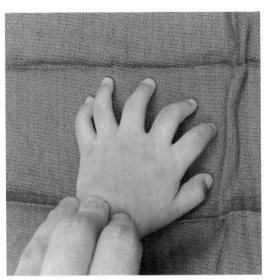

Fig. 8. Patient with a well-developed postaxial polydactyly (type A).

digits instead of using the aforementioned systems. Surgeons describe the duplicated digit anatomically (location, size, degree of individual component development) and functionally (mobility, stability), which is often thought to be a stronger basis for surgical planning.

Preaxial polydactyly is most often due to sporadic mutations resulting in a unilateral presentation of the malformation.[33] However, an exception exists, because triphalangeal thumb duplications are often inherited in an autosomal-dominant pattern.[38] Triphalangeal thumb duplication is associated with Blackfan-Diamond anemia, Holt-Oram syndrome, Bloom syndrome, Carpenter syndrome, and Ullrich-Feichtiger syndrome and should prompt a referral to a geneticist.[31,39] Postaxial polydactyly is also inherited in an autosomal-dominant pattern with variable penetrance particularly in blacks. When postaxial polydactyly is present in whites, it can be associated with Trisomy 13, Ellis-van Creveld syndrome, Laurence-Moon-Bardet-Biedle syndrome, and Meckel syndrome, which can manifest with cardiac and renal malformations. Therefore, these children may require a referral to a geneticist for an echocardiogram or renal ultrasound. In general, polydactyly of the hand is more commonly associated with other musculoskeletal abnormalities (ie, polydactyly of toes) than with other organ system abnormalities.[12,33–36]

Surgical Procedure

Surgical treatment of polydactyly is inherently complex. Careful consideration of the anatomic

level of duplication, musculoskeletal components involved, stability, balanced motor function, developmental stage (pinch grasp in children), and cosmetic outcomes all must be incorporated into the surgical plan of care. Patients with duplications at the joint level will require joint narrowing and collateral ligament preservation, whereas duplications at the bony level often result in deformity that needs to be addressed with osteotomy. The goal is to produce a digit that is aligned along the mechanical axis with a central pull of the extensor and flexor tendons.

Preoperative Planning

- Preaxial polydactyly patients should be assessed to determine which thumb is better suited for reconstruction. Typically, the ulnar thumb is more functional and less angulated, resulting in the need for ablation of the radial thumb (**Fig. 9**).
- Postaxial type B digits with narrow stalks can be ligated at birth or treated with simple amputation at the bedside under local anesthesia with pressure hemostasis; however, this may result in neuroma formation and persistent scarring.
- Alternatively, many surgeons recommend that postaxial type B digits be treated with elliptical excision, proximal amputation of the neurovascular bundle, and primary closure.

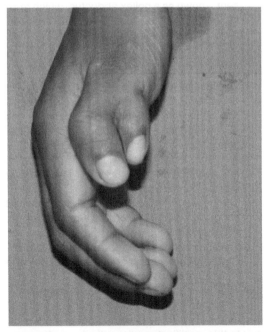

Fig. 9. Patient demonstrating that the radial thumb duplication is less developed and less functional than the ulnar thumb.

- In patients with preaxial and type A postaxial polydactyly, preoperative radiographs should be assessed before reconstruction to identify bone and joint duplication level in order to decide on the best treatment strategy.

Surgical Procedure: Preaxial Polydactyly Reconstruction

- In the case of symmetric components, the ulnar thumb is typically preserved to maintain the ulnar collateral ligament for pinch, unless the Bilhaut-Cloquet procedure is performed (see later discussion).
- A large, radial-sided flap with zigzag incisions is drawn along the radial thumb that will be ablated. This flap should be drawn larger than expected, and can be trimmed later if not needed.
- Care is taken to preserve the radial collateral ligament attachment to a small piece of articular cartilage at the base of the proximal phalanx. This piece of articular cartilage is sutured or pinned to the proximal phalanx base of ulnar thumb to reconstruct the deficient collateral ligament.
- Further extra-articular malalignment requires corrective osteotomy, with either a closing- or an opening-wedge osteotomy parallel to the joint surface, and stabilization with a K-wire.
- In some cases, an anomalous connection between the flexor and extensor tendons is present, known as a pollex abductus, which must be released before centralizing the terminal flexor and extensor tendons (**Fig. 10**).

Surgical Procedure: Bilhaut-Cloquet Procedure

- The Bilhaut-Cloquet procedure, which was designed to decrease thumb size mismatch, can be performed for Wassel types I, II, and III, when there is minimal size mismatch between the 2 thumbs (**Fig. 11**).
- A central wedge of tissue including pulp tissue, nail bed, and distal phalanx up to the articular surface of the distal phalanx is excised.
- The round convex surface of the nail bed should be reapproximated via rotation of the separated distal phalanges.
- The nail bed is reapproximated with 6-0 absorbable suture, and the skin is closed with 5-0 absorbable suture.
- Alternatively, Baek and colleagues[40,41] described an extra-articular and extraphyseal modification to the Bilhaut-Cloquet procedure.
- In this modification, the articular surface and physis of the ulnar thumb is kept intact, while the distal, radial aspect of the distal phalanx is

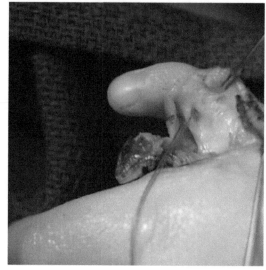

Fig. 10. Patient with preaxial polydactyly demonstrating (via suture) an anomalous connection between the extensor and flexor pollicis longus tendons.

divided and combined with the distal, ulnar aspect of the radial thumb.
- In addition, the radial collateral ligament of the interphalangeal (IP) joint is kept with the radial thumb distal phalanx piece to provide thumb stability.

Surgical Procedure: Postaxial Polydactyly Reconstruction Type A

- Well-developed, postaxial, supranumerary digits require excision of the hypoplastic digit and reconstruction of a single, stable,

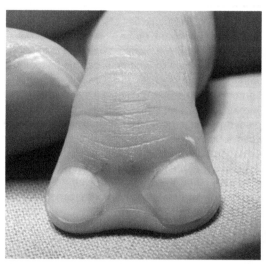

Fig. 11. Patient with Wassel-Flatt type I polydactyly with near symmetric bifurcation of the distal phalanx.

functional digit, abiding by similar principles as in preaxial digit reconstruction.

- A large, ulnar-sided flap with zigzag incisions is drawn along the supranumerary ulnar digit; this should be drawn larger than expected and can be trimmed later.
- The ulnar collateral ligament to the excised digit is spared, and the articular surface of the metacarpal may need to be trimmed similar to treatment of a duplicated thumb (see earlier discussion).
- In cases of coronal plane deformity, corrective osteotomy should be performed via opening- or closing-wedge osteotomy and stabilized with a K-wire.

Complications and Management

Suture ligation for type B polydactyly can be associated with complications, such as bleeding, scarring, skin cracking, residual growth (**Fig. 12**), neuroma, infection, and incomplete excision.[35,42] Rayan and Frey[43] sutured ligated digits on 105 infants and found that the most significant complication was unacceptable cosmetic result/tender digit occurring in 16% of patients, whereas bleeding was reported to occur in 1% and infection in 6% of patients. Several authors have reported small series of patients treated with excision of the stalk or revision surgery following previous suture ligation with overall good outcomes.[44–46]

The most common complication following type A reconstruction is a zigzag deformity, which

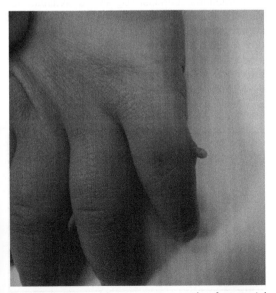

Fig. 12. Patient with recurrent growth of postaxial polydactyly type B after suture ligation in the newborn nursery.

results from residual deformity or imbalanced growth of the thumb. Prevention of this deformity is difficult in some cases with significant preoperative deformity, but is best ameliorated via strict adherence to the above-mentioned reconstruction principles including the creating of parallel joint surfaces, centralizing the pull of all tendons, and limiting longitudinal scar formation. The Bilhaut-Cloquet procedure is complicated by joint stiffness, growth arrest, asymmetric growth, and longitudinal nail-bed deformities.[47] Using the Baek modification, joint stiffness and growth arrest can be limited by staying extraphyseal and extra-articular with the osteotomy, although nail-bed abnormalities are still possible, but were not noted in their series.[40,41]

Postoperative Care

In patients without corrective osteotomy or joint realignment, dressings are maintained for 10 to 14 days and then removed to allow for ROM exercises. Patients who undergo ligament reconstruction or corrective osteotomy with temporary pin fixation will benefit from cast or splint treatment to allow for full healing. After 4 weeks, if bony union is achieved, ROM exercises are begun under the supervision of an occupational therapist. Patients should be monitored yearly to biannually until skeletal maturity to evaluate for worsening deformity.

Outcomes

Watson and Hennrikus[35] performed suture ligation on 21 infants with type B postaxial polydactyly. They reported no complications in regard to infection or bleeding; however, one child required operative intervention to remove a digit that failed to auto-amputate. Forty-three percent had a noticeable bump from 1 to 6 mm in size. Katz and Linder[44] performed excision of 15 type B digits using topical anesthetic, scalpel excision at base of the stalk, and subsequent pressure to control bleeding. Good cosmetic appearance was reported in all patients with no complications noted at follow-up. Leber and Gosain[46] performed 12 primary elliptical excisions of supernumerary digits without residual deformity and re-excision of 5 traumatic amputation neuromas resultant from treatment in the nursery. Mullick and Borschel[48] presented 13 hands that underwent previous string ligation, producing either an unsightly incomplete amputation or a tender neuroma, or both. In the series, patients were all successfully treated with completion amputation of the residual stump combined with proximal ligation of the supernumerary digital nerves.

In patients with type A polydactyly, the decision to perform surgery is the first priority. If ablation and reconstruction are indicated or requested, care must be taken to maintain joint stability and motion of the remaining small finger. Complications are relatively low when treated surgically, Rayan and Frey[43] reported 1 complication (infection) in 27 patients treated surgically for type A postaxial polydactyly.

Lee and colleagues[49] reviewed 139 cases of Wassel type IV duplications and found 44 cases of postsurgical Z deformity, defined as joint angulation greater than 20° at MCP and IP. Yen and colleagues[45] reported joint instability in 25 of 36 and joint deformity in 10 of 36 surgically treated thumbs. Stutz and colleagues[50] evaluated 41 patients with 43 surgically reconstructed thumbs at greater than 10 years (mean 17 years) and noted that 10 revision surgeries were required, most commonly for IP joint deformity and pain. The rate of revision surgery increased over time, indicating that long-term follow-up is recommended for patients with these deformities.

There are few isolated reports of outcomes for the Bilhaut-Cloquet procedure, often intermixed with other techniques for thumb polydactyly reconstruction. Most demonstrate good results, and outcomes scores are equivalent among most groups.[45,47,51] In a small sample size of 7 patients, Baek and colleagues[40] demonstrated satisfactory functional and cosmetic results with preserved preoperative ROM in type III, improved ROM in type II thumbs, and no cases of nail deformities or growth arrest.

THUMB HYPOPLASIA

Hypoplasia of the thumb occurs within a spectrum of hypoplasia along the radial side of the entire upper extremity. This radial longitudinal deficiency can be mild, involving only mild size discrepancy to the thumb, or severe and include global shoulder hypoplasia and instability along with elbow deficiency, and complete thumb and radius absence. The estimated incidence of radial longitudinal deficiency is approximately 1:30,000 live births[52]; however, this frequency may be underestimated because mild deformity may be missed due to excellent function and cosmesis. Thumb hypoplasia can occur in isolation but is almost always noted with underlying radial longitudinal deficiency. Male patients and female patients are equally affected, and the incidence of bilaterality is approximately 50%, although asymmetrical presentation is commonly seen.[53]

Radial longitudinal deficiency was initially classified radiographically by the severity of radial deformity by Bayne and Klug,[54] and this classification has been modified by James and Bednar[55] to include thumb hypoplasia and abnormalities of the radial carpus (**Table 3**). Blauth[56] classified thumb hypoplasia by the severity of clinical deformity from type I, mild decrease in thumb size with intact intrinsic and extrinsic function, to type V, complete thumb absence. This classification was modified by Manske[57] to include a differentiation in type III, which included the stability of the trapeziometacarpal joint (type IIIA) or lack thereof (type IIIB) (**Table 4**). In patients with trapeziometacarpal joint instability (type IIIB or more severe), reconstruction of a stable, useful thumb is exceedingly difficult, and most surgeons would consider these patients appropriate for thumb ablation and index finger pollicization.

Patients with radial and thumb deficiency commonly have other musculoskeletal and systemic abnormalities. Scoliosis is the most common musculoskeletal abnormality noted with radial deficiency. The most common systemic associations are Holt-Oram syndrome, thrombocytopenia absent radius (TAR) syndrome, Fanconi anemia, and VACTERL (Vertebral defects, Anal atresia, Cardiac malformations, Tracheoesophageal fistula, Esophageal atresia, Renal anomalies, and Limb anomalies) association.[53,58] The treating surgeon may be the first person to recognize these associations and should initiate further diagnostic steps. A referral to a pediatric geneticist may be of benefit, but if one is not available, the hand surgeon should order spine radiographs to screen for scoliosis, renal ultrasound to evaluate for kidney malformations, echocardiogram to evaluate for cardiac malformations such as atrial or ventral septal defect commonly seen in Holt-Oram syndrome, and a complete blood count and chromosomal breakage test to evaluate for thrombocytopenia and Fanconi anemia, respectively. Patients with TAR syndrome have complete

Table 3
Modified Bayne and Klug classification of radial longitudinal deficiency

Type N	Isolated thumb hypoplasia/absence
Type 0	Type N with anomaly of radial carpus
Type 1	Shortened distal radius
Type 2	Hypoplastic radius
Type 3	Partial absence of radius
Type 4	Complete absence of radius

From James MA, McCarroll HR Jr, Manske PR. The spectrum of radial longitudinal deficiency: a modified classification. J Hand Surg Am 1999;24(6):1147.

Table 4 Modified Blauth classification of thumb hypoplasia	
Type I	Slight decrease in thumb size
Type II	Narrowed first web space, hypoplastic thenar musculature, unstable MCP joint

Type III	Features of type II hypoplasia, including
	    IIIA: Extrinsic muscle abnormalities, metacarpal hypoplasia
	    IIIB: Extrinsic muscle abnormalities, partial aplasia of metacarpal, unstable
	        carpometacarpal joint

Type IV	Pouce flottant with only soft tissue connection to hand (floating thumb)
Type V	Complete absence of thumb

From Manske PR, McCarroll HR Jr, James M. Type III-A hypoplastic thumb. J Hand Surg Am 1995;20(2):246.

radius aplasia, but always have thumbs present with varying degrees of hypoplasia.

Surgical Procedure

Patients with thumb hypoplasia should be evaluated for concomitant finger abnormalities and for radial longitudinal deficiency. The treatment for these patients is based on the severity of the hypoplasia. In patients with mild hypoplasia, including type I, and mild variations of type II with some opposition function, no surgical treatment is indicated. Patients with type II and IIIA hypoplasia often benefit from opponensplasty, stabilization of the radial and ulnar collateral ligaments of the thumb MCP, and web space deepening. This treatment is best done with a single tendon transfer from the ring or middle finger flexor digitorum superficialis (FDS) tendon; however, this will not restore thenar bulk. Opponensplasty using the abductor digiti minimi (ADM) via a Huber transfer helps to restore the thenar contour and function, but does not have sufficient length to restore the collateral ligaments of the thumb MCP joint. In patients with Blauth type IIIB, IV, and V thumbs, pollicization with ablation of the thumb remnant is the procedure of choice (**Fig. 13**).

In patients with thumb hypoplasia and underlying severe radial longitudinal deficiency, the treatment is somewhat controversial. Most of these patients have significant thumb hypoplasia and stiffness of the radial digits, with relatively good function to the small finger. These patients may have functional postaxial pinch patterns present and may lose function with correction of the wrist deformity and subsequent index pollicization, especially when the index finger is hypoplastic or syndactylized to the middle finger. In addition, in patients with severe radial deficiency and limited elbow motion, correction of wrist radial deviation will limit useful hand-to-mouth function.

Preoperative Planning

- Careful clinical and radiographic examination should be performed in order to establish the exact degree of thumb hypoplasia.

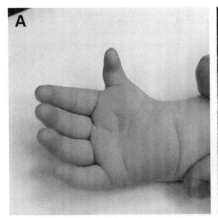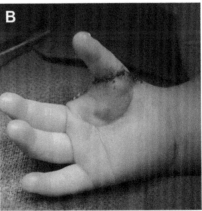

Fig. 13. Patient with (*A*) Blauth type IIIB thumb hypoplasia and (*B*) following thumb ablation and index finger pollicization.

- In general, a patient will bypass a thumb with an unstable trapeziometacarpal joint and prefer a scissor pinch between the index and middle fingers.

Surgical Procedure: Opponensplasty, Ligament Reconstruction, Web Space Deepening

- A transverse incision is made over the proximal interphalangeal joint crease of the ring finger along with a longitudinal volar incision over the flexor carpi ulnaris (FCU) tendon.
- Both slips of the FDS tendon are divided at the chiasm, passed through a loop created from the FCU tendon and then passed through a subcutaneous tunnel to a longitudinal incision along the radial border of the thumb MCP joint (**Fig. 14**).
- The thumb web space is deepened with a 4-flap Z-plasty, which is left open until collateral ligament reconstruction is performed (**Fig. 15**).
- In cases of MCP joint instability, a drill hole is made through the metacarpal head at the level of the collateral ligament origin. One slip of the FDS is passed through the tunnel to the 4-flap Z-plasty and then secured to the ulnar volar aspect of the proximal phalanx base, whereas the other slip is used to reconstruct the radial collateral ligament (see **Fig. 14**).
- Alternatively, in the Huber transfer, the ADM muscle can be harvested and transferred on its neurovascular pedicle to the thumb APB tendon insertion via a wide subcutaneous tunnel. The ADM muscle can be taken with a skin paddle to provide additional skin contouring.

In patients with unstable MCP joints following Huber transfer, collateral ligament reconstruction is performed with free tendon grafts or the joint can be stabilized with chondrodesis between the metacarpal head and epiphysis of the proximal phalanx.

Surgical Procedure: Pollicization

- Drawing appropriate skin incisions is crucial to successfully performing a pollicization. There are 2 main variations described.[58–60]
- The volar neurovascular bundle is isolated and, along with the periadventitial fat, dissected free from the underlying flexor tendon sheath to allow for mobilization to the thumb position without kinking the vessels.
- The dorsal skin incision is made making sure to preserve as many dorsal veins as possible. These veins are dissected proximally and distally to allow for easy transposition to the thumb position without kinking.
- The metacarpal is dissected extraperiosteally from the origin of interosseous muscles and surrounding tissues and removed from the metaphyseal flare to the epiphysis.
- The shortened index metacarpal is rotated 100 to 120° and placed into 45° of palmar abduction and 15° of radial abduction to recreate the normal thumb position.
- The skin incisions are inset with absorbable sutures. The volar skin flap is advanced into the new thumb/long finger web space, taking care not to place any suture line through the web space to minimize later scar contracture.
- The patient is observed for 23 hours postoperatively to ensure that vascularity remains intact and pain is well controlled before discharge home.

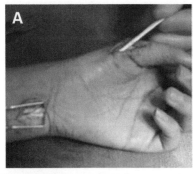
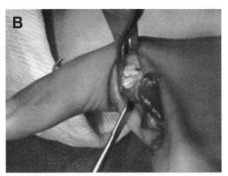

Fig. 14. (*A*) Ring FDS opponensplasty demonstrating line of pull after passing the FDS tendon through a pulley created by a slip of the FCU tendon. (*B*) Reconstruction of the ulnar collateral ligament of the MCP joint with a slip of the FDS tendon passed through the metacarpal head into the web space z-plasty incision. In this case, the proximal phalanx physis was closed, allowing drill holes in the proximal phalanx base; however, in younger children, the FDS tendon can be sutured to the periosteum at the proximal phalanx base.

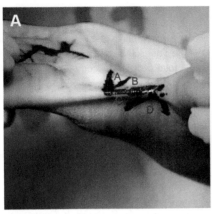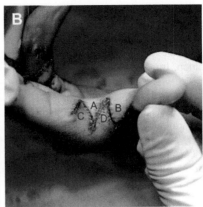

Fig. 15. Patient with thumb-index web space contracture demonstrating a 4-flap Z Plasty (*A*) before separation and (*B*) after closure. Note how the letters corresponding to each flap are reorganized from A-B-C-D to C-A-D-B.

Postoperative Care

Postoperatively, the patient is casted for 4 weeks, and the stabilizing pin is removed as needed. Occupational therapy is then begun to retrain the patient for use of the reconstructed thumb. This therapy often lasts for 2 to 3 months postoperatively and can be discontinued when the patient has maximized function and the family is sufficiently versed in a home exercise program to continue at home. The patients are followed monthly for the first 3 to 4 months and then yearly to ensure that function has been maintained and to evaluate for long-term complications.

Complications and Management

Complications are infrequent during reconstruction of a hypoplastic thumb as long as the correct surgical indications are met and the surgical techniques are carefully followed. In general, if a child ignores a thumb that does not have a stable base, they will likely continue to ignore that thumb if it is reconstructed. Conversely, a patient who tries to use a hypoplastic thumb but struggles due to opposition weakness and MCP joint instability will likely benefit greatly from opponensplasty and ligament reconstruction. Therefore, preoperative assessment and patient selection are critical to a functional thumb reconstruction. Occupational therapy evaluation preoperatively and postoperatively is very helpful in determining the surgical goals and assisting the patient in functional recovery.

The most significant complication following pollicization is poor vascular inflow or outflow, which can result in loss of the digit if not treated immediately. If the new thumb does not turn pink immediately, vasospasm may be the cause, which should resolve with observation and/or warming. If

vascularity does not return in 5 minutes, the arteries should be explored for damage and freed of any soft tissue tether. Venous congestion is more frequently encountered, which can be ameliorated by loosening dressings or removing tight sutures that may be compressing the dorsal veins.

Long-term complications, such as malrotation, excessive length, or web contracture of the new thumb, are due to technical failures and are best prevented by meticulous attention to the steps involved in surgical correction. Lack of opposition following pollicization is seen in approximately 10% to 20% of patients and is likely due to an underlying deficiency in intrinsic muscles; this can be successfully treated by subsequent opponensplasty as described previously.[61]

Outcomes

In most cases, improved outcomes are achieved following reconstruction in patients with hypoplastic thumbs as long as the surgical plan addresses the deficient components for each patient. Abdel-Ghani and Amro[62] reported on 9 patients who underwent FDS opponensplasty and web space deepening. All patients had improved function, and 8 of 9 achieved thumb opposition to the small finger, whereas only 71% achieved full stabilization of the MCP joint. Graham and Louis[63] reported on the functional results of 14 patients with hypoplastic thumbs with all achieving functional improvement and only 2 of 14 noting mild instability of the thumb MP joint. Upton and Taghinia[64] reported on 14 patients who underwent ADM opponensplasty for type II and IIIA thumb hypoplasia and noted improved function and no loss of function during growth.

Manske and colleagues[65] evaluated index finger pollicization at an average of 8 years postoperatively and demonstrated that the new thumb has a total active motion of 98° (approximately 50% of the normal thumb). These reconstructed thumbs exhibited approximately 20% of normal key pinch, tripod pinch, grip, and opposition strength and were consistently (92% of the time) used for grasping large objects, as compared with small objects (77%). Lightdale-Miric and colleagues[66] reported on 8 patients at an average of 9 years postoperatively following index finger pollicization (10 total hands) and noted that grip, lateral pinch, and tripod pinch were greater than 3 standard deviations below normal and scored below average in all functional tests. However, 6 hands had normal scores for dexterity and 7 had normal scores on the Pediatric Outcomes Data Collection Instrument. They also reported that older age at surgery and increasing severity of radial dysplasia correlated with worse strength and functional outcomes.

SUMMARY

Although congenital hand anomalies are relatively rare, pediatric othropedic surgeons and hand surgeons will frequently see them during the course of clinical practice. The clinician should be aware of the associated malformations and conditions that may, in some cases, be fatal if not recognized and treated appropriately. The goals of surgery are to improve hand function and cosmesis while limiting complications that could impair function long term. The surgeon must balance functional, cosmetic, and cultural goals and align those goals with the proper surgical techniques in order to maximize patient and parent satisfaction following surgical intervention.

REFERENCES

1. Ekblom AG, Laurell T, Arner M. Epidemiology of congenital upper limb anomalies in 562 children born in 1997 to 2007: a total population study from Stockholm, Sweden. J Hand Surg Am 2010;35(11): 1742–54.
2. Lamb DW, Wynne-Davies R. Incidence and genetics. In: Buck-Gramcko D, editor. Congenital malformations of the hand and forearm. London: Churchill Livingstone; 1998. p. 21–7.
3. Andersson GB, Gillberg C, Fernell E, et al. Children with surgically corrected hand deformities and upper limb deficiencies: self-concept and psychological well-being. J Hand Surg Eur Vol 2011;36(9): 795–801.
4. Koskimies E, Lindfors N, Gissler M, et al. Congenital upper limb deficiencies and associated malformations in Finland: a population-based study. J Hand Surg Am 2011;36(6):1058–65.
5. Giele H, Giele C, Bower C, et al. The incidence and epidemiology of congenital upper limb anomalies: a total population study. J Hand Surg Am 2001;26A: 628–33.
6. Watts AC, Hooper G. (iii) Congenital hand anomalies. Curr Orthop 2006;20:266–73.
7. Swanson AB. A classification for congenital malformations of the hand. N J Bull Acad Med 1964;10:166–9.
8. Oberg KC, Feenstra JM, Manske PR, et al. Developmental biology and classification of congenital anomalies of the hand and upper extremity. J Hand Surg Am 2010;35(12):2066–76.
9. Gallant GG, Bora FW Jr. Congenital deformities of the upper extremity. J Am Acad Orthop Surg 1996; 4(3):162–71.
10. Johnson RL, Riddle RD, Tabin CJ. Mechanisms of limb patterning. Curr Opin Genet Dev 1994;4(4): 535–42.
11. Riddle RD, Tabin C. How limbs develop. Sci Am 1999;280(2):74–9.
12. Biesecker LG. Polydactyly: how many disorders and how many genes? 2010 update. Dev Dyn 2011; 240(5):931–42.
13. Riddle RD, Johnson RL, Laufer E, et al. Sonic Hedgehog mediates polarizing activity of the ZPA. Cell 1993;75(7):1401–16.
14. Bouldin CM, Gritli-Linde A, Ahn S, et al. Shh pathway activation is present and required within the vertebrate limb bud apical ectodermal ridge for normal autopod patterning. Proc Natl Acad Sci U S A 2010;107(12):5489–94.
15. Lu P, Yu Y, Perdue Y, et al. The apical ectodermal ridge is a timer for generating distal limb progenitors. Development 2008;135(8):1395–405.
16. VanderMeer JE, Ahituv N. cis-regulatory mutations are a genetic cause of human limb malformations. Dev Dyn 2011;240(5):920–30.
17. Charite J, McFadden DG, Olson EN. The bHLH transcription factor dHAND controls Sonic hedgehog expression and establishment of the zone of polarizing activity during limb development. Development 2000;127(11):2461–70.
18. Chow CS, Ho PC, Tse WL, et al. Reconstruction of hypoplastic thumb using hemi-longitudinal metatarsal transfer. J Hand Surg Eur Vol 2012;37(8): 738–44.
19. Kozin SH. Syndactyly. J Am Soc Surg Hand 2001;1: 1–13.
20. Eaton CJ, Lister GD. Syndactyly. Hand Clin 1990;6: 555–75.
21. Kozin SH. Upper-extremity congenital anomalies. J Bone Joint Surg Am 2003;85-A(8):1564–76.
22. Temtamy SA, McKusick VA. The genetics of hand malformations. Birth Defects Orig Artic Ser 1978; 14(3):i–xviii, 1–619.

23. Malik S. Syndactyly: phenotypes, genetics and current classification. Eur J Hum Genet 2012;20(8): 817–24.

24. Ghani HA. Modified dorsal rotation advancement flap for release of the thumb web space. J Hand Surg Br 2006;31(2):226–9.

25. Barabás AG, Pickford MA. Results of syndactyly release using a modification of the Flatt technique. J Hand Surg Eur Vol 2014;39(9):984–8.

26. Vekris MD, Lykissas MG, Soucacos PN, et al. Congenital syndactyly: outcome of surgical treatment in 131 webs. Tech Hand Up Extrem Surg 2010;14(1):2–7.

27. Lumenta DB, Kitzinger HB, Beck H, et al. Long-term outcomes of web creep, scar quality, and function after simple syndactyly surgical treatment. J Hand Surg Am 2010;35(8):1323–9.

28. Ekerot L. Syndactyly correction without skin-grafting. J Hand Surg Br 1996;21(3):330–7.

29. Bandoh Y, Yanai A, Seno H. The three-square-flap method for reconstruction of minor syndactyly. J Hand Surg Am 1997;22(4):680–4.

30. Sahin C, Ergun O, Kulahci Y, et al. Bilobed flap for web reconstruction in adult syndactyly release: a new technique that can avoid the use of skin graft. J Plast Reconstr Aesthet Surg 2014;67(6):815–21.

31. Graham TJ, Ress AM. Finger polydactyly. Hand Clin 1998;14(1):49–64.

32. McCarroll HR. Congenital anomalies: a 25-year overview. J Hand Surg Am 2000;25(6):1007–37.

33. Temtamy SA, McKusick VA. Polydactyly as an isolated malformation. Birth Defect 1978;14:364–92.

34. Lamb DW, Wynne-Davies R, Soto L. An estimate of the population frequency of congenital malformations of the upper limb. J Hand Surg Am 1982; 7(6):557–62.

35. Watson BT, Hennrikus WL. Postaxial type-B polydactyly. Prevalence and treatment. J Bone Joint Surg Am 1997;79(1):65–8.

36. Zhao H, Tian Y, Breedveld G, et al. Postaxial polydactyly type A/B (PAP-A/B) is linked to chromosome 19p13.1-13.2 in a Chinese kindred. Eur J Hum Genet 2002;10(3):162–6.

37. Wassel HD. The results of surgery for polydactyly of the thumb. Clin Orthop Relat Res 1969;64:175–93.

38. Farooq M, Troelsen JT, Boyd M, et al. Preaxial polydactyly/triphalangeal thumb is associated with changed transcription factor-binding affinity in a family with a novel point mutation in the long-range cis-regulatory element ZRS. Eur J Hum Genet 2010;18(6):733–6.

39. Zuidam JM, Selles RW, Ananta M, et al. A classification system of radial polydactyly: inclusion of triphalangeal thumb and triplication. J Hand Surg Am 2008;33(3):373–7.

40. Baek GH, Gong HS, Chung MS, et al. Modified Bilhaut-Cloquet procedure for Wassel type-II and III polydactyly of the thumb. J Bone Joint Surg Am 2007;89(3):534–41.

41. Baek GH, Gong HS, Chung MS, et al. Modified Bilhaut-Cloquet procedure for Wassel type-II and III polydactyly of the thumb. Surgical technique. J Bone Joint Surg Am 2008;90(Suppl 2 Pt 1):74–86.

42. Abzug JM, Kozin SH. Treatment of postaxial polydactyly Type B. J Hand Surg Am 2013;38(6):1223–5.

43. Rayan GM, Frey B. Ulnar polydactyly. Plast Reconstr Surg 2001;107(6):1449–54.

44. Katz K, Linder N. Postaxial type B polydactyly treated by excision in the neonatal nursery. J Pediatr Orthop 2011;31(4):448–9.

45. Yen CH, Chan WL, Leung HB, et al. Thumb polydactyly: clinical outcome after reconstruction. J Orthop Surg (Hong Kong) 2006;14(3):295–302.

46. Leber GE, Gosain AK. Surgical excision of pedunculated supernumerary digits prevents traumatic amputation neuromas. Pediatr Dermatol 2003; 20(2):108–12.

47. Tonkin MA, Bulstrode NW. The Bilhaut-Cloquet procedure for Wassel types III, IV and VII thumb duplication. J Hand Surg Eur Vol 2007;32(6):684–93.

48. Mullick S, Borschel GH. A selective approach to treatment of ulnar polydactyly: preventing painful neuroma and incomplete excision. Pediatr Dermatol 2010;27(1):39–42.

49. Lee CC, Park HY, Yoon JO, et al. Correction of Wassel type IV thumb duplication with zigzag deformity: results of a new method of flexor pollicis longus tendon relocation. J Hand Surg Eur Vol 2013;38(3): 272–80.

50. Stutz C, Mills J, Wheeler L, et al. Long-term outcomes following radial polydactyly reconstruction. J Hand Surg Am 2014;39(8):1549–52.

51. Maillet M, Fron D, Martinot-Duquennoy V, et al. Results after surgical treatment of thumb duplication: a retrospective review of 33 thumbs. J Child Orthop 2007;1(2):135–41.

52. James MA, Bednar MS. Deformities of the wrist and forearm. In: Green DP, Hotchkiss RN, Pederson WC, et al, editors. Operative hand surgery. 5th edition. New York: Churchill Livingstone; 2005. p. 1469–506.

53. Goldfarb CA, Wall L, Manske PR. Radial longitudinal deficiency: the incidence of associated medical and musculoskeletal conditions. J Hand Surg Am 2006; 31(7):1176–82.

54. Bayne LG, Klug MS. Long-term review of the surgical treatment of radial deficiencies. J Hand Surg Am 1987;12(2):169–79.

55. James MA, McCarroll HR Jr, Manske PR. The spectrum of radial longitudinal deficiency: a modified classification. J Hand Surg Am 1999;24(6): 1145–55.

56. Blauth W. The hypoplastic thumb. Arch Orthop Unfallchir 1967;62(3):225–46 [in German].

57. Manske PR, McCarroll HR Jr, James M. Type III-A hypoplastic thumb. J Hand Surg Am 1995;20(2): 246–53.

58. Bednar MS, James MA, Light TR. Congenital longitudinal deficiency. J Hand Surg Am 2009;34(9): 1739–47.

59. Buck-Gramcko D. Pollicization of the index finger: method and results in aplasia and hypoplasia of the thumb. J Bone Joint Surg Am 1971;53(8):1605–17.

60. Kozin SH. Pollicization: the concept, technical details, and outcome. Clin Orthop Surg 2012;4(1):18–35.

61. Goldfarb CA, Monroe E, Steffen J, et al. Incidence and treatment of complications, suboptimal outcomes, and functional deficiencies after pollicization. J Hand Surg Am 2009;34(7):1291–7.

62. Abdel-Ghani H, Amro S. Characteristics of patients with hypoplastic thumb: a prospective study of 51 patients with the results of surgical treatment. J Pediatr Orthop B 2004;13(2):127–38.

63. Graham TJ, Louis DS. A comprehensive approach to surgical management of the type IIIA hypoplastic thumb. J Hand Surg Am 1998;23(1):3–13.

64. Upton J, Taghinia AH. Abductor digiti minimi myocutaneous flap for opponensplasty in congenital hypoplastic thumbs. Plast Reconstr Surg 2008;122(6): 1807–11.

65. Manske PR, Rotman MB, Dailey LA. Long-term functional results after pollicization for the congenitally deficient thumb. J Hand Surg Am 1992;17(6): 1064–72.

66. Lightdale-Miric N, Mueske NM, Lawrence EL, et al. Long term functional outcomes after early childhood pollicization. J Hand Ther 2015;28(2): 158–66.

Upper Extremity

Preface

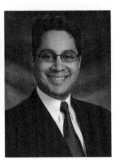

Asif M. Ilyas, MD
Editor

This is the last issue of the *Orthopedic Clinics of North America* I will be overseeing as the section editor of Upper Extremity. It has truly been an honor and privilege to oversee this dynamic and diverse section for the past several years. Below is a brief preface of what this issue discusses.

Both rotator cuff tears and instability are common upper extremity complaints that often warrant surgical repair. Unfortunately, recurrent tears following repairs are common, too. There are a number of potential causes for recurrent rotator cuff tears, including the timing and duration of immobilization. Hsu and colleagues present an evidence-based review of the effect, if any, on late or early mobilization after surgery on retearing. Similarly, Chang and colleagues review posterior shoulder instability in overhead throwing athletes.

Distal biceps tendon tears are common and potentially debilitating conditions most commonly presenting in middle age. When surgery has been indicated, a number of techniques are available. Stoll and Huang present an evidence-based review on the pathology and available surgical repairs for these common injuries.

Although total joint arthroplasty is commonly utilized for a number of joints with great success, its application in the wrist for advanced arthritis has been limited. However, with newer implants, there has been renewed interest in the potential utilization of total wrist arthroplasty. Kennedy and Huang review the current available systems and review the latest outcomes of total wrist arthroplasty.

Fowler and colleagues take on a review of two very common but challenging conditions of the hand and wrist: flexor tendon injuries and scapholunate advanced collapse (SLAC) wrist. Specifically, they provide a review of both the ever-improving understanding of flexor tendon healing biology and repair and the motion-sparing procedures for SLAC wrists.

Finally, in this last issue I will have the pleasure to edit, I am proud to present two articles I have coauthored with my colleagues that challenge current dogma in hand surgery. In the first, Vosbikian and colleagues review volar plate fixation of distal radius fractures with specific consideration of the late loss of volar tilt following fixation. What we introduce is the concept of the DDD, the "Distal Dorsal cortical Distance," which is a measurement that can be readily utilized by surgeons intraoperatively to optimize subchondral screw positioning relative to the articular surface, analogous to the "Tip-Apex" distance used in the hip. In the second article, Tulipan and I review the unique features of open fractures of the hand, distal to the distal radius, and discuss the inapplicability of the current Gustilo-Anderson classification to the hand. Subsequently, we present to the reader a new straightforward classification specifically for open hand fractures, which can potentially guide treatment and provide prognostic information.

Asif M. Ilyas, MD
Rothman Institute
Thomas Jefferson University
925 Chestnut Street
Philadelphia, PA 19107, USA

E-mail address:
asif.ilyas@rothmaninstitute.com

Orthop Clin N Am 47 (2016) xxv
http://dx.doi.org/10.1016/j.ocl.2015.10.007

orthopedic.theclinics.com

Immobilization After Rotator Cuff Repair
What Evidence Do We Have Now?

Jason E. Hsu, MD[a], John G. Horneff, MD[b],
Albert O. Gee, MD[a],*

KEYWORDS

- Rotator cuff tear • Rotator cuff repair • Tendon healing • Mechanobiology • Immobilization
- Early mobilization • Postoperative rehabilitation

KEY POINTS

- Tendon is a mechanically sensitive tissue. Biochemical and biomechanical properties of the repair site are altered by mechanical load.
- Tendon-to-bone healing likely responds best to controlled loading. Complete removal of load may understimulate the healing process, while excessive loading can cause microtrauma, gap formation, and repair failure.
- Clinically, numerous randomized controlled trials have shown no difference in healing rates between early mobilization and delayed rehabilitation protocols.
- In the early postoperative period, range of motion and function may be better with early mobilization compared with delayed rehabilitation. However, this benefit is transient, and there is no difference 1 year after surgery.

INTRODUCTION

The rate of rotator cuff tears is high in the increasingly aging population, and rotator cuff repair has become one of the most commonly performed orthopedic procedures.[1–3] However, re-tear rates after rotator cuff repair is reported to be around 20%[4–6] and even greater than 90% in massive tears.[7] Age, tear size, and chronicity are all important factors affecting healing rates after repair but are inherent to the patient and disease. Two important and modifiable factors that the surgeon can control are the surgical technique and the postoperative rehabilitation protocol. There is an abundance of literature concerning surgical approach and techniques for rotator cuff repair.[4,8,9] Unfortunately, despite advances in both techniques and technology, the rate of recurrent tearing after rotator cuff repair remains substantial.[6] Surgeons

may potentially improve outcomes after rotator cuff repair by controlling and optimizing the mechanical environment after rotator cuff repair, but until recently, literature regarding postoperative rehabilitation and mobilization was relatively scarce.

There is significant variation in the postoperative rehabilitation for patients undergoing rotator cuff repair. Some surgeons may choose to immobilize the shoulder for a period of time after surgery. Immobilization protects the repair site from excessive force that may damage the repair construct and lead to early failure. This approach, however, risks increased postoperative shoulder stiffness and decreased shoulder function. Other surgeons prefer to mobilize early in order to improve early shoulder function. Early mobilization may potentially put the repair construct and tendon-to-bone healing potential at risk.

a Department of Orthopaedics and Sports Medicine, University of Washington, Seattle, WA 98195, USA;
b Department of Orthopaedic Surgery, University of Pennsylvania, 2 Silverstein Pavilion, 3400 Spruce Street, Philadelphia, PA 19104, USA
* Corresponding author. 1959 NE Pacific Street, Box 356500, Seattle, WA 98195, USA.
E-mail address: ag112@uw.edu

orthopedic.theclinics.com

In the past decade, in vitro studies, animal studies, and clinical investigations have helped to guide the understanding of the role of mechanobiology, early mobilization, and immobilization after rotator cuff repair. The objective of this article is to review the basic science and clinical evidence behind mobilization after rotator cuff repair. The effects of mechanical loading on tendon-to-bone healing are outlined. The most recent evidence investigating the effects of immobilization on tendon healing in animal models are reviewed. Finally, recent high-quality randomized clinical trials are summarized. This information can help surgeons formulate a postoperative rehabilitation protocol.

BASIC SCIENCE EVIDENCE
Tendon-to-Bone Healing

The tendon-bone junction represents a crucial area that is most commonly affected in rotator cuff disease. The structural and mechanical properties in this complex area of transition are the focus of both laboratory and clinical investigations on rotator cuff healing. The rotator cuff has a direct fibrocartilaginous insertion that incorporates 4 different but continuous zones of tissue composition (**Fig. 1**). Zone 1 is predominantly type I collagen similar to that found in the midsubstance of the tendon. The transition from zone 1 to 2 constitutes a change in the collagen composition (predominantly types II and III) as well as a change in extracellular matrix composition. In zone 3, the collagen and extracellular matrix composition is similar to cartilage. Zone 4 completes the transition with constituents similar to bone. This gradation from tendon to fibrocartilaginous tissue to bone assists in efficiently transferring and

dissipating load between 2 tissue structures with very different mechanical properties.

In some patients, tearing at this tendon-bone junction causes shoulder pain and dysfunction and necessitates repair. After a torn rotator cuff is repaired back down to its insertion, a scar-forming process ensues. However, the healing process does not recapitulate the normal transition from tendon to bone, and therefore, even a healed rotator cuff repair is structurally and mechanically inferior to a healthy native enthesis. The enthesis of a normal rotator cuff insertion is already typically weaker in tension than the midsubstance of a healthy tendon. The significant re-tear rate seen after repair may be due to formation of disorganized reactive scar tissue rather than organized tendon with a fibrocartilaginous intermediary zone.

Tendon healing follows 3 phases. During the first 4 to 7 days, inflammatory cells including macrophages and neutrophils remove tissue debris. Callous is formed through deposition of types I and III collagen. The second phase is the proliferative or reparative phase in which collagen and other extracellular matrix components are deposited. The last phase is the remodeling phase, which starts approximately 6 to 8 weeks after injury. This phase is characterized by increased order of collagen structure in a linear orientation, presumably in response to stress along the longitudinal axis of the tendon.

During this remodeling phase, mechanical traction, in addition to many other elements such as growth factors, plays a role in the generation of organized tissue at the repaired tendon site. Tendon-to-bone healing, like healing of many other musculoskeletal tissues such as bone and ligament, is affected by an increased transmission of force across the healing interface. This force

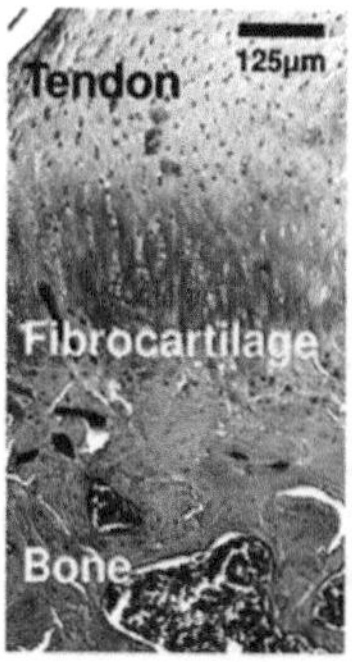

	Tissue Region	Cell Type	Major Matrix Component
Tendon	Tendon	Fibroblasts	Collagen types I, III (Diameter: 40–400 nm)
	Nonmineralized Fibrocartilage	Fibrochondrocytes	Collagen types I, II, III
Fibrocartilage	Mineralized Fibrocartilage	Hypertrophic Fibrochondrocytes	Collagen types I, II, X
Bone	Bone	Osteoblasts Osteocytes Osteoclasts	Collagen type I (Diameter: 34.5–39.5 nm)

Fig. 1. Structure and composition of tendon-to-bone insertion site with Masson trichrome staining in a rat. (*Adapted from* Zhang X, Bogdanowicz D, Erisken C, et al. Biomimetic scaffold design for functional and integrative tendon repair. J Shoulder Elbow Surg 2012;21(2):268; with permission.)

transmission may promote the formation of collagen in a more organized fashion and may increase the strength of the repair over time.

Mechanobiology in Tendon Healing

Rotator cuff healing is a mechanosensitive process and therefore can be altered by adjusting the mechanical load to the repair site. Tendons have biochemical and biomechanical properties that respond and adjust to mechanical loading.[10–13] Many studies have supported the theory that appropriate exercise-related loading can enhance tendon mechanical properties, while removal of load from the tendon can lead to deterioration.[14–17] Adequate mechanical loading can also help to reverse deteriorating mechanical properties in aging tendon.[18]

When mechanical load is imparted onto tendon, biochemical changes within tenocytes are evident, along with increased collagen deposition and up-regulation of growth factors important in collagen synthesis. Expression of transforming growth factor-β and scleraxis, both of which are involved in differentiation and proliferation, is altered with varying mechanical load.[19–21] On the other hand, chronic, repetitive loads on tendon (overuse/overload) can lead to microtrauma and production of inflammatory mediators, including prostaglandin 2 and leukotriene 4[22–24]; this can lead to further degeneration of tendon and soft tissue edema. Literature suggests that repetitive mechanical load can have 2 opposite effects that are dependent on the magnitude of load.[25] A smaller magnitude decreases matrix metalloproteinase-1 (MMP-1), cyclo-oxygenase-2, and interleukin1β and has an anti-inflammatory effect, while the opposite is seen with larger magnitudes.

Disuse and immobilization can decrease stiffness and tensile strength of tendon. Deprivation of stress at the repair site can induce a catabolic state. Arnoczky and colleagues[26] have shown that mRNA expression of collagenase (MMP-1) is markedly increased in load-deprived tendon cells but significantly inhibited with increasing load to the tendon cells. This finding suggests that upregulation of MMP-1 expression can be inhibited through a cytoskeletally based mechanotransduction pathway. A subsequent study by the same group has suggested that load deprivation decreases the mechanoresponsiveness of tendon cells.[27]

Animal Studies of Immobilization and Load Removal

A large portion of the literature pertaining to tendon-to-bone healing has been carried out in the rat rotator cuff model initially described by Soslowsky and colleagues.[28] Subsequent studies using the rat animal model have been shown to be a good animal model to evaluate overuse activity and treatment modalities of rotator cuff injuries.[29–32] Because of the similarities in soft tissue and bony anatomy between the rat and the human, the rat model has been one of the primary animal models to study rotator cuff disease and tendon-to-bone healing.

The rat rotator cuff model has been commonly used to investigate the role of immobilization on rotator cuff healing. Thomopoulos and colleagues[30] initially investigated tendon-to-bone healing under a variety of loading conditions. After detachment and immediate repair of the supraspinatus tendon, rats were divided into 3 different groups based on activity level: immobilization in a cast, cage activity, and exercise. At 8 weeks, they noted that the tendons in the immobilized group had superior material properties, better tendon organization, and higher type I to type III collagen ratio when compared with the exercise group. These results supported the clinical practice of decreased activity and immobilization after surgical repair. In a subsequent study, Gimbel and colleagues[33] investigated the length of immobilization and activity on the mechanical properties of the supraspinatus tendon of the rat using a similar method. They found that decreased activity level had the greatest positive effect on elastic properties over time. Further studies by the same group have shown that the joint stiffness that resulted from immobilization was only transient[34] and that exercise after a short period of immobilization was detrimental to tendon properties.[35]

Subsequent studies by other groups have shown that complete removal of load from the repair site is detrimental to healing. By using botulunim toxin (Botox) to inhibit contraction of skeletal muscle, multiple investigators have shown that completely unloading the repair site is deleterious to the healing tendon.[15,36] This finding was investigated by Galatz and colleagues[15] using the same rat rotator cuff model. Cuff healing in 3 different groups were investigated: Botox and immobilization, Botox and free range of motion, and saline-injected and immobilization. Rats that were immobilized and injected with botulinum toxin A into the supraspinatus muscle belly had inferior structural properties compared with saline-injected, immobilized rats. Hettrich and colleagues[36] performed a similar study using Botox without immobilization and suggested that stress deprivation from the tendon-bone interface leads to decreased mechanical properties. It should be noted that in the study by Galatz and colleagues, the material properties were not different between any of the groups; the increased structural properties in the saline/casted group were due to increased volume of scar tissue formation. This finding suggests that, regardless of method for load removal, reparative rather than regenerative scar tissue is generated. Leading the repair site down a regenerative pathway rather than a reparative pathway remains a challenge.

Both complete removal of load and chronic overload are detrimental to tendon healing. Removing load will understimulate the repair site, whereas chronic overload can damage the repair site and may activate a catabolic environment that is detrimental to healing. Clinically, controlled mobilization after rotator cuff repair must balance between understimulation and overload of the repair site.

Clinical Evidence

Until recently, clinicians relied heavily on personal experience and intuition when formulating postoperative rehabilitation protocols after rotator cuff repair; literature on this topic was almost nonexistent. Fortunately, multiple prospective, randomized trials investigating various postoperative rehabilitation protocols have recently been published. A summary of the characteristics and results of these studies are summarized in **Tables 1** and **2**, respectively. The data from these studies pertaining to healing of the rotator cuff, pain, range of motion, strength, and function have been helpful in formulating postoperative rehabilitation protocols. Although the important details of each study are summarized in this section, it is important to realize that the postoperative protocols in each of these studies vary greatly, and the reader should be familiar with the details and variations of each of the randomized studies in order to draw his or her own conclusion regarding the role of immobilization after repair.

Randomized Controlled Trials on Postoperative Mobilization

Lee and colleagues[37] treated 64 patients with arthroscopic single-row repair for medium- to large-sized full-thickness cuff tears and randomized them to 2 different rehabilitation protocols. One group received aggressive early passive motion, which included manual therapy by a therapist without limitation and unlimited self-directed passive stretching. In the second group, a continuous passive motion (CPM) machine was used to 90° of elevation twice daily for 3 weeks. After 3 weeks, the passive forward flexion range was increased as tolerated, and passive external rotation was

initiated. Both groups did not start active exercises until 6 weeks. Patients were evaluated at 3, 6, and 12 months. The aggressive early motion group had better range of motion at 3 months, but there were no differences by 1 year. Between 6 to 12 months after surgery (mean of 7.6 months), the integrity of the repair was evaluated with MRI. The aggressive motion group had a higher re-tear rate (23.3%) than the limited exercise group (8.8%), but this was not statistically significant.

Cuff and Pupello[38] randomized 68 patients that underwent arthroscopic suture-bridge repair of full-thickness supraspinatus tears. The early group performed therapist-directed passive forward elevation and external rotation starting on day 2 after surgery, while the delayed therapy performed pendulums for the first 6 weeks, followed by formal therapy. Patients were followed clinically for 12 months. The groups had similar satisfaction, range of motion, American Shoulder and Elbow Surgeons (ASES) scores, and Simple Shoulder Test (SST) scores. Ultrasound imaging at a minimum of 9 months showed no differences in rotator cuff healing.

Kim and colleagues[39] randomized 105 patients with small- to medium-sized full-thickness rotator cuff tears to early and delayed passive motion. Small tears were repaired with a single-row technique, while medium tears were primarily fixed with double-row or suture bridge techniques. In the early motion group, passive motion was started the day after surgery. In the delayed motion group, passive motion was started at 4 weeks for a small tear and 5 weeks for a medium tear. Range-of-motion and VAS pain scores were similar between the 2 groups at 3, 6, and 12 months. Constant, SST, and ASES scores were all similar as well at all time points. Re-tear rates at 1 year were similar in the 2 groups: 12% in the early group and 18% in the delayed group.

Keener and colleagues[40] similarly randomized 124 patients that were treated with double-row repairs for small- or medium-sized full-thickness rotator to 2 different motion protocols. A traditional rehabilitation protocol consisted of pendulums starting immediately postoperatively and therapist-guided passive range of motion 1 week after surgery. Pain, range of motion, and functional outcomes were collected at 6, 12, and 24 months postoperatively, and range of motion was additionally reviewed at 3 months. Range of motion was significantly worse in the immobilized group at 3 months, but this resolved in the later time points. There were no significant differences in the 2 groups in any other parameter. Healing rates were similar between the 2 groups with an overall healing rate of 92%.

Table 1
Characteristics of randomized prospective trials investigating mobilization after rotator cuff repair

Study	Rehabilitation Protocol	No. of Patients	Average Age (y)	Tear Size	Repair Technique	Key Elements of Rehabilitation Protocol	Follow-Up (mo)	% Follow-up
Lee et al, 2012	Early aggressive therapy	30	54.5	21 medium, 8 large	Single row	0–6 wk: manual therapy w/out limitation & self-directed passive ROM	12	70% (30/43)
	Early limited therapy	34	55.2	20 medium, 14 large		0–3 wk: FE <90° w/CPM 3–6 wk: FE >90° w/CPM & passive ER	12	81% (34/42)
Cuff and Pupello, 2012	Early therapy	33	63.0	N/A	Suture bridge	0–6 wk: pendulums & therapist-guided passive FE/ER	12	N/A
	Delayed therapy	35	63.5	N/A		0–6 wk: pendulums only	12	N/A
Kim et al, 2012	Early passive motion	56	60.1	All <3 cm	9 single row 1 double row 46 suture bridge	0 to 4–5 wk: passive FE, abduction, ER day after surgery	12	93% (56/60)
	Immobilization × 4–5 wk	49	60.0	All <3 cm	8 single row 1 double row 40 suture bridge	0 to 4–5 wk: no passive ROM	12	86% (49/57)
Keener et al, 2014	Early passive motion	61	56.1	All <3 cm	Double row	0–1 wk: pendulums only 2–6 wk: therapist-guided passive ROM 7–12 wk: active & active-assist ROM	24	91% (61/67)
	Immobilization × 6 wk	53		All <3 cm		0–6 wk: immobilization 6–12 wk: therapist-guided passive ROM	24	85% (53/62)
Koh et al, 2014	Immobilization × 4 wk	40	59.9	2–4 cm	Single row	0–4 wk: immobilization 5–10 wk: gentle passive ROM, progression to active, & active-assist ROM	24	85% (40/47)
	Immobilization × 8 wk	48		2–4 cm		0–8 wk: immobilization 9–14 wk: gentle passive ROM, progression to active, & active-assist ROM	24	91% (48/53)

Abbreviations: ER, external rotation; FE, forward elevation; IR, internal rotation; N/A, not reported; ROM, range of motion.
Data from Refs.[37–41]

Table 2
Results of randomized prospective trials investigating mobilization after rotator cuff repair

Study	Rehabilitation Protocol	Re-Tear Rate	Pain	ROM	Score	Strength
Lee et al, 2012	Early aggressive therapy Early limited therapy	23.3% (7/30) 8.8% (3/34)	VAS similar at all time points	Better in all planes in early aggressive group at 3 mo No difference at 12 mo	UCLA score better in early aggressive at 3 mo only	FE, ER, IR strength no difference at 1 y
Cuff and Pupello, 2012	Early therapy Delayed therapy	15% (5/33) 9% (3/35)	N/A	FE statistically better in early therapy at 6 mo but not 1 y ER and IR similar at all time points	ASES, SST scores similar at 1 y	N/A
Kim et al, 2012	Early passive motion Immobilization × 4–5 wk	12% (7/56) 18% (9/49)	VAS similar at all time points	FE, ER, IR similar at all time points	ASES, Constant, SST scores similar at all time points	N/A
Keener et al, 2014	Early passive motion Immobilization × 6 wk	10% (6/63) 6% (3/53)	VAS similar at all time points	FE, ER better in early passive motion at 3 mo ROM similar at all other time points	ASES, relative Constant, SST scores similar at all time points	Abduction and ER strength similar at all time points
Koh et al, 2014	Immobilization × 4 wk Immobilization × 8 wk	12.5% (5/40) 8.3% (4/48)	VAS similar at all time points	Avg FE/ER/IR similar at all time points % of pts with stiffness in at least one plane higher in 8-wk than 4-wk group	ASES, Constant scores similar at all time points	N/A

Abbreviations: ER, external rotation; FE, forward elevation; IR, internal rotation; N/A, not reported; ROM, range of motion; VAS, visual analog scale.
Data from Refs.[37–41]

Koh and colleagues[41] investigated the effect of increased immobilization time on healing rates after rotator cuff repair. In 100 patients that had a single-row repair of 2- to 4-cm full-thickness rotator cuff tears, patients were randomized to either 4 weeks or 8 weeks of immobilization with no passive or active range-of-motion exercises. Five tears occurred in the 4-week immobilization group, and 4 tears occurred in the 8-week immobilization group. Range-of-motion and clinical scores were no different between groups at the time of final follow-up, but a higher proportion of the 8-week immobilized patients (38%) was stiff compared with the 4-week group (18%). Stiffness was defined as any one of the following 3 criteria: forward elevation less than 120°, internal rotation less than the L3 spinal level, and external rotation with the arm at the side less than 20°. A subgroup analysis demonstrated that patients in the 8-week group without preoperative stiffness or diabetes had a higher percentage of postoperative stiffness at 24 months (37.5%) than patients in the 4-week group (4.0%). The authors conclude that increased immobilization period does not improve healing rates at 2 years. Additional immobilization after 4 weeks leads to more stiffness without an increased healing rate.

These 5 randomized, prospective controlled trials have given important information that can help surgeons formulate a postoperative rehabilitation plan. Data from these studies do not suggest any differences in healing rates when comparing an early passive motion protocol to a protocol incorporating 4 to 6 weeks of immobilization. Early motion protocols may improve range of motion early, but follow-up at more than 1 year does not show any advantage to early motion. In 3 of the 5 studies, range of motion was improved at an early time point in the group with the more aggressive motion protocol. However, in all 3 of these studies, this benefit was not seen at longer follow-up periods.

At a minimum of 1 year, the aggregate healing rate from these 5 studies is approximately 88%, which is higher than that reported in most systematic reviews on rotator cuff healing.[6] However, there was a relatively higher re-tear rate in one of the groups described by Lee and colleagues.[37] This group had patients that were assigned to early aggressive therapy whereby therapist-guided manual therapy without limitation was allowed for the first 6 weeks. For most surgeons, this protocol would be considered more aggressive than a more traditional rehabilitation protocol. It is possible that mechanical overload to the repair site could explain the 23.3% repair failure rate in this group. The other group in this study

had limited passive range of motion in the form of CPM machine for 3 weeks followed by the addition of passive external rotation for the next 3 weeks. This group had a significantly lower re-tear rate of 8.8%, suggesting that a protocol that is too aggressive may not adequately protect the repair in the early postoperative period.

This brings into question whether the gentle motion using a CPM machine without therapist-guided exercises would be adequate postoperatively. The use of a CPM machine was investigated by Garofalo and colleagues.[42] They randomized 100 patients to one group receiving therapist-guided passive range of motion with CPM and a second group without CPM. Similar to findings in the randomized studies, they found that there was a short-term motion benefit to CPM use for 4 weeks. The group using CPM had improved forward flexion, abduction, and external rotation in abduction up to 6 months, but by 1 year, there was no significant difference between groups. They did not report healing rates after rotator cuff repair.

Patient-reported outcome scores were consistently similar between the comparative groups of each study. Lee and colleagues[37] noted a slightly better University of California—Los Angeles (UCLA) score in an early aggressive therapy group, but this difference was no longer significant at longer follow-up. ASES, Constant, and SST scores were used in the other 4 randomized studies.[38–41] In these studies, there was no benefit to early mobilization at any time point.

Although these 5 studies represent high-level quality randomized trials, one major difficulty with carrying out such trials is the ability to document patient compliance with rehabilitation protocols. Patients assigned to early motion may not always be consistent with their assigned exercises or physical therapy, and patients assigned to delayed therapy may participate in activities that make them noncompliant with immobilization instructions. Both motion and healing rates would be affected by noncompliance. Unfortunately, it is not possible for the investigators to document and analyze protocol noncompliance. Koh and colleagues[41] did report on patient compliance and found a high rate of compliance with 4 weeks of immobilization, but only a 63% compliance rate in patients randomized to an 8-week immobilization period. Therefore, although some of these trials were adequately powered to show no difference, the 2 various rehabilitation protocols may be more similar due to patient noncompliance.

The results of these randomized trials can be interpreted and used differently. In young patients with small- or medium-sized tears, early mobilization may result in better function at earlier time points without risking re-tear. On the other hand, patients with risk factors for re-tearing, such as older age, larger tears, or revision repairs, may benefit from a delayed rehabilitation protocol in which the repair site is protected. From a socioeconomic standpoint, the cost of multiple physical therapy visits early in the postoperative period is significant, and there likely is a large cost-savings benefit with delayed rehabilitation. However, therapist-guided visits early in the postoperative period seem to result in better early range of motion and function. Although transient, this early functional improvement is not inconsequential to the patient.

SUMMARY

Tendon-to-bone healing is a mechanically sensitive process. Complete removal of load may under-stimulate the repair site, whereas repetitive overload can cause gap formation and repair site failure. Tendon healing responds best to controlled loading. Recent high-quality studies comparing various post-operative rehabilitation protocols have suggested that early passive range of motion does not risk failure of the repair unless the protocol is too aggressive. Early therapist-guided exercises may result in better range of motion in the short term, but none of these studies have shown a long-term benefit.

REFERENCES

1. Yamaguchi K, Ditsios K, Middleton WD, et al. The demographic and morphological features of rotator cuff disease. A comparison of asymptomatic and symptomatic shoulders. J Bone Joint Surg Am 2006; 88(8):1699–704.
2. Ensor KL, Kwon YW, Dibeneditto MR, et al. The rising incidence of rotator cuff repairs. J Shoulder Elbow Surg 2013;22(12):1628–32.
3. Colvin AC, Egorova N, Harrison AK, et al. National trends in rotator cuff repair. J Bone Joint Surg Am 2012;94(3):227–33.
4. Millett PJ, Warth RJ, Dornan GJ, et al. Clinical and structural outcomes after arthroscopic single-row versus double-row rotator cuff repair: a systematic review and meta-analysis of level I randomized clinical trials. J Shoulder Elbow Surg 2014;23(4): 586–97.
5. Russell RD, Knight JR, Mulligan E, et al. Structural integrity after rotator cuff repair does not correlate with patient function and pain: a meta-analysis. J Bone Joint Surg Am 2014;96(4):265–71.
6. McElvany MD, McGoldrick E, Gee AO, et al. Rotator cuff repair: published evidence on factors associated with repair integrity and clinical outcome. Am J Sports Med 2015;43(2):491–500.
7. Galatz LM, Ball CM, Teefey SA, et al. The outcome and repair integrity of completely arthroscopically repaired large and massive rotator cuff tears. J Bone Joint Surg Am 2004;86A(2):219–24.
8. Chen M, Xu W, Dong Q, et al. Outcomes of single-row versus double-row arthroscopic rotator cuff repair: a systematic review and meta-analysis of current evidence. Arthroscopy 2013;29(8):1437–49.
9. DeHaan AM, Axelrad TW, Kaye E, et al. Does double-row rotator cuff repair improve functional outcome of patients compared with single-row technique? A systematic review. Am J Sports Med 2012; 40(5):1176–85.
10. Thomopoulos S, Genin GM, Galatz LM. The development and morphogenesis of the tendon-to-bone insertion—what development can teach us about healing. J Musculoskelet Neuronal Interact 2010; 10(1):35–45.
11. Killian ML, Cavinatto L, Galatz LM, et al. The role of mechanobiology in tendon healing. J Shoulder Elbow Surg 2012;21(2):228–37.
12. Banes AJ, Horesovsky G, Larson C, et al. Mechanical load stimulates expression of novel genes in vivo and in vitro in avian flexor tendon cells. Osteoarthritis and cartilage/OARS. Osteoarthritis Cartilage 1999;7(1):141–53.
13. Wang JH. Mechanobiology of tendon. J Biomech 2006;39(9):1563–82.
14. Uchida H, Tohyama H, Nagashima K, et al. Stress deprivation simultaneously induces over-expression of interleukin-1beta, tumor necrosis factor-alpha, and transforming growth factor-beta in fibroblasts and mechanical deterioration of the tissue in the patellar tendon. J Biomech 2005;38(4):791–8.
15. Galatz LM, Charlton N, Das R, et al. Complete removal of load is detrimental to rotator cuff healing. J Shoulder Elbow Surg 2009;18(5):669–75.
16. Thomopoulos S, Zampiakis E, Das R, et al. The effect of muscle loading on flexor tendon-to-bone healing in a canine model. J Orthop Res 2008; 26(12):1611–7.
17. Woo SL, Gomez MA, Amiel D, et al. The effects of exercise on the biomechanical and biochemical properties of swine digital flexor tendons. J Biomech Eng 1981;103(1):51–6.
18. Narici MV, Maganaris CN. Adaptability of elderly human muscles and tendons to increased loading. J Anat 2006;208(4):433–43.
19. Pryce BA, Watson SS, Murchison ND, et al. Recruitment and maintenance of tendon progenitors by TGFbeta signaling are essential for tendon formation. Development (Cambridge, England) 2009; 136(8):1351–61.
20. Schweitzer R, Chyung JH, Murtaugh LC, et al. Analysis of the tendon cell fate using Scleraxis, a specific

marker for tendons and ligaments. Development (Cambridge, England) 2001;128(19):3855–66.

21. Murchison ND, Price BA, Conner DA, et al. Regulation of tendon differentiation by scleraxis distinguishes force-transmitting tendons from muscle-anchoring tendons. Development (Cambridge, England) 2007; 134(14):2697–708.

22. Li Z, Yang G, Khan M, et al. Inflammatory response of human tendon fibroblasts to cyclic mechanical stretching. Am J Sports Med 2004;32(2):435–40.

23. Woo SL, Gomez MA, Sites TJ, et al. The biomechanical and morphological changes in the medial collateral ligament of the rabbit after immobilization and remobilization. J Bone Joint Surg Am 1987;69(8): 1200–11.

24. Woo SL, Gomez MA, Woo YK, et al. Mechanical properties of tendons and ligaments. II. The relationships of immobilization and exercise on tissue remodeling. Biorheology 1982;19(3):397–408.

25. Yang G, Im HJ, Wang JH. Repetitive mechanical stretching modulates IL-1beta induced COX-2, MMP-1 expression, and PGE2 production in human patellar tendon fibroblasts. Gene 2005;363:166–72.

26. Arnoczky SP, Tian T, Lavagnino M, et al. Ex vivo static tensile loading inhibits MMP-1 expression in rat tail tendon cells through a cytoskeletally based mechanotransduction mechanism. J Orthop Res 2004;22(2):328–33.

27. Arnoczky SP, Lavagnino M, Egerbacher M, et al. Loss of homeostatic strain alters mechanostat "set point" of tendon cells in vitro. Clin Orthop Relat Res 2008;466(7):1583–91.

28. Soslowsky LJ, Carpenter JE, DeBano CM, et al. Development and use of an animal model for investigations on rotator cuff disease. J Shoulder Elbow Surg 1996;5(5):383–92.

29. Soslowsky LJ, Thomopoulos S, Tun S, et al. Neer Award 1999. Overuse activity injures the supraspinatus tendon in an animal model: a histologic and biomechanical study. J Shoulder Elbow Surg 2000; 9(2):79–84.

30. Thomopoulos S, Williams GR, Soslowsky LJ. Tendon to bone healing: differences in biomechanical, structural, and compositional properties due to a range of activity levels. J Biomech Eng 2003;125(1):106–13.

31. Carpenter JE, Flanagan CL, Thomopoulos S, et al. The effects of overuse combined with intrinsic or extrinsic alterations in an animal model of rotator cuff tendinosis. Am J Sports Med 1998;26(6):801–7.

32. Carpenter JE, Thomopoulos S, Flanagan CL, et al. Rotator cuff defect healing: a biomechanical and histologic analysis in an animal model. J Shoulder Elbow Surg 1998;7(6):599–605.

33. Gimbel JA, Van Kleunen JP, Williams GR, et al. Long durations of immobilization in the rat result in enhanced mechanical properties of the healing supraspinatus tendon insertion site. J Biomech Eng 2007;129(3):400–4.

34. Sarver JJ, Peltz CD, Dourte L, et al. After rotator cuff repair, stiffness–but not the loss in range of motion–increased transiently for immobilized shoulders in a rat model. J Shoulder Elbow Surg 2008;17(Suppl 1): 108S–13S.

35. Peltz CD, Sarver JJ, Dourte LM, et al. Exercise following a short immobilization period is detrimental to tendon properties and joint mechanics in a rat rotator cuff injury model. J Orthop Res 2010;28(7): 841–5.

36. Hettrich CM, Rodeo SA, Hannafin JA, et al. The effect of muscle paralysis using Botox on the healing of tendon to bone in a rat model. J Shoulder Elbow Surg 2011;20(5):688–97.

37. Lee BG, Cho NS, Rhee YG. Effect of two rehabilitation protocols on range of motion and healing rates after arthroscopic rotator cuff repair: aggressive versus limited early passive exercises. Arthroscopy 2012;28(1):34–42.

38. Cuff DJ, Pupello DR. Prospective randomized study of arthroscopic rotator cuff repair using an early versus delayed postoperative physical therapy protocol. J Shoulder Elbow Surg 2012;21(11):1450–5.

39. Kim YS, Chung SW, Kim JY, et al. Is early passive motion exercise necessary after arthroscopic rotator cuff repair? Am J Sports Med 2012;40(4):815–21.

40. Keener JD, Galatz LM, Stobbs-Cucchi G, et al. Rehabilitation following arthroscopic rotator cuff repair: a prospective randomized trial of immobilization compared with early motion. J Bone Joint Surg Am 2014;96(1):11–9.

41. Koh KH, Lim TK, Shon MS, et al. Effect of immobilization without passive exercise after rotator cuff repair: randomized clinical trial comparing four and eight weeks of immobilization. J Bone Joint Surg Am 2014;96(6):e44.

42. Garofalo R, Conti M, Notarnicola A, et al. Effects of one-month continuous passive motion after arthroscopic rotator cuff repair: results at 1-year follow-up of a prospective randomized study. Musculoskelet Surg 2010;94(Suppl 1):S79–83.

Posterior Shoulder Instability in Overhead Athletes

Edward S. Chang, MD[a],*, Nicholas J. Greco, MD[b],
Michael P. McClincy, MD[b], James P. Bradley, MD[c]

KEYWORDS

- Posterior shoulder instability • Throwers • Overhead athletes • Zone-specific repair
- Surgical technique • Arthroscopic posterior capsulolabral reconstruction

KEY POINTS

- Overhead-throwing athletes are at a risk for injury to the posterior glenolabral complex from repetitive microtrauma.
- The examiner must differentiate between adaptive capsular laxity and pathologic instability.
- Repair constructs using suture anchors improves the athlete's prospect in returning to throwing activities.
- Knotless fixation should be used above the glenoid equator to minimize iatrogenic humeral head abrasion from suture knots.
- The overhead athlete's kinetic chain and throwing mechanics must be analyzed and corrected to decrease the risk of reinjury.

INTRODUCTION

Overhead, or throwing, athletes are a distinct group of patients with unique injuries to the shoulder. Much attention has been placed on superior labral anterior to posterior tears and undersurface rotator cuff tears in the overhead athlete. Posterior shoulder instability in throwers, although less common than the previously mentioned conditions, can lead to similar symptoms as well as decreased performance.[1,2]

Three general etiologies of posterior instability of the shoulder exist: acute traumatic, repetitive microtrauma, and atraumatic or ligamentous laxity. In athletes, the most common cause of posterior instability is from repetitive microtrauma to the posterior capsulolabral complex.[3,4] This is especially well documented in football lineman, weight lifters, and rowers. Recent studies have shown these athletes return to preinjury level of competition following arthroscopic capsulolabral reconstruction.[5]

Posterior shoulder instability in overhead athletes presents a unique and difficult challenge. Often, this group has an inherent capsular laxity and/or humeral retroversion to accommodate the range of motion (ROM) necessary to throw.[6] This adaptation makes the diagnosis of posterior capsulolabral pathology challenging, as the examiner must differentiate between adaptive capsular laxity and pathologic instability. Further complicating matters, the intraoperative surgeon must

[a] Department of Orthopaedic Surgery, Sports Medicine Institute at Inova Medical Group, Inova Health System, 8501 Arlington Boulevard, Suite 200, Fairfax, VA 22031, USA; [b] Department of Orthopaedic Surgery, University of Pittsburgh Medical Center, 3200 South Water Street, Pittsburgh, PA 15203, USA; [c] Department of Orthopaedic Surgery, University of Pittsburgh Medical Center, 200 Delafield Road, 200 Medical Arts Building, Suite 4010, Pittsburgh, PA 15125, USA
* Corresponding author.
E-mail address: Chang.edward@gmail.com

Orthop Clin N Am 47 (2016) 179–187
http://dx.doi.org/10.1016/j.ocl.2015.08.026
0030-5898/16/$ – see front matter © 2016 Elsevier Inc. All rights reserved.

find the delicate balance of achieving stability while still allowing the necessary ROM. To our knowledge, there have been only 2 studies documenting the results of arthroscopic posterior capsulolabral reconstruction in overhead athletes.[1,2]

INDICATIONS AND CONTRAINDICATIONS

Initial nonoperative management consists of cessation of throwing activities for a minimum of 4 to 6 weeks. This is followed by intensive muscle strengthening about the shoulder, along with analyzing and correcting throwing mechanics and deficits along the kinetic chain.

For patients who fail nonoperative treatment, wish to continue overhead athletics, and are willing to adhere to the lengthy postoperative rehabilitation protocol, arthroscopic posterior capsulolabral reconstruction is indicated.

SURGICAL TECHNIQUE
Preoperative Planning

At our institution, we generally use magnetic resonance arthrography (MRA) to aid in the diagnosis as well as for preoperative planning. MRA allows the surgeon to identify anatomic pathologies, namely posterior labral tears, patulous posterior capsule, and, on rare occasions, posterior humeral avulsion of the glenohumeral ligament. We find MRA especially useful in the diagnosis of incomplete and concealed posterior labral tears (Kim lesion) that would otherwise appear benign on diagnostic arthroscopy.

Patient Positioning

Following administration of general anesthesia, the patient is positioned in the lateral decubitus position. An inflatable beanbag is used to hold the patient in place. All bony prominences are well padded and an axillary gel roll is placed under the nonoperative arm.

A lateral arm positioner is used on the operative arm and 10 pounds of traction is added. The arm is then positioned in 45° of abduction and 20° of forward flexion.

DIAGNOSTIC ARTHROSCOPY

We begin with a standard diagnostic arthroscopy from the posterior portal. This portal, which later becomes a working portal, is slightly lateral than the traditional portal, allowing a less acute trajectory to the posterior glenoid.

An anterior portal is then made within the rotator interval and a 6-mm cannula (Arthrex, Naples, FL) is placed. The arthroscope is then placed through the anterior cannula to evaluate the posterior capsulolabral complex. We typically use a 70° arthroscope to aid in visualization (Fig. 1) and place an 8.25-mm cannula (Arthrex).

GLENOID AND LABRUM PREPARATION

Once the labral tear has been identified, the labrum is sharply lifted off the glenoid using an elevator from the posterior portal (Figs. 2 and 3). We then perform a meticulous glenoid preparation, using a combination of a shaver, bur, and rasp to produce a fresh, bleeding surface for the labrum to heal to (Fig. 4).

ZONE-SPECIFIC REPAIR

Once the labrum and glenoid are adequately prepared, we use a zone-specific capsulolabral reconstruction centered around the glenoid equator (Fig. 5). Below the equator (9 o'clock to 6 o'clock), we use 2.4-mm SutureTak anchors

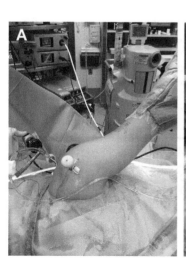
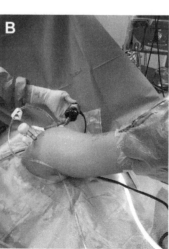

Fig. 1. (A, B) The patient is positioned in a lateral decubitus position with the arm abducted 45° and flexed 20°.

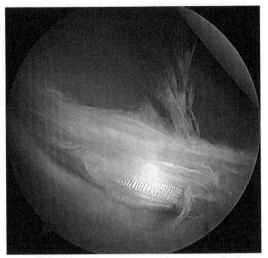

Fig. 2. Arthroscopic view of a posterior labral tear from the posterior portal.

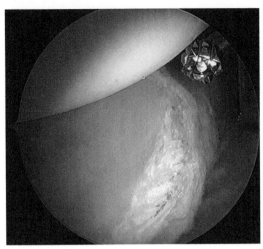

Fig. 4. Instruments are brought in from the posterior portal for glenoid and labral preparation.

(Arthrex), securing the labrum to the glenoid via suture knots.

Superior to the equator, we use knotless labral fixation with 2.9-mm Short PushLock anchors and 1.5-mm LabralTape (Arthrex). The advantage of knotless fixation above the equator include minimizing the potential risk of postoperative iatrogenic humeral head chondral injury from suture knot abrasion. The broader surface area of the LabralTape versus traditional suture may also have a biomechanical advantage, with a larger maximum load to failure.

SUBEQUATORIAL REPAIR

A percutaneous posterolateral portal at the 7 o'clock position is confirmed with a spinal needle. This portal is typically 2 cm lateral to the posterolateral acromion. A stab incision is made and followed by the insertion of the 2.4-mm SutureTak anchor (**Figs. 6** and **7**). If placement of a second anchor is anticipated, the drill guide should not be removed to prevent multiple iatrogenic holes into the capsule.

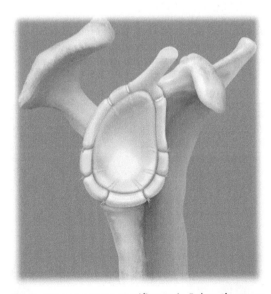

Fig. 5. We use a zone-specific repair. Below the equator (9 o'clock to 6 o'clock), suture knots are used to secure the labrum. Above the equator (9 o'clock to 12 o'clock), knotless fixation is used to avoid iatrogenic chondral injury to the humeral head.

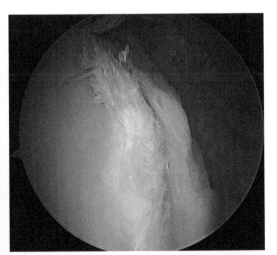

Fig. 3. The posterior labral tear is visualized from the anterior portal using a 70° arthroscope.

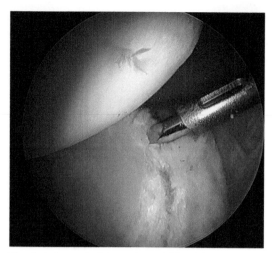

Fig. 6. Subequatorial repair: a drill guide is inserted percutaneously.

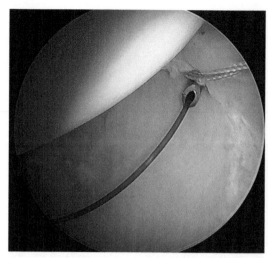

Fig. 8. A curved suture passer is introduced through the posterior cannula and passed behind the labrum just inferior to the anchor.

The sutures are retrieved through the posterior cannula. A curved suture passer is then introduced through the same cannula and passed behind the labrum just inferior to the anchor. The suture closest to the labrum is identified and eventually passed around the labrum. We then secure the labrum with a sliding Weston knot, followed by 3 alternating half-hitches (**Figs. 8–10**). These steps can be repeated if another anchor is indicated below the glenoid equator.

SUPRAEQUATORIAL REPAIR

The curved suture passer is reintroduced into the posterior cannula and passed through the labrum just inferior to the anticipated anchor location. A free LabralTape is then passed around the labrum (**Figs. 11** and **12**). The 2 free ends of the labral tape are then placed through the 2.9-mm PushLock anchor eyelet. Following drilling of the glenoid, the 2.9-mm PushLock anchor is slid down the Labral-Tape and inserted into the pilot hole, while maintaining gentle tension on the limbs. The anchor is then malleted into the glenoid and the limbs are cut flush (**Figs. 13–15**). These steps can be repeated through the same cannula (**Fig. 16**).

POSTERIOR CAPSULE CLOSURE

Following any posterior labral repair, we close the posterior capsule using a No. 1 Polydioxanone (PDS) suture as described by Schneeberger and Yian (**Fig. 17**).[7]

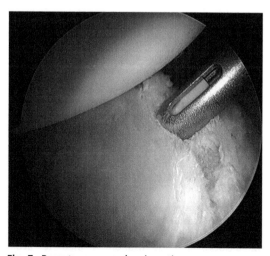

Fig. 7. Percutaneous anchor insertion.

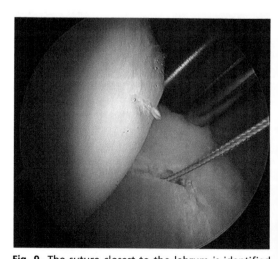

Fig. 9. The suture closest to the labrum is identified and eventually shuttled behind the labrum.

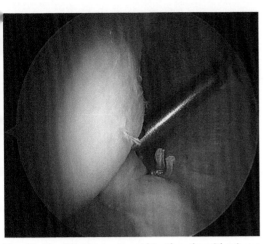

Fig. 10. The labrum is secured to the glenoid using a sliding Weston knot, followed by 3 half-hitches.

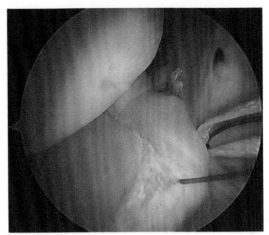

Fig. 12. A 2-mm LabralTape (Arthrex) is shuttled behind the labrum. The LabralTape is then fed through the eyelet of the 2.9-mm PushLock anchor (Arthrex).

POSTOPERATIVE CARE

Following surgery, the patient is placed in an Ul-traSling (DonJoy, Carlsbad, CA), which immobilizes the shoulder in 30° abduction while preventing internal rotation. Patients are permitted to perform active elbow and wrist motion along with passive scaption exercises.

Once the sling is discontinued, active-assisted ROM and isometric internal and external exercises are initiated. By 2 to 3 months postoperatively, the patient should achieve full passive and active motion.

An interval throwing program is initiated 4 months postoperatively. The first phase consists of flat ground throwing with an emphasis on mechanics and strengthening. The goal of the graduated program is for the athlete to throw pain free at a specified number of feet before progressing to the next distance.

The second phase emphasizes throwing from the mound. The athlete begins throwing fastballs at 50%, progressing to 75% and 100%. At this time, breaking balls can be initiated in a similar fashion. Once the athlete is throwing pain-free simulated innings for 2 weeks, he or she is permitted to return to competition.

OUTCOMES

Posterior shoulder instability is an increasingly recognized pathology among athletes, and

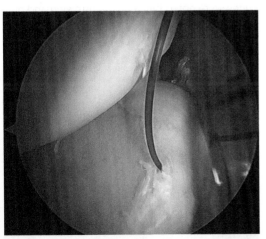

Fig. 11. Supraequatorial repair. The curved suture passer is first introduced and passed around the labrum just inferior to the anticipated anchor location.

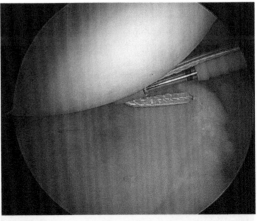

Fig. 13. Following drilling of the glenoid, the anchor slides down the LabralTape and into the joint.

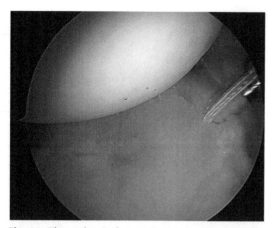

Fig. 14. The anchor is then malleted into the drill hole.

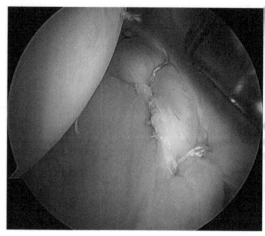

Fig. 16. Final labral repair construct following insertion of a third anchor to secure the labrum in a knotless fashion.

numerous recent studies have documented the effectiveness of arthroscopic capsulolabral reconstruction in returning these injured athletes to their preinjury sports activities.[1,2,8–18] The significant demands placed on the glenohumeral joint in overhead throwing sports put these athletes at a significant risk for developing posterior shoulder instability. Despite the heightened risks for injury to the posterior glenolabral complex in these overhead-throwing athletes, there has been a relative paucity in data detailing their recovery after operative intervention until recently. **Table 1** displays the available posterior shoulder instability literature that specifically mentioned the inclusion of overhead athletes. Most of these studies are extremely variable with regard to surgical technique.

The treatment of posterior shoulder instability in all athletes has evolved with time and with growing surgeon experience with arthroscopic techniques. Through this change, there has been a transition from open to arthroscopic-based surgical approaches as well as a shift from nonanatomic to anatomic repairs. In considering these modern treatment strategies, there have been 2 studies detailing the outcomes of posterior shoulder instability in throwers following arthroscopic capsulolabral repair.

Radkowski and colleagues[1] compared a group of 27 throwers to 71 nonthrowing athletes across all levels of competition following arthroscopic capsulolabral repair. The results indicated that 55% of throwing athletes were able to return to their preinjury level of performance. Another 30% of the athletes returned to competition but did not achieve the same level of performance. When considering postoperative American Shoulder and Elbow Surgeons (ASES) scores, stability scores, strength, and ROM, no substantial differences were noted between the throwing and nonthrowing athletes.

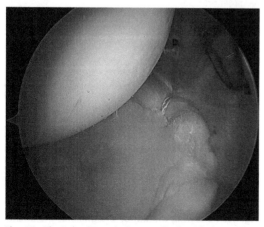

Fig. 15. The LabralTape is then cut flush with the anchor.

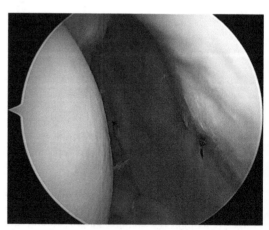

Fig. 17. The posterior portal is closed with a No. 1 PDS suture.

Table 1
Available posterior shoulder instability literature that specifically mentions the inclusion of overhead athletes

Authors	No. Patients/ Shoulders	Surgical Technique	No./ Percentage of Throwers	Mean Follow-up, mo	Instability Recurrence Rate, %	Outcome in Throwers
Tibone & Ting,[12] 1990	20/20	Plication with staple	9/45%	69	30.0	4/9 throwers unsatisfied
Bradley & Tibone,[18] 1993	40/40	Posterior suture/staple	23/57%	48	27.5	28% of overhead athletes return to preinjury competition level
Bigliani et al,[17] 1995	34/35	Posterior capsular shift	5/14.3%	60	11.4	All 5 throwers noted impairment
Wolf & Eakin,[16] 1998	14/14	Capsular plication with suture anchor	>1	33	7.1	No individual results on throwers
Misamore & Facibene,[13] 2000	14	Posterior capsular shift	3/21.4%	45	7.1	No individual results on throwers
Kim et al,[10] 2003	27/27	Capsular plication with suture anchor	3/11.1%	39	3.7	No individual results on throwers
Williams et al,[15] 2003	26/27	Bioabsorbable tack	3/11.5%	61	7.7	1 of 3 failed, requiring revision surgery
Radkowski et al,[1] 2008	98/107	Capsulolabral reconstruction with suture anchor	27/25%	27	10.2	23/27 (85%) returned to sport, 15/27 (56%) returned to preinjury level
McClincy et al,[2] 2015	96/96	Capsulolabral reconstruction with suture anchor	48/50%	37	4	41/48 (85%) returned to sport, 29/60 (48%) returned to preinjury level

Data from Refs. [1,2,10,12,13,15–18]

The study by McClincy and colleagues[2] served as a continuation of the data of Radkowski and colleagues.[1] The benefit of an expanded population of throwing athletes who had undergone arthroscopic capsulolabral reconstruction, it was possible to analyze the postoperative outcomes between throwers and nonthrowers in a case-matched fashion. This study included 48 competitive throwers and matched them pairwise based on age, gender, and level of competition to a non-throwing athlete.

At a mean of 37 months, no differences were noted between the ASES scores, stability scores, ROM, strength, or return to play rates between the throwing and nonthrowing cohorts. When considering the throwing athletes, clinically and statistically significant improvements were noted in ASES scores (both pain and functional domains) and stability scores between the preoperative and latest follow-up values. Sixty percent of throwing athletes were able to return to their preinjury level of throwing competition postoperatively; 25% of throwers were able to return to sport but did not achieve their preinjury level of performance. When considering a cohort of 18 pitchers, 50% of these athletes returned to their preinjury performance level. This study also noted that the inclusion of suture anchors into the glenolabral repair construct significantly improved the likelihood of an athlete returning to competitive throwing activities. They concluded that anchor-based repairs likely improved the stability of the repair construct to withstand the throwing-specific forces generated by these athletes. The suture anchor constructs did not appear to influence return to play rates in nonthrowing populations.

Surgical pearls and pitfalls

1. The initial posterior portal should be placed lateral to the traditional portal to allow a less acute trajectory for anchor placement.

2. Meticulous bony glenoid preparation is critical to provide the optimal healing environment for the labrum.

3. Knotless labral fixation above the glenoid equator minimizes the risk of iatrogenic humeral head abrasion from suture knots.

4. The greatest challenge lies in finding the delicate balance between achieving glenohumeral stability while preserving the necessary capsular laxity for the overhead athlete to achieve his or her "slot" position.

5. The posterior portal should be closed to prevent an unnecessary stress on the repair.

SUMMARY

Overhead-throwing athletes are at risk for injury to the posterior glenolabral complex from repetitive microtrauma. The examiner must differentiate between adaptive capsular laxity and pathologic instability. Repair constructs using suture anchors improves the athlete's prospect in returning to throwing activities. However, knotless fixation should be used above the glenoid equator to minimize iatrogenic humeral head abrasion from suture knots. However, it is imperative that the overhead athlete's kinetic chain and throwing mechanics are analyzed and corrected to decrease the risk of reinjury.

REFERENCES

1. Radkowski CA, Chhabra A, Baker CL, et al. Arthroscopic capsulolabral repair for posterior shoulder instability in throwing athletes compared with nonthrowing athletes. Am J Sports Med 2008;36:693–9.

2. McClincy MP, Arner JW, Bradley JP. Posterior shoulder instability in throwing athletes: a case-matched comparison of throwers and non-throwers. Arthroscopy 2015;31:1041–51.

3. Provencher MT, LeClere LE, King S, et al. Posterior instability of the shoulder: diagnosis and management. Am J Sports Med 2011;39:874–86.

4. Robinson CM, Aderinto J. Recurrent posterior shoulder instability. J Bone Joint Surg Am 2005; 87:883–92.

5. Arner JW, McClincy MP, Bradley JP. Arthroscopic stabilization of posterior shoulder instability is successful in American football players. Arthroscopy 2015. http://dx.doi.org/10.1016/j.arthro.2015.02.022.

6. Kinsella SD, Thomas SJ, Huffman GR, et al. The thrower's shoulder. Orthop Clin North Am 2014;45: 387–401.

7. Schneeberger AG, Yian EH. Arthroscopic posterior portal closure. Arthroscopy 2004;20(Suppl 2):110–2.

8. Bradley JP, Baker CL, Kline AJ, et al. Arthroscopic capsulolabral reconstruction for posterior instability of the shoulder: a prospective study of 100 shoulders. Am J Sports Med 2006;34:1061–71.

9. Bradley JP, McClincy MP, Arner JW, et al. Arthroscopic capsulolabral reconstruction for posterior instability of the shoulder: a prospective study of 200 shoulders. Am J Sports Med 2013;41: 2005–14.

10. Kim S-H, Ha K-I, Park J-H, et al. Arthroscopic posterior labral repair and capsular shift for traumatic unidirectional recurrent posterior subluxation of the shoulder. J Bone Joint Surg Am 2003;85-A:1479–87.

11. Savoie FH, Holt MS, Field LD, et al. Arthroscopic management of posterior instability: evolution of technique and results. Arthroscopy 2008;24:389–96.

12. Tibone J, Ting A. Capsulorrhaphy with a staple for recurrent posterior subluxation of the shoulder. J Bone Joint Surg Am 1990;72:999–1002.

13. Misamore GW, Facibene WA. Posterior capsulorrhaphy for the treatment of traumatic recurrent posterior subluxations of the shoulder in athletes. J Shoulder Elbow Surg 2000;9:403–8.

14. Fuchs B, Jost B, Gerber C. Posterior-inferior capsular shift for the treatment of recurrent, voluntary posterior subluxation of the shoulder. J Bone Joint Surg Am 2000;82:16–25.

15. Williams RJ, Strickland S, Cohen M, et al. Arthroscopic repair for traumatic posterior shoulder instability. Am J Sports Med 2003;31:203–9.

16. Wolf EM, Eakin CL. Arthroscopic capsular plication for posterior shoulder instability. Arthroscopy 1998;14:153–63.

17. Bigliani LU, Pollock RG, McIlveen SJ, et al. Shift of the posteroinferior aspect of the capsule for recurrent posterior glenohumeral instability. J Bone Joint Surg Am 1995;77:1011–20.

18. Tibone JE, Bradley JP. The treatment of posterior subluxation in athletes. Clin Orthop Relat Res 1993;(291):124–37.

Surgical Treatment of Distal Biceps Ruptures

Laura E. Stoll, MD, Jerry I. Huang, MD*

KEYWORDS

- Distal biceps rupture • Distal biceps repair • Fixation method • Surgical techniques • Treatment

KEY POINTS

- Distal biceps ruptures usually occur with eccentric extension loading of a flexed elbow.
- Surgical approaches include 1-incision or 2-incision techniques, with recent studies showing more anatomic repair and improved supination strength with a 2-incision technique.
- Fixation techniques include bone tunnels, cortical buttons, suture anchors, and biotenodesis screws, with cadaveric studies demonstrating the highest load to failure with the button technique.
- Chronic distal biceps ruptures may require reconstruction with tendon allograft due to proximal retraction, and often, poor tissue quality.
- Complications include elbow stiffness, heterotopic ossification, rerupture, and nerve injury, with transient neurapraxia of the lateral antebrachial cutaneous nerve being the most common.

INTRODUCTION

Distal biceps ruptures occur at an incidence of 1.2 per 100,000 persons per year, representing 10% of all biceps injuries.[1] They are most common in the dominant arm of men in their fifth and sixth decades of life. Other risk factors include smoking, anabolic steroid use, and weight-lifting.[1–3] The mechanism of injury is most commonly forceful eccentric extension of a flexed elbow. Proposed etiologies of distal biceps ruptures include decreased vascularity,[4] impingement of the tendon against the radial tuberosity,[4,5] and degenerative changes due to radial bursitis.[6] There is a 2-cm hypovascular zone in the distal biceps between the perforators from branches of the posterior interosseous recurrent artery distally and the brachial artery proximally.[4] With forearm rotation from supination to pronation, there is a 50% reduction of the space in the proximal radioulnar joint, with the distal biceps occupying 85% of the space in full forearm pronation.

ANATOMY

The biceps functions as the primary supinator of the forearm and also contributes to elbow flexion, along with the brachialis muscle. The biceps muscle is innervated by a single branch of the musculocutaneous nerve 61% of the time at an average of 134 mm distal to the acromion.[7] The biceps is formed by 2 muscular bellies, the long head and the short head, whose corresponding tendons continue as discrete units with well-defined attachments to the bicipital tuberosity.[8,9] At the musculotendinous junction, the short head is medial to the long head. The distal biceps externally rotates as it approaches the radial tuberosity (right distal biceps spirals counterclockwise, whereas the left spirals clockwise) (**Fig. 1**A).[8–10] The long head, which is more radial, inserts proximally on the bicipital tuberosity, and makes up the bulk of the distal biceps tendon and functions as a powerful supinator. The short head inserts distally as it fans out over a larger surface area, allowing it

The authors have no financial interests in any of the products or techniques mentioned and have received no external support related to this study.
Department of Orthopaedics and Sports Medicine, University of Washington Medical Center, Seattle, WA 98105, USA
* Corresponding author. 4245 Roosevelt Way Northeast, Box 354740, Seattle, WA 98105.
E-mail address: jihuang@uw.edu

Orthop Clin N Am 47 (2016) 189–205
http://dx.doi.org/10.1016/j.ocl.2015.08.025

A   B

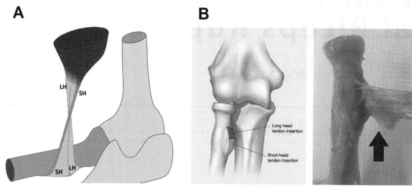

Fig. 1. (A) The distal biceps externally rotates as it approaches the radial tuberosity with distinct long head (LH) and short head (SH) tendon insertions. (B) The long head, which is more radial, inserts proximally on the bicipital tuberosity, and makes up the bulk of the distal biceps tendon and functions as a powerful supinator. Patients can have a partial rupture involving only the short head of the biceps (*arrow*). (*From* [A] Schmidt CC, Jarrett CD, Brown BT. The distal biceps tendon. J Hand Surg Am 2013;38A:811–21, with permission; and [B] Athwal GS, Steinmann SP, Rispoli DM. The distal biceps tendon: footprint and relevant clinical anatomy. J Hand Surg Am 2007;32A:1226–7; with permission.)

to serve more as an elbow flexor.[11] A bursa lies between the tendon and volar radius. The bicipital aponeurosis, or lacertus fibrosis, is a broad sheet of connective tissue that originates from the short head of the biceps and fans out medially to blend with the deep anterior forearm fascia, inserting onto the ulna. An intact lacertus fibrosis prevents proximal retraction of the distal biceps tendon.

The distal biceps footprint is on the posterior and ulnar aspect of the bicipital tuberosity, centered 30 to 65° anterior to the coronal plane with forearm fully supinated, allowing the tuberosity to increase the moment arm as well as serve as a cam with the forearm pronated (**Fig. 1**B).[12,13] The bicipital tuberosity has a mean length of 22 to 24 mm and width of 15 to 18 mm, whereas the distal biceps tendon inserts in a ribbon-shaped configuration with mean dimensions ranging from 18 to 21 mm in length and 3 to 7 mm in width.[8,13,14] Therefore, the footprint occupies only 63% of the length and 13% of the width of the biceps tuberosity.

CLINICAL EVALUATION

Diagnosis begins with a thorough history and physical. Distal biceps ruptures usually occur from a single traumatic event with sudden eccentric contraction while the elbow is flexed. Patients report a sudden sharp pain and sometimes an audible "pop." Those with acute ruptures will demonstrate ecchymosis in the antecubital fossa with pain and weakness with resisted forearm supination. Patients may note some weakness with flexion, but this is more subtle, as the brachialis and brachioradialis are still competent to provide

strong elbow flexion. In complete ruptures, there is a palpable absence of the distal biceps tendon with a hook test. O'Driscoll and colleagues[15] described the hook sign, which is the inability to hook the examiner's finger under the lateral edge of the intact biceps tendon when the elbow is flexed to 90° and the forearm is supinated. The hook test is reported to have a sensitivity and specificity of 100%. It is important to hook under the lateral edge of the tendon, as one could mistake the lacertus fibrosus as intact tendon. The squeeze test, as described by Ruland and colleagues,[16] is 96% sensitive for diagnosing a complete distal biceps rupture. The patient sits relaxed with the elbow flexed at 60° and the forearm in slight pronation. When the examiner squeezes the biceps with both hands, the forearm should supinate if the biceps is intact. One may also note a "reverse Popeye sign," from proximal retraction of the biceps muscle (**Fig. 2**).

Partial ruptures can be difficult to diagnose. Those with partial ruptures will have pain with palpation over the distal biceps tendon and pain with resisted supination, but will have a palpably intact tendon. Ruch and colleagues[17] found that partial distal biceps tears tended to involve disruption of the lateral side of the tendon insertion involving the short head of the biceps. The lateral portion of the tendon is more of the gliding portion and abuts the bursa and thus chronic inflammation of the bursa may make the lateral portion of the tendon more prone to rupture.[18]

Plain radiographs will often be normal, but are important to obtain to assess for other elbow trauma. MRI is not necessary for a diagnosis in acute ruptures, but may be helpful in chronic

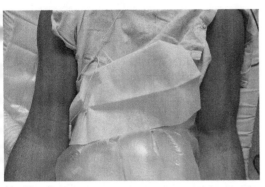

Fig. 2. Patient with a "reverse Popeye" sign in the injured, right arm compared with the uninjured contralateral left arm.

ruptures to determine the level of retraction of the biceps tendon, in diagnosing partial ruptures, and in determining if the tear is at the insertion or at the musculotendinous junction. It is best if a FABS (flexed, abducted, and supinated) view is obtained,[19] as this gives the clearest view of the longitudinal course of the biceps tendon and allows for optimal fat-suppressed images. The patient lies prone with the shoulder abducted 180°, the elbow flexed, and the forearm supinated. Ultrasound also can be used to diagnose distal biceps tears, but does not give the same level of detail as MRI.[20,21]

MANAGEMENT

As patients lose a significant amount of supination strength without repair, surgery is recommended for those with complete distal biceps ruptures as long as they are fit to undergo an operation. With nonoperative management of a complete rupture, patients will lose 21% to 55% of supination strength, 79% of supination endurance, 10% to 40% of flexion strength, and 30% of flexion endurance.[2,22–24] In a study of 22 middle-aged active men, Hetsroni and colleagues[25] compared the outcome of 12 patients managed with early repair with those managed nonoperatively. Although there was no significant difference in functional outcomes, with 9 of 10 nonoperative patients reporting good to excellent outcomes, there was a mean loss of 20% of maximum flexion strength, 35% maximum supination strength, and 40% loss of supination endurance. Patients are often pain free but complain of weakness and easily fatigue with activities requiring forearm supination, such as use of a screwdriver. Acute repair should occur within 2 to 3 weeks of injury. Delay can lead to need for more extensile exposure as well as difficulties with mobilization and reduction of the tendon due to adhesion formation and loss of

elasticity. With the 2-incision technique, complications are more common in repairs performed after 2 to 3 weeks.[26,27]

Low-demand patients or those with significant medical comorbidities are not candidates for distal biceps repair. Patients with associated neurologic deficits that would inhibit a functional recovery would also not benefit from a repair. In addition, patients should be able to comply with the postoperative rehabilitation protocol and be willing to abide by activity limitations. Patients receiving workers compensation take longer to return to work and have worse Disabilities of the Arm, Shoulder, and Hand (DASH) scores.[28]

In partial distal biceps ruptures, patients with high-grade tears (>50%) or those with persistent pain following conservative management also may benefit from surgical repair, although the management of partial tears is debatable. Debriding the distal biceps tendon in partial tears has been described,[29] but most advocate for complete detachment and debridement, followed by reattachment of the distal biceps tendon.[30–32]

SURGICAL APPROACH

The 2-incision technique was initially described by Boyd and Anderson[33] in an attempt to minimize anterior dissection and avoid complications associated with a large single incision. It went on to be modified by Kelly and colleagues,[27] whereby the extensor carpi ulnaris (ECU) muscle is split and dissection of the supinator muscle and subperiosteal dissection of the ulna is minimized in an attempt to decrease the risk of radioulnar synostosis. With the development of new fixation techniques, such as suture anchors,[34] cortical buttons,[35] and biotenodesis screws,[36] there has been a trend toward single-incision repairs in the past decade to limit the theoretic complications of heterotopic ossification and bridging radioulnar synostosis thought to be associated with the 2-incision technique.

Single-Incision Technique

For the anterior approach, either a longitudinal or transverse incision can be used. Longitudinally, the incision begins 1 to 2 cm distal to the elbow crease, medial to the brachioradialis muscle, and extends distally. A transverse incision, centered over the bicipital tuberosity, is more cosmetic and can be used in acute ruptures, but limits extension of the incision. For more extensive exposure in chronic cases or tendon reconstruction, a long S-shaped incision is typically used.

After incision through skin and subcutaneous tissue, care must be taken to identify and protect the lateral antebrachial cutaneous (LABC) nerve (**Fig. 3**A). Proximally the interval is between the brachioradialis and brachialis, whereas more distally the interval is between the brachioradialis and pronator teres. The distal biceps tendon stump can be found proximally in a bursal sac. After control of the tendon is gained, the biceps tuberosity is exposed. The leash of radial recurrent vessels overlies the proximal radius and frequently needs to be ligated to expose the bicipital tuberosity and avoid a postoperative hematoma. The superficial radial nerve is deep to the brachioradialis muscle (**Fig. 3**B). The posterior interosseous nerve pierces the supinator muscle to lie on the dorsal radial cortex. It is important to keep the forearm fully supinated to protect the PIN when working around the bicipital tuberosity from the anterior approach.

Two-Incision Technique

In the 2-incision technique, the same anterior incision is used. The dorsal incision is made over the bicipital tuberosity, found by pronating and supinating the arm or using a blunt instrument through the anterior incision to tent the skin. Dissection is carried down through the common extensors, preferably the ECU, and the supinator is split, taking care to avoid exposure of the ulna. The forearm is placed in pronation for preparation of the bicipital tuberosity.

Single-Incision Posterior Technique

Kelly and colleagues[37] described a single-incision technique using a posterior incision for partial distal biceps ruptures. This involves making an incision centered over the mobile wad centered over the tuberosity. The extensor digitorum communis fascia is split in line with the skin incision. With the forearm pronated, the supinator is split longitudinally over the radial tuberosity, exposing the biceps tendon at its insertion. Partial tears usually occur on the undersurface of the tendon. A stay suture is placed and the tendon is pulled out of the wound to expose the torn undersurface of the tendon. The intact tendon is then detached,

any degenerative tissue is debrided, and the tendon is then repaired.

SURGICAL PROCEDURE
Exposure and Mobilization of the Biceps Tendon

In acute ruptures, the tendon can be identified in the proximal portion of the wound. In subacute ruptures, a pseudosheath can form as the tendon retracts. The tendon stump should be freed from scarring and adhesions to allow for full mobilization of the tendon. In chronic ruptures, tendon retraction can be limited by an intact lacertus fibrosis. However, with significant retraction, a second transverse incision proximally may be necessary to allow for extraction and mobilization of the tendon. In partial ruptures, the intact tendon can be traced down to its insertion on the tuberosity. Tourniquet deflation can aid in tendon retrieval in cases in which the tendon has retracted proximally. Endoscopic visualization has been described for visualization of the distal biceps tendon in partial ruptures to determine the extent of the tear.[38]

Bicipital Tuberosity Preparation

No matter the fixation technique, the bicipital tuberosity is exposed and prepared. The forearm should be held at 90° of supination to minimize the risk to the PIN. The location of the drill hole for the suture anchor, cortical button, or tenodesis screw is determined. Fluoroscopy can aid in determining the correct location. All bony debris should be removed with judicious irrigation, and there should be minimal trauma to the periosteum to help prevent heterotopic ossification formation.

Tendon Preparation

Use a running, locking, braided, synthetic suture such as No. 2 FiberWire (Arthrex Inc., Naples, FL) to prepare the tendon, incorporating 3 to 4 cm of the distal tendon. Any degenerative distal tendon stumps should be debrided back to healthy fibers.

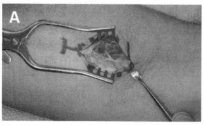 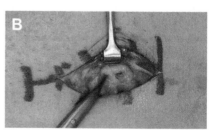

Fig. 3. Surgical approach through anterior incision demonstrating the location of the LABC adjacent to the mobile wad (*A*) as well as the superficial radial nerve, which lies deep to the brachioradialis muscle (*B*).

FIXATION TECHNIQUES
Bone Tunnel Fixation

Before the advent of more advanced fixation techniques, bone tunnel fixation using a 2-incision exposure was the standard of treatment.[2] The distal biceps tendon is prepared as described previously through the anterior approach. With the forearm supinated, a hemostat is advanced along the medial border of the radius and into the dorsolateral forearm to help identify the site for the posterolateral incision. The forearm is pronated, which helps protect the PIN and brings the bicipital tuberosity into view. Through the posterolateral incision, the tuberosity is prepared by first inserting a guide pin, then drilling out the cortex so it can accommodate the tendon (usually a 10–15-mm oval-shaped hole). Next, 2 or 3, 2-mm holes are drilled through the lateral side of the radius. The sutures attached to the biceps tendon are shuttled into the posterior incision and then passed from the cavitation in the tuberosity and out the drill holes. The sutures are then tied across the bone bridges with the forearm in pronation.

Suture Anchors

This technique is performed through a single anterior incision. After exposure of the bicipital tuberosity, 2 suture anchors are placed ulnarly over the tuberosity to reproduce the insertion footprint of the biceps tendon. The advantage of suture anchors is that there is a reduced risk of PIN injury, as the posterior cortex is not drilled. However, biomechanical studies suggest that there is a lower load to failure (see later in this article). In addition, there is a risk of gapping between the distal biceps tendon and the bicipital tuberosity, as the tendon is not pulled into a bone tunnel.

Biotenodesis Screw

This technique also uses a single-incision approach. After exposure of the bicipital tuberosity, a guide pin is drilled through the tuberosity. The tendon width is measured and a drill hole is made in the bicipital tuberosity with a cannulated drill to accommodate the tendon in addition to the biotenodesis screw. The tendon is prepared with a No. 2 nonabsorbable suture, which is then passed through the biotenodesis screw. The distal end of the tendon is passed to the screw tip. The screw and the tendon are advanced into the hole and screwed flush with the tuberosity.

Cortical Button

Bain and colleagues[35] first described the use of a suspensory cortical button for distal biceps repair.

After exposure and mobilization of the tendon, the bicipital tuberosity is prepared. In the technique originally described by Bain and colleagues,[35] a slotted Beath pin is drilled from anterior to posterior through the bicipital tuberosity. Drilling should be slightly ulnarly to minimize risk of injury to the posterior interosseous nerve. Care also must be taken to avoid overdrilling beyond the far cortex, as to avoid damage to the dorsal soft tissues, in particular, the PIN. A cannulated drill is then used to overdrill both cortices to accommodate the button. The anterior hole is enlarged with a surgical burr or an appropriately sized cannulated drill (typically 7–9 mm) to accommodate the width of the tendon. The tendon is prepared with a running, locking synthetic suture with the 2 tails placed through the 2 middle holes of the cortical button. Note that 2 to 3 mm of suture must be left between the distal tendon stump and the cortical button as to allow the button to pass through the dorsal cortex and be flipped. Two separate sutures are passed through the 2 outer holes of the cortical button; these will act as control sutures. The Beath pin is then passed through the drill hole and out the dorsal forearm soft tissue. The sutures are then toggled and pulled to flip and lock the button over the dorsal radial cortex. An appropriately tensioned biceps tendon will feel taut with the elbow extended. Fluoroscopy is used to confirm the cortical button is secured against the dorsal radial cortex. Gapping between the cortical button and the dorsal cortex can lead to entrapment of dorsal compartment soft tissues, including the PIN.

Sethi and Tibone[39] described the "tension-slide" use of the cortical button. This obviates the need to predetermine the length of suture between the button and the biceps. It also eliminates the need to pass a Beath pin or needle through the dorsal forearm, thereby decreasing the risk of injury to the PIN. After tendon preparation, one strand of suture is threaded through the left and then back up through the right hole of the cortical button. Similarly, another suture is threaded in the opposite direction, through the right and then back up the left hole of the cortical button, so that the suture ends face the biceps tendon. The guide pin is drilled from anterior to posterior over the radial tuberosity. The anterior cortex is prepared with a cannulated drill after sizing the diameter of the distal biceps tendon (**Fig. 4**A). The button inserter is used to push the button with an attached distal biceps tendon through the prepared radial tuberosity hole (**Fig. 4**B). Tension is pulled on the strands to secure the button down (**Fig. 4**C). Fixation can be supplemented with an interference screw to push the distal biceps insertion ulnarly, in a more anatomic position (**Fig. 4**D).

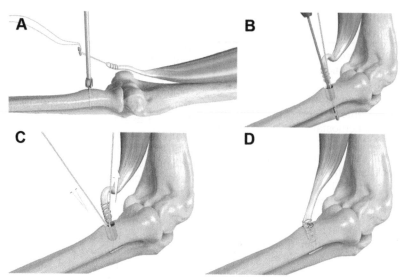

Fig. 4. Tension slide technique for distal biceps repair. A 3.2-mm guide pin is drilled bicortically over the bicipital tuberosity, followed by overdrilling of the near cortex (*A*). The cortical button is then pushed through the far cortex (*B*) and flipped to sit flush against the dorsal cortex by toggling the 2 suture ends (*C*). A biotenodesis screw can be placed to seat the distal biceps tendon more ulnarly, in a more anatomic position (*D*). (*Courtesy of* Arthrex, Inc, Naples, FL, USA; with permission.)

The "tension slide" technique with a cortical button has been shown to lead to less gap formation,[40] but this has not translated into clinical outcome improvements.[41,42]

Siebenlist and colleagues[43,44] reported good outcomes when using intramedullary cortical button fixation, which, in theory, minimizes the risk of PIN injury. In addition, by using double intramedullary buttons, more anatomic repair of both heads of the distal biceps can be performed to its footprint.[45]

Single-Incision Power Optimizing Cost-effective Technique

Tanner and colleagues[46] recently reported on the SPOC (single-incision power optimizing cost-effective) method of distal biceps repair. This technique is thought to reattach the biceps tendon onto the more anatomic posterior and ulnar surface of the radius, thereby maximizing supination strength, but using a standard single anterior incision (**Fig. 5**). This is an intraosseous suture technique using two 2.5-mm drill holes over the bicipital tuberosity. Using suture shuttles, the distal biceps tendon is repaired down to the posterior aspect of the drill hole over the tuberosity, back to its more anatomic and biomechanically advantageous position.

COMPARISON OF FIXATION TECHNIQUES
Biomechanical Comparison

The repaired distal biceps needs to allow for early active range of motion in the postoperative period.

The mean force required to actively flex the elbow ranges from 25 N at 30°, up to 67 N at 130° of elbow flexion. The force required to rupture the intact distal biceps is approximately 200 N.[47,48] Current fixation methods include bone tunnels, suture anchors, biotenodesis screws, and cortical buttons. Traditional bone tunnel techniques fail through fracture between the bone tunnels, suture breakage, and the suture cutting. A systematic review in 2008 found that the cortical button had the best pullout strength.[41] However, most current repair techniques approach native tendon strength (**Table 1**).[42,47,49–53] Adding an interference screw to the cortical button construct does not add strength to the construct. However, it enables a more anatomic construct by pushing the distal biceps more ulnarly, closer to the anatomic footprint on the bicipital tuberosity, which may improve clinical outcomes.[40,54]

With regard to displacement of the repair after cyclical loading, Mazzocca and colleagues[42] also found that the cortical button had the highest load to failure, but had the second highest displacement (3.42 mm) as compared with bone tunnel (3.55 mm), suture anchor (2.33 mm), and interference screw (2.14 mm) fixation. Thirty-percent of suture anchor repairs failed during this series, with no failures seen in the cortical button specimen. The theoretic clinical significance of displacement is loss of fixation and altered healing in the setting of early postoperative range of motion. Displacement and pistoning of the tendon during early motion could inhibit tendon-bone healing.

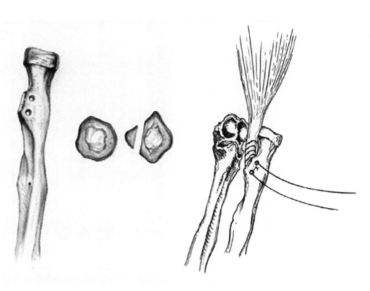

Fig. 5. The SPOC distal biceps repair technique described by Tanner and colleagues[46] uses two 2.5-mm drill holes and suture shuttles, which allows for repair of the distal biceps in a more anatomic posterior position using a standard anterior incision. (*From* Tanner C, Johnson T, Muradov P, et al. Single incision power optimizing cost-effective (SPOC) distal biceps repair. J Shoulder Elbow Surg 2013;22(3):306–7; with permission.)

Clinical Outcomes Comparison

Although cortical button fixation is stronger than suture anchor techniques biomechanically, Olsen and colleagues[55] recently looked at functional outcomes between repairs performed with a cortical button and interference screw versus a suture anchor (**Table 2**).[46,56–63] They found that those who underwent suture anchor repair had slightly better DASH scores at 6 months, but had more subjective weakness (although quantitative flexion and supination strength were similar). The cortical button group had slightly better pronation, whereas the suture anchor group had slightly better flexion and supination. All of these differences were small. Potapov and colleagues[64] reported a case series raising the concern of possible osteolysis of the radius after distal biceps tendon repair with a bioabsorbable screw. Eighteen of 19 patients treated with a bioabsorbable screw developed osteolysis,

but there was no clear clinical correlation. Cain and colleagues[61] found that neurapraxias were more common with cortical button fixation, and rerupture rates were greater with suture anchors. They did not find a significant difference in the overall complication rate among fixation methods. However, this study was underpowered and included some chronic ruptures. Interestingly, there was no difference in complication rates when repair occurred more than 4 weeks after surgery.

In their systematic review of 498 elbows that underwent acute repair, Watson and colleagues[65] found that bone tunnel (20.4%) and cortical button (0%) methods had significantly lower complication rates than did suture anchors (26.4%) or intraosseous screws (44.8%). However, the sample size for cortical button fixation lacked the statistical power to say that this method is superior to the others.

Table 1
Biomechanical comparison of fixation techniques

Study	Bone Tunnel	Suture Anchor	Interference/ Tenodesis Screw	Cortical Button
Greenberg et al,[49] 2003	178N	254N (Mitek G4 Super)	—	584N
Lemos et al,[50] 2004	203N	263N (Super Mitek × 2)	—	—
Idler et al,[47] 2006	125N	—	178N	—
Spang et al,[51] 2006	—	230N (5 mm × 2)	—	275N
Krushinski et al,[52] 2007	—	147N (3.5 mm × 2)	192N (8 mm)	—
Kettler et al,[53] 2007	210N	196–225N (Various)	131N (5.5 mm)	259N
Mazzocca et al,[42] 2007	310N	381N	232N	440N

Data from Refs.[42,47,49–53]

Table 2
Outcomes table (literature review past 5 years)

Reference	Elbows	Fixation	Incisions	Functional Outcomes	Complications
Recordon et al,[56] 2015	19	Cortical button	2	4.8/5 satisfaction score 53% with subjective weakness. Supination 81°, Pronation 72° Extension −3° Flexion 129° 95% low-speed torque. 103% high-speed torque. 4.5% reduction in endurance.	30% with some degree of LABC paresthesias in the 2 groups, only 2 did not resolve 3 asymptomatic HO
	27	Bone tunnels	2	4.4/5 satisfaction score 55% with subjective weakness Supination 82°, Pronation 70° Extension −2° Flexion 125° 90% low-speed torque. 101% high-speed torque. 3.4% reduction in endurance	1 HO with reduced motion, 3 with asymptomatic HO
Shields et al,[57] 2015	20	Cortical button	1	DASH 4.5 Loss of flexion of 1.8 lb Loss of supination of 6.8 lb Loss of flexion 3.4° Loss of supination 7.4° Loss of pronation 0.4°	2 superficial infections, 4 SRN paresthesias
	21	Bone tunnels	2	DASH 5.7 Loss of flexion of 1.96 lb Loss of supination of 11.2 lb Loss of flexion 1.8° Loss of supination 10.8° Loss of pronation 11.3°	1 SRN paresthesia

Study	N	Technique		Outcomes	Complications
Hansen et al,[58] 2014	27	Suture anchor	1	DASH 10.7 97–106% flexion strength 80–86% supination strength 66–75% supination work	Not reported
Olsen et al,[55] 2014	20	Cortical button with interference screw	1	DASH 4.5 Loss of elbow flex-ext 3° Loss of supination 7° No loss of pronation No difference in strength	2 superficial infections 4 SRN paresthesias
	17	Suture anchor	—	DASH 10.3 Gain of elbow flexion-extension 2° Loss of supination 2° Loss of pronation 4°	1 SRN paresthesia 3 LABC paresthesias 1 ulnar nerve paresthesia
Siebenlist et al,[59] 2014	49	Suture anchor	1	DASH 7.9 86% satisfied or highly satisfied Loss of supination 3°	HO in 39%, but no significant difference in functional outcome 4 suture anchor failures
Banerjee et al,[60] 2013	27	Cortical button	1	DASH 1.9 Elbow flexion 91.7% Supination 87.8%	4 transient PIN palsies, 2 persistent SRN palsies 1 HO 1 disengaged button
Tanner et al,[46] 2013	30	Bone tunnels (SPOC technique)	1	93% of patients no pain and returned to normal activities Supination strength 91%	1 partial laceration LABC 1 transient cubital tunnel syndrome 1 repair failure
Cain et al,[61] 2012	10	Bone tunnels	2	Not reported	1 LABC palsy 1 superficial infection 30 LABC palsies 9 SRN palsies 3 PIN palsies 4 HO
	119	Suture anchor	1	Not reported	
	69	Cortical button	1	Not reported	4 reruptures 2 superficial infections 21 LABC palsies 2 SRN palsies 4 PIN palsies 2 HO

(continued on next page)

Table 2
(continued)

Reference	Elbows	Fixation	Incisions	Functional Outcomes	Complications
Grewal et al,[62] 2012	47	Suture anchors	1	No difference in DASH scores No difference in isometric extension, pronation, or supination strength. 10% advantage in flexion strength bone tunnels compared with suture anchors	19 LABC palsies 2 nerve deficits requiring reoperation 3 reruptures 1 HO
	43	Bone tunnels	2		3 LABC palsies 1 rerupture 1 HO
Citak et al,[63] 2011	15	Intraosseous screws	1	No difference in DASH scores, duration of surgery, or ROM	2 LABC palsies
	24	Suture anchors	1		3 LABC palsies 3 reruptures 2 with postoperative stiffness, 1 wound problem
	25	Bone tunnels	2		1 LABC palsies

Abbreviations: DASH, disabilities of the arm, shoulder and hand; HO, heterotopic ossification; LABC, lateral antebrachial cutaneous; PIN, posterior interosseous nerve; SPOC, single-incision power optimizing cost-effective.

Data from Refs.[46,55–63]

CLINICAL OUTCOMES OF SINGLE-INCISION VERSUS 2-INCISION TECHNIQUES

It has long been thought that the 2-incision technique hampers forearm motion and leads to an increased risk of synostosis. This has been perpetuated throughout the years with limited recent evidence to support this hypothesis.[41,66] Karunaker and colleagues,[67] published a study of 21 distal biceps ruptures repaired using the original Boyd-Anderson technique, and showed loss of rotation in 19% of elbows and loss of flexion in 5% of elbows. Thirty-eight percent of elbows showed loss of supination endurance and 33% had loss of flexion endurance. This study reported a 35% complication rate, with heterotopic ossification (HO) being the most common complication. In 2008, Chavan and colleagues[41] performed a systematic review of single-incision versus double-incision repairs. There were more unsatisfactory results in the double-incision group compared with the single-incision group, with most unsatisfactory results in the double-incision group being related to loss of forearm motion and strength. These results were likely biased, though, as the analysis included older studies that used the original Boyd-Anderson approach, which has been replaced by the muscle-splitting posterior approach, with less soft tissue stripping and trauma. However, multiple more recent studies have failed to show a difference in functional outcomes after single-incision versus double-incision repairs.[57,62,63] El-Hawary and colleagues[68] prospectively compared 9 patients who had undergone a 2-incision technique with those who had undergone a single-incision technique. At 1 year, the single-incision group had 11.7 more degrees of elbow flexion than the 2-incision group (142.8 vs 131.1°). There was no difference in supination strength or motion or in flexion strength.

Grewal and colleagues[62] examined the clinical outcomes of 91 patients randomized to either a single-incision repair with 2 suture anchors or a 2-incision repair with transosseous drill holes. There was no difference in isometric strength relative to the uninvolved arm at 1 year between the 2 groups in extension (104% vs 106%), pronation (99% vs 103%), or supination (98% vs 92%). There was a 10% advantage in isometric flexion strength at 1 year when the 2-incision technique was used (104% vs 94%). There was no difference in functional outcome scores both at short-term and long-term follow-up or in range of motion. However, there was a significantly higher complication rate, primarily neuropraxias of the LABC, in the single-incision technique. There was no difference in incidence of HO formation.

Three reruptures occurred in the single-incision technique and 1 in the 2-incision technique. The investigators noted that these reruptures were due to noncompliance rather than fixation technique.

A recent systematic review by Watson and colleagues[65] reviewed 22 studies (498 elbows) of primary repairs of acute distal biceps tendon ruptures. Overall, the complication rate was 24.5%, with no difference between single-incision or 2-incision techniques. The most common complication was LABC neurapraxia (9.6%), which was higher for single-incision approaches. There were 4.4% of patients who developed HO, with 3.1% for single-incision and 7.0% for 2-incision techniques (P = .06). Stiffness was more common in the 2-incision technique (5.7% for 2-incision vs 1.8% for single-incision technique). Rerupture rate was 1.8% for the single-incision and 1.2% for the 2-incision technique. Synostosis occurred at a rate of 2.3% for the 2-incision technique, whereas there were no reported cases for the single-incision technique.

TUNNEL PLACEMENT

Anatomic tunnel placement and repair has become the subject of recent distal biceps repair research. The biceps tendon inserts eccentrically onto the tuberosity, which, when combined with the height of the tuberosity, increases the supinator vector and allows for a cam effect.[13,14,54]

Incision technique may affect the ability to obtain anatomic tunnel placement. Jobin and colleagues[69] reported a more anatomic position of the tunnel using a 2-incision technique compared with a single-incision technique. Hasan and colleagues[70] also looked at cadaveric models of tunnel placement and found a larger percentage of the footprint was covered when using a 2-incision technique compared with a single-incision technique (73.4% vs 9.7%, P = .002).

Henry and colleagues[71] looked at the biomechanical effects of different attachment sites of the tendon and found a trend toward loss of supination when the tendon was placed in a more anterior position on the bicipital tuberosity. Prud'homme-Foster and colleagues[72] and Schmidt and colleagues,[73] had similar findings. Using MRI to study single-incision repairs with a cortical button, they found all tendons to be healed, but the repair was often nonanatomic, being on average 73° radial compared with the uninjured controls. There was a significant loss (67%) of supination strength with the forearm in 60° of supination compared with the uninjured side. They concluded that with anterior nonanatomic repairs, the tendon unwraps as the forearm supinates, losing its ability to generate torque.[54,73]

Hansen and colleagues[58] reviewed computed tomography scans in 27 patients who underwent single-incision distal biceps repairs with suture anchors and found that on average anchor placement was 50° radial to the apex of the tuberosity. Patients in this study had significantly decreased supination strength and work (80%–86% and 66%–75% of the contralateral side, respectively). Therefore, when the tendon is repaired in a nonanatomic position anteriorly and more radially, the biceps cannot generate a supination force when the forearm is supinated.

A study by Forthman and colleagues[12] measured the bicipital tuberosity to be, on average, in 65° of pronation relative to the coronal plane of the radius. They also estimated that the maximum angle of tuberosity orientation to allow for operative instrumentation using an anterior approach is 60° of pronation. Thirty-five percent of their specimens had the bicipital tuberosity oriented in greater than 60° of pronation, inferring that anatomic repair could not be achieved, suggesting that use of a single-incision technique may lead to nonanatomic and hence less biomechanically favorable repairs.

Chronic Ruptures

When the biceps tendon has been retracted proximally into the arm for a prolonged period, surgical options include reconstruction using grafts or direct repair while keeping the elbow in flexion. Reconstruction techniques include using interposing tendon autografts, such as semitendinosus,[74] flexor carpi radialis,[75] and hamstring,[76] as well as use of Achilles,[77,78] semitendinosus,[79,80] and tibialis tendon allografts. The tendon graft is interwoven into the retracted biceps tendon in a Pulvertaft fashion or directly sutured into the distal biceps muscle belly and remaining tendon as an onlay tendon graft[77,81] Snir and colleagues[79] reported on 18 patients who underwent reconstruction with allograft. All patients had full range of motion, with reported 4.7/5 strength in elbow flexion and forearm supination.

Bosman and colleagues[82] reported good outcomes with direct repair of distal biceps ruptures without interposition grafts in patients with delayed presentation with mean time to repair of 79 days (range 35–116 days) using a cortical button technique and immediate mobilization. Morrey and colleagues[83] recently reviewed their experience with 188 distal biceps repairs and described a series of 23 cases in which acute repair was performed in greater than 60° of flexion with a 2-incision technique without need for tendon allograft. Allograft augmentation with Achilles was used in cases in which there was no distinct tendon stump. Intraoperatively, the amount of tensioning with elbow passive extension guided postoperative care and slow increase in elbow extension to allow for stress relaxation of the muscle. All patients reported that they were subjectively "very satisfied" or "satisfied," although 3 patients reported fatigue. The average flexion-extension arc was 3 to 138° with 82° of pronation and 78° of supination. Compared with matched controls, there was no difference in pain, range of motion, satisfaction, return to work, strength, or complications. The authors feel that use of a tendon graft in reconstruction does not restore the proper muscle-tendon length, and thus does not restore normal elbow active muscle function and mechanics.

COMPLICATIONS AND MANAGEMENT

Minor complications following distal biceps repair are not uncommon, with reported rates as high as 36%.[61] Complications include LABC, PIN, and radial sensory nerve injuries, infection, HO, radioulnar synostosis, hematoma, and tendon rerupture. In a systematic review by Chavan and colleagues,[41] the total complication rate for single-incision repairs was 18%, whereas that of double-incision repairs was 16% (P = .88). The more recent systematic review by Watson and colleagues[65] reported a 23.9% complication rate for the single-incision technique compared with 25.7% for the 2-incision technique (P = .32).

Nerve injuries are the most common complication of distal biceps repairs.[26,62,66] The rate of LABC neuropraxia has been reported to be 3% to 26%.[26,27,61,62,66,84] PIN palsy has been reported in up to 9% of patients undergoing distal biceps repair, but is usually transient and resolves spontaneously.[27,61,66,85,86] In a review of 9 patients of 280 who developed a postoperative PIN palsy, all had complete resolution of symptoms at an average of 3 months.[86] The PIN, which courses around the radial neck to enter the supinator, can be injured from retraction, direct injury from the guide wire or drill, or placement of the cortical button itself. The PIN is located on average 10 to 14 mm from a Kirschner-wire pointed in an ulnar-only trajectory on the bicipital tuberosity, with the distance dramatically decreasing when pointing in the distal or radial direction (**Table 3**).[87–90]

HO and radioulnar synostosis result in loss of motion (**Fig. 6**A, B). The prevalence of HO has been reported to be 2% to 10%.[26,27,62,68] The risk of HO formation was higher with repairs

Table 3
Drill trajectory during distal biceps repairs and proximity of the posterior interosseous nerve

Drill Trajectory	90° to Axis of Radius	30° Ulnar-Distal	30° Ulnar	30° Distal	30° Radial
Thumm et al,[87] 2015	—	8.0 mm	14.0 mm	1.0 mm	—
Duncan et al,[88] 2013	8.9 mm	—	—	0.6 mm	—
Lo et al,[89] 2011	11.2 mm	—	16.0 mm	2.0 mm (45° distal)	4.2 mm
Saldua et al,[90] 2008	10.86 mm	—	16.28 mm	—	—

Data from Refs.[87–90]

performed via a traditional Boyd-Anderson technique, which stripped the soft tissues off of the ulna posteriorly. The incidence has decreased since the advent of the double-incision muscle-splitting approach.[27,91] In an MRI study by Schmidt and colleagues,[54] 42% of repairs had bone formation within the repaired tendon; however, this did not correlate with significant differences in outcome scores. Similarly, Greenberg and colleagues[49] reported an asymptomatic HO rate of 36%. In a small study of patients who had HO excision, Wysocki and Cohen[92] found a loss of 9° of forearm pronation compared with the uninvolved side. Compared with a matched cohort that had an uncomplicated distal biceps repair, there were no differences in isokinetic torque, endurance strength, or DASH scores, or arc of motion, although this study was a small sample size. Prophylaxis against HO has been reported, but there are no studies that prove its efficacy in preventing HO formation.[62] Radioulnar synostosis initially presents as pain and swelling that eventually leads to loss of rotation, especially supination. If radioulnar synostosis occurs, surgical resection and radiotherapy can help improve motion and prevent recurrence, but should be performed once the soft tissue has become quiescent.[93]

Rerupture rates have been reported to be as high as 4.4%.[27,61,62,84,94] In the recent systematic review by Watson and colleagues,[65] the rerupture rate was 1.6% overall. Reruptures occur more frequently with suture anchor repairs compared with use of cortical buttons, bone tunnels, or intraosseous screws.[63,84] In the series of Cain and colleagues,[61] all 4 reruptures occurred in the suture-anchor group, whereas Cusick and colleagues[84] also reported reruptures only in the suture anchor patients.

POSTOPERATIVE CARE

A bulky splint with the elbow flexed to 90° and the forearm supinated can be applied postoperatively but should be removed within 1 to 2 weeks. Motion begins at this point. Some surgeons prefer to place the patient in a Bledsoe brace after splint removal; however, studies have shown great recovery of motion without increased complications using an unbraced, immediate motion protocol.[35,39,91,95,96] Terminal extension should be avoided for 6 weeks postoperatively. Early range of motion should be performed, emphasizing forearm rotation. If a brace is used, it is discontinued at 6 weeks postoperatively. Resistive strengthening

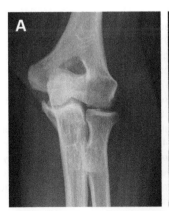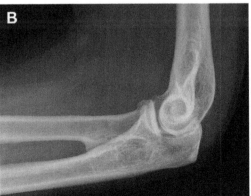

Fig. 6. AP (*A*) and Lateral (*B*) radiographs demonstrate bridging heterotopic ossification with complete proximal radioulnar synostosis following a 2-incision distal biceps repair with limited forearm rotation.

should not begin until 10 to 12 weeks postoperatively. Patients should be counseled that it will be 3 to 5 months before they can return to heavy activities.

SUMMARY

Active patients benefit from distal biceps repair to restore full function. Partial tears can be treated nonoperatively, but those involving more than 50% of the tendon benefit from repair. Both single-incision and 2-incision techniques have successful outcomes, but can be complicated by nerve injuries, HO formation, and radioulnar synostosis. Ultimately, the surgeon should proceed with whatever approach he or she feels most comfortable with; however, anterior approach–only repairs may make restoration of the anatomic footprint difficult. Biomechanical studies suggest that cortical button fixation is the strongest fixation method. However, future randomized studies are needed to examine fixation methods, as they relate to anatomic repair and in vivo strength, as well as functional outcomes. There is a lack of controlled prospective studies in the literature and, thus, one technique of fixation cannot be recommended.

REFERENCES

1. Safran MR, Graham SM. Distal biceps tendon ruptures: incidence, demographics, and the effect of smoking. Clin Orthop 2002;404:275–83.
2. Morrey BF, Askew LJ, An KN, et al. Rupture of the distal tendon of the biceps brachii. A biomechanical study. J Bone Joint Surg Am 1985;67:418–21.
3. Visuri T, Lindholm H. Bilateral distal biceps tendon avulsions with use of anabolic steroids. Med Sci Sports Exerc 1994;26:941–4.
4. Seiler JG, Parker LM, Chamberland P. The distal biceps tendon: two potential mechanisms involved in its rupture: arterial supply and mechanical impingement. J Shoulder Elbow Surg 1995;4:149–56.
5. Davis WM, Yassine Z. An etiological factor in tear of the distal tendon of the biceps brachii. J Bone Joint Surg Am 1956;38–A:1365–8.
6. Hughes JS, Morrey BF. Injury of the flexors of the elbow: biceps tendon injury. In: Morrey BF, Sanchez-Sotelo J, editors. The elbow and its disorders. 4th edition. Philadelphia: Elsevier Health Sciences; 2009. p. 518–35.
7. Vicente DP, Calvet PF, Burgaya AC, et al. Innervation of biceps brachii and brachialis: anatomical and surgical approach. Clin Anat 2005;18:186–94.
8. Athwal GS, Steinmann SP, Rispoli DM. The distal biceps tendon: footprint and relevant clinical anatomy. J Hand Surg Am 2007;32:1225–9.
9. Eames MHA, Bain GI, Fogg QA, et al. Distal biceps tendon anatomy: a cadaveric study. J Bone Joint Surg Am 2007;89:1044–9.
10. Kulshreshtha R, Singh R, Sinha J, et al. Anatomy of the distal biceps brachii tendon and its clinical relevance. Clin Orthop 2007;456:117–20.
11. Jarrett CD, Weir DM, Stuffmann ES, et al. Anatomic and biomechanical analysis of the short and long head components of the distal biceps tendon. J Shoulder Elbow Surg 2012;21:942–8.
12. Forthman CL, Zimmerman RM, Sullivan MJ. Cross-sectional anatomy of the bicipital tuberosity and biceps brachii tendon insertion: relevance to anatomic tendon repair. J Shoulder Elbow Surg 2008;17:522–6.
13. Hutchinson HL, Gloystein D, Gillespie M. Distal biceps tendon insertion: an anatomic study. J Shoulder Elbow Surg 2008;17:342–6.
14. Mazzocca AD, Cohen M, Berkson E. The anatomy of the bicipital tuberosity and distal biceps tendon. J Shoulder Elbow Surg 2007;16:122–7.
15. O'Driscoll SW, Goncalves LBJ, Dietz P. The hook test for distal biceps tendon avulsion. Am J Sports Med 2007;35:1865–9.
16. Ruland CRT, Dunbar CSRP, Bowen CJD. The biceps squeeze test for diagnosis of distal biceps tendon ruptures. Clin Orthop 2005;437:128–31.
17. Ruch DS, Watters TS, Wartinbee DA, et al. Anatomic findings and complications after surgical treatment of chronic, partial distal biceps tendon tears: a case cohort comparison study. J Hand Surg Am 2014;39:1572–7.
18. Kannus P, Józsa L. Histopathological changes preceding spontaneous rupture of a tendon. A controlled study of 891 patients. J Bone Joint Surg Am 1991;73:1507–25.
19. Giuffre BM, Moss MJ. Optimal positioning for MRI of the distal biceps brachii tendon: flexed abducted supinated view. AJR Am J Roentgenol 2004;182: 944–6.
20. Belli P, Costantini M, Mirk P, et al. Sonographic diagnosis of distal biceps tendon rupture: a prospective study of 25 cases. J Ultrasound Med 2001;20:587–95.
21. Brigido MK, De Maeseneer M, Morag Y. Distal biceps brachii. Semin Musculoskelet Radiol 2013;17: 20–7.
22. Baker BE, Bierwagen D. Rupture of the distal tendon of the biceps brachii. Operative versus nonoperative treatment. J Bone Joint Surg Am 1985; 67:414–7.
23. Freeman CR, McCormick KR, Mahoney D. Nonoperative treatment of distal biceps tendon ruptures compared with a historical control group. J Bone Joint Surg Am 2009;91:2329–34.
24. Nesterenko S, Domire ZJ, Morrey BF. Elbow strength and endurance in patients with a ruptured distal

biceps tendon. J Shoulder Elbow Surg 2010;19: 184–9.

25. Hetsroni I, Pilz-Burstein R, Nyska M, et al. Avulsion of the distal biceps brachii tendon in middle-aged population: is surgical repair advisable? A comparative study of 22 patients treated with either nonoperative management or early anatomical repair. Injury 2008;39:753–60.

26. Bisson L, Moyer M, Lanighan K, et al. Complications associated with repair of a distal biceps rupture using the modified two-incision technique. J Shoulder Elbow Surg 2008;17:S67–71.

27. Kelly EW, Morrey BF, O'Driscoll SW. Complications of repair of the distal biceps tendon with the modified two-incision technique. J Bone Joint Surg Am 2000;82A:1575–81.

28. Atanda A, O'Brien DF, Kraeutler MJ, et al. Outcomes after distal biceps repair in patients with workers' compensation claims. J Shoulder Elbow Surg 2013;22:299–304.

29. Dürr HR, Stäbler A, Pfahler M, et al. Partial rupture of the distal biceps tendon. Clin Orthop 2000;374: 195–200.

30. Bourne MH, Morrey BF. Partial rupture of the distal biceps tendon. Clin Orthop 1991;271:143–8.

31. Dellaero DT, Mallon WJ. Surgical treatment of partial biceps tendon ruptures at the elbow. J Shoulder Elbow Surg 2006;15:215–7.

32. Vardakas DG, Musgrave DS, Varitimidis SE. Partial rupture of the distal biceps tendon. J Shoulder Elbow Surg 2001;10:377–9.

33. Boyd HB, Anderson LD. A method for reinsertion of the distal biceps brachii tendon. J Bone Joint Surg Am 1961;43:1041–3.

34. Khan AD, Penna S, Yin Q, et al. Repair of distal biceps tendon ruptures using suture anchors through a single anterior incision. Arthroscopy 2008;24:39–45.

35. Bain GI, Prem H, Heptinstall RJ, et al. Repair of distal biceps tendon rupture: a new technique using the Endobutton. J Shoulder Elbow Surg 2000; 9:120–6.

36. Khan W, Agarwal M, Funk L. Repair of distal biceps tendon rupture with the Biotenodesis screw. Arch Orthop Trauma Surg 2004;124:206–8.

37. Kelly EW, Steinmann S, O'Driscoll SW. Surgical treatment of partial distal biceps tendon ruptures through a single posterior incision. J Shoulder Elbow Surg 2003;12:456–61.

38. Bain GI, Johnson LJ, Turner PC. Treatment of partial distal biceps tendon tears. Sports Med Arthrosc 2008;16:154–61.

39. Sethi PM, Tibone JE. Distal biceps repair using cortical button fixation. Sports Med Arthrosc 2008; 16:130–5.

40. Sethi P, Obopilwe E, Rincon L, et al. Biomechanical evaluation of distal biceps reconstruction with cortical button and interference screw fixation. J Shoulder Elbow Surg 2010;19:53–7.

41. Chavan PR, Duquin TR, Bisson LJ. Repair of the ruptured distal biceps tendon: a systematic review. Am J Sports Med 2008;36:1618–24.

42. Mazzocca AD, Burton KJ, Romeo AA, et al. Biomechanical evaluation of 4 techniques of distal biceps brachii tendon repair. Am J Sports Med 2007;35: 252–8.

43. Siebenlist S, Lenich A, Buchholz A, et al. Biomechanical in vitro validation of intramedullary cortical button fixation for distal biceps tendon repair: a new technique. Am J Sports Med 2011;39:1762–8.

44. Siebenlist S, Buchholz A, Zapf J, et al. Double intramedullary cortical button versus suture anchors for distal biceps tendon repair: a biomechanical comparison. Knee Surg Sports Traumatol Arthrosc 2013;23:926–33.

45. Schmidt CC, Jarrett CD, Brown BT. The distal biceps tendon. J Hand Surg Am 2013;38:811–21.

46. Tanner C, Johnson T, Muradov P, et al. Single incision power optimizing cost-effective (SPOC) distal biceps repair. J Shoulder Elbow Surg 2013;22: 305–11.

47. Idler CS, Montgomery WH III, Lindsey DP, et al. Distal biceps tendon repair: a biomechanical comparison of intact tendon and 2 repair techniques. Am J Sports Med 2006;34:968–74.

48. Pereira DS, Kvitne RS, Liang M, et al. Surgical repair of distal biceps tendon ruptures: a biomechanical comparison of two techniques. Am J Sports Med 2002;30:432–6.

49. Greenberg JA, Fernandez JJ, Wang T. EndoButton-assisted repair of distal biceps tendon ruptures. J Shoulder Elbow Surg 2003;12:484–90.

50. Lemos SE, Ebramzedeh E, Kvitne RS. A new technique: in vitro suture anchor fixation has superior yield strength to bone tunnel fixation for distal biceps tendon repair. Am J Sports Med 2004;32: 406–10.

51. Spang JT, Weinhold PS, Karas SG. A biomechanical comparison of EndoButton versus suture anchor repair of distal biceps tendon injuries. J Shoulder Elbow Surg 2006;15:509–14.

52. Krushinski EM, Brown JA, Murthi AM. Distal biceps tendon rupture: biomechanical analysis of repair strength of the Bio-Tenodesis screw versus suture anchors. J Shoulder Elbow Surg 2007;16:218–23.

53. Kettler M, Lunger J, Kuhn V, et al. Failure strengths in distal biceps tendon repair. Am J Sports Med 2007; 35:1544–8.

54. Schmidt CC, Diaz VA, Weir DM, et al. Repaired distal biceps magnetic resonance imaging anatomy compared with outcome. J Shoulder Elbow Surg 2012;21:1623–31.

55. Olsen JR, Shields E, Williams RB, et al. A comparison of cortical button with interference

screw versus suture anchor techniques for distal biceps brachii tendon repairs. J Shoulder Elbow Surg 2014;23:1607–11.

56. Recordon JAF, Misur PN, Isaksson F, et al. Endobutton versus transosseous suture repair of distal biceps rupture using the two-incision technique: a comparison series. J Shoulder Elbow Surg 2015; 24:928–33.

57. Shields E, Olsen JR, Williams RB, et al. Distal biceps brachii tendon repairs: A single-incision technique using a cortical button with interference screw versus a double-incision technique using suture fixation through bone tunnels. Am J Sports Med 2015; 43:1072–6.

58. Hansen G, Smith A, Pollock JW, et al. Anatomic repair of the distal biceps tendon cannot be consistently performed through a classic single-incision suture anchor technique. J Shoulder Elbow Surg 2014;23:1898–904.

59. Siebenlist S, Fischer SC, Sandmann GH, et al. The functional outcome of forty-nine single-incision suture anchor repairs for distal biceps tendon ruptures at the elbow. Int Orthop 2014;38:873–9.

60. Banerjee M, Shafizadeh S, Bouillon B, et al. High complication rate following distal biceps refixation with cortical button. Arch Orthop Trauma Surg 2013;133:1361–6.

61. Cain RA, Nydick JA, Stein MI, et al. Complications following distal biceps repair. J Hand Surg Am 2012;37:2112–7.

62. Grewal R, Athwal GS, MacDermid JC, et al. Single versus double-incision technique for the repair of acute distal biceps tendon ruptures. J Bone Joint Surg Am 2012;94:1166–74.

63. Citak M, Backhaus M, Seybold D, et al. Surgical repair of the distal biceps brachii tendon: a comparative study of three surgical fixation techniques. Knee Surg Sports Traumatol Arthrosc 2011;19: 1936–41.

64. Potapov A, Laflamme YG, Gagnon S, et al. Progressive osteolysis of the radius after distal biceps tendon repair with the bioabsorbable screw. J Shoulder Elbow Surg 2011;20:819–26.

65. Watson JN, Moretti VM, Schwindel L. Repair techniques for acute distal biceps tendon ruptures: a systematic review. J Bone Joint Surg Am 2014;96: 2086–90.

66. McKee MD, Hirji R, Schemitsch EH, et al. Patient-oriented functional outcome after repair of distal biceps tendon ruptures using a single-incision technique. J Shoulder Elbow Surg 2005;14:302–6.

67. Karunakar MA, Cha P, Stern PJ. Distal biceps ruptures: a followup of Boyd and Anderson repair. Clin Orthop 1999;363:100–7.

68. El-Hawary R, MacDermid JC, Faber KJ. Distal biceps tendon repair: comparison of surgical techniques. J Hand Surg Am 2003;28:496–502.

69. Jobin CM, Kippe MA, Gardner TR, et al. Distal biceps tendon repair: a cadaveric analysis of suture anchor and interference screw restoration of the anatomic footprint. Am J Sports Med 2009;37: 2214–21.

70. Hasan SA, Cordell CL, Rauls RB, et al. Two-incision versus one-incision repair for distal biceps tendon rupture: a cadaveric study. J Shoulder Elbow Surg 2012;21:935–41.

71. Henry J, Feinblatt J, Kaeding CC. Biomechanical analysis of distal biceps tendon repair methods. Am J Sports Med 2007;35:1950–4.

72. Prud'homme-Foster M, Louati H, Pollock JW. Proper placement of the distal biceps tendon during repair improves supination strength—a biomechanical analysis. J Shoulder Elbow Surg 2015;24: 527–32.

73. Schmidt CC, Weir DM, Wong AS, et al. The effect of biceps reattachment site. J Shoulder Elbow Surg 2010;19:1157–65.

74. Wiley WB, Noble JS, Dulaney TD, et al. Late reconstruction of chronic distal biceps tendon ruptures with a semitendinosus autograft technique. J Shoulder Elbow Surg 2006;15:440–4.

75. Levy HJ, Mashoof AA, Morgan D. Repair of chronic ruptures of the distal biceps tendon using flexor carpi radialis tendon graft. Am J Sports Med 2000; 28:538–40.

76. Hallam P, Bain GI. Repair of chronic distal biceps tendon ruptures using autologous hamstring graft and the Endobutton. J Shoulder Elbow Surg 2004; 13:648–51.

77. Darlis NA, Sotereanos DG. Distal biceps tendon reconstruction in chronic ruptures. J Shoulder Elbow Surg 2006;15:614–9.

78. Sanchez-Sotelo J, Morrey BF, Adams RA. Reconstruction of chronic ruptures of the distal biceps tendon with use of an Achilles tendon allograft. J Bone Joint Surg Am 2002;84A:999–1005.

79. Snir N, Hamula M, Wolfson T, et al. Clinical outcomes after chronic distal biceps reconstruction with allografts. Am J Sports Med 2013;41:2288–95.

80. McCarty LP III, Alpert JM, Bush-Joseph C. Reconstruction of a chronic distal biceps tendon rupture 4 years after initial injury. Am J Orthop 2008;37: 579–82.

81. Patterson RW, Sharma J, Lawton JN. Distal biceps tendon reconstruction with tendoachilles allograft: a modification of the endobutton technique utilizing an ACL reconstruction system. J Hand Surg Am 2009;34:545–52.

82. Bosman HA, Fincher M, Saw N. Anatomic direct repair of chronic distal biceps brachii tendon rupture without interposition graft. J Shoulder Elbow Surg 2012;21:1342–7.

83. Morrey ME, Abdel MP, Sanchez-Sotelo J. Primary repair of retracted distal biceps tendon ruptures in

extreme flexion. J Shoulder Elbow Surg 2014;23:
679–85.

84. Cusick MC, Cottrell BJ, Cain RA, et al. Low incidence of tendon rerupture after distal biceps repair by cortical button and interference screw. J Shoulder Elbow Surg 2014;23:1532–6.

85. Cohen MS. Complications of distal biceps tendon repairs. Sports Med Arthrosc 2008;16:148–53.

86. Nigro PT, Cain R, Mighell MA. Prognosis for recovery of posterior interosseous nerve palsy after distal biceps repair. J Shoulder Elbow Surg 2013;22:70–3.

87. Thumm N, Hutchinson D, Zhang C, et al. Proximity of the posterior interosseous nerve during cortical button guidewire placement for distal biceps tendon reattachment. J Hand Surg Am 2015;40:534–6.

88. Duncan D, Lancaster G, Marsh SG, et al. Anatomical evaluation of a cortical button for distal biceps tendon repairs. Hand 2013;8:201–4.

89. Lo EY, Li C-S, Van den Bogaerde JM. The effect of drill trajectory on proximity to the posterior interosseous nerve during cortical button distal biceps repair. Arthroscopy 2011;27:1048–54.

90. Saldua N, Carney J, Dewing C, et al. The effect of drilling angle on posterior interosseous nerve safety during open and endoscopic anterior single-incision repair of the distal biceps tendon. Arthroscopy 2008;24:305–10.

91. Hartman MW, Merten SM, Steinmann SP. Mini-open 2-incision technique for repair of distal biceps tendon ruptures. J Shoulder Elbow Surg 2007;16:616–20.

92. Wysocki RW, Cohen MS. Radioulnar heterotopic ossification after distal biceps tendon repair: results following surgical resection. J Hand Surg Am 2007;32:1230–6.

93. Sotereanos DG, Sarris I, Chou KH. Radioulnar synostosis after the two-incision biceps repair: a standardized treatment protocol. J Shoulder Elbow Surg 2004;13:448–53.

94. Hinchey JW, Aronowitz JG, Sanchez-Sotelo J. Rerupture rate of primarily repaired distal biceps tendon injuries. J Shoulder Elbow Surg 2014;23:850–4.

95. Cil A, Merten S, Steinmann SP. Immediate active range of motion after modified 2-incision repair in acute distal biceps tendon rupture. Am J Sports Med 2009;37:130–5.

96. Cheung EV, Lazarus M, Taranta M. Immediate range of motion after distal biceps tendon repair. J Shoulder Elbow Surg 2005;14:516–8.

Prosthetic Design in Total Wrist Arthroplasty

Colin D. Kennedy, MD[a], Jerry I. Huang, MD[b],*

KEYWORDS

- Wrist replacement • Arthroplasty • Implant • Prosthesis • Arthritis

KEY POINTS

- Total wrist arthroplasty provides a motion-preserving alternative to wrist arthrodesis for low-demand patients with debilitating, painful pancarpal arthritis.
- Technical advancement in implant design promotes osteointegration and preserves motion with the goal of reducing torque transmission to the carpal component.
- Current generation implants have reduced rates of dislocation and instability but reoperation rates remain high and further long-term evaluation of survivability and complications are necessary.
- Long-term, prospective, randomized trials comparing total wrist arthroplasty with wrist arthrodesis are needed to understand which patients receive the greatest benefit with the lowest failure and complications.

INTRODUCTION

Total wrist arthroplasty (TWA) provides a motion-preserving alternative to total wrist arthrodesis for low-demand patients with debilitating arthritis. Palmer and Werner[1] determined the functional range of motion of the wrist to be 30° of extension and 5° of flexion. To perform most activities of daily living, including hygiene and food preparation, Ryu and colleagues[2] suggested that wrist flexion and extension of 40° are required. The first description of a wrist prosthesis was by Gluck, who placed an ivory wrist implant for tuberculosis of the wrist in 1891.[3] Swanson introduced the first commercially available total wrist implant with a hinged silicone interpositional spacer prosthesis in 1967.[4] Significant improvements have been made with TWA prosthesis design over the past 2 decades, which has simultaneously allowed for both improvements in clinical outcomes with TWA, and the expansion of clinical indications for this procedure.

INDICATIONS AND CONTRAINDICATIONS

TWA is classically described for patients with rheumatoid arthritis, especially those with bilateral wrist involvement. Its use has expanded to pancarpal wrist arthritis in patients with nonrheumatoid inflammatory arthritis, posttraumatic arthritis, osteoarthritis and avascular necrosis. Ideal surgical candidates are patients who have failed nonoperative management with persistent debilitating pain that limits the ability to perform activities of daily living, have low-demand lifestyles, and are seeking a pain-free wrist with preservation of moderate motion. Patients with arthritis involving multiple joints of the upper extremity, including limitations in elbow motion or forearm rotation, often find activities of daily living easier when some wrist motion is preserved and thus may have greater benefit from a TWA over a wrist arthrodesis.[5]

Absolute contraindications include a lack of neuromuscular control of the hand, laborers, those

The authors have nothing to disclose.

[a] Department of Orthopaedics and Sports Medicine, University of Washington Medical Center, 4245 Roosevelt Way Northeast, Box 354740, Seattle, WA 98105, USA; [b] UW Combined Hand Fellowship, Department of Orthopaedics and Sports Medicine, University of Washington Medical Center, 4245 Roosevelt Way Northeast, Box 354740, Seattle, WA 98105, USA

* Corresponding author.

E-mail address: jihuang@uw.edu

Orthop Clin N Am 47 (2016) 207–218
http://dx.doi.org/10.1016/j.ocl.2015.08.018

with high-demand use of the upper extremity for ambulation and transfer, previous surgery with implant or bone loss that limit adequate carpal or radial fixation, and patients with an active infection. One relative contraindication is inadequate carpal bone stock to support the implants from severe erosions or osteopenia.[5,6] In addition, inadequate treatment of soft tissue contractures or imbalance can lead to persistent instability or motion restriction after TWA.

OPERATIVE PROCEDURE

A dorsal longitudinal midline incision is made over the wrist. Full-thickness skin flaps are raised with attention paid to protecting the branches of the radial sensory and dorsal ulnar cutaneous nerves. The retinaculum over the sixth dorsal compartment is incised followed by elevation of the flap radially to the septum between the first and second extensor compartments.[3] The dorsal capsule is raised as a broad, distally based flap off the distal radius from proximal to distal, through the floors of the first and sixth extensor compartments.[7] Care is taken to elevate full-thickness capsular flaps to allow for closure. Alternatively, the distal portion of the extensor retinaculum can be placed under the finger extensors to augment the capsular closure.

Once the dorsal capsule is raised, the wrist can be flexed to expose the joint and perform synovectomies if necessary. A distal ulnar resection can now be performed if there is an arthritic distal radioulnar joint. The order of preparation of the carpus and radius varies. The distal radius is cut, broached, and trialed according to the specific implant, and care is taken to protect the volar radiocarpal ligaments. The technique for carpal bone preparation varies among implants, and Kirschner wires are often used to temporarily pin the carpal bones to facilitate the carpal bone cuts. The distal radius cut is usually made perpendicular to the long axis of the forearm while the carpal cut is made perpendicular to the axis of the third metacarpal. Care is taken to protect the volar capsule and radiocarpal ligaments. Soft tissue balance is extremely important. With the trial radial component in place, trial polyethylene carpal components can be introduced so that both stability and range of motion can be assessed and adjustments made as necessary. Intraoperatively, there should be wrist flexion and extension of 30° in each direction. With limited wrist extension, more distal radius should be resected. If there is volar instability, a larger polyethylene should be used. Repair of the volar radiocarpal ligaments can also be considered. Patients with

severe wrist flexion contractures may benefit from step cut lengthening of the wrist flexors.

PROSTHETIC DESIGN

Themistocles Gluck performed the TWA using an ivory implant in a 19-year-old patient with tuberculosis of the wrist in 1890.[8] This subsequently developed a chronic fistula and was recognized as a failure despite reported good range of motion. Since then, there have been significant advances in prosthetic design, materials, fixation, and surgical techniques that have led to remarkable improvements in clinical outcome and implant survivorship and decreased complications. Newer implants have more anatomic design, involve minimal bony resection, and have more stable fixation.

First-generation Implants

Often described as a first-generation implant, the first commercially available Swanson implant was designed in 1967 as a silicone rubber, 1-piece, flexible, hinged implant that primarily serves as an interpositional implant (**Fig. 1**). The implant stems are mobile in the medullary canals, fitting into the radius proximally and passing through the capitate and seats in the third metacarpal distally.[9] Long-term follow-up studies have demonstrated prosthetic fracture, implant subsidence, silicone synovitis, and progressive radiologic and clinical deterioration.

Fatti and colleagues[10,11] retrospectively reviewed 47 patients with Swanson TWA and found that at average follow-up of 5.8 years postoperatively, only 51% of patients reported pain relief compared with their initial 1986 review of the same cohort demonstrating pain relief in 67% at average follow-up of 4.8 years, suggestive of continued clinical deterioration. Long-term studies have shown considerable problems with implant fracture, which most often occurs at the distal stem and barrel junction.[12] Jolly and colleagues[13] found an implant fracture rate of 52% and also showed a trend toward progressive radiologic and clinical deterioration at an average follow-up of 6 years. Silicone synovitis is a well-documented complication of the Swanson implant, with studies reporting rates of radiologic silicone synovitis as high as 30%.[13]

In 2005, Kistler and colleagues[14] reviewed 12 patients with rheumatoid arthritis treated with the Swanson implant with a minimum 10-year follow-up. Interestingly, they reported good to very good subjective results in 75% of patients despite a high number of implant fractures and expected silicone synovitis, suggesting that the correlation between clinical results and implant

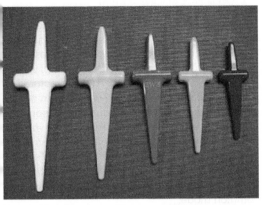

Fig. 1. The Swanson silicone prosthesis was introduced in 1967 and became the foundation for modern designs in total wrist implants. (*From* Lawler EA, Paksima N. Total wrist arthroplasty. Bull NYU Hosp Jt Dis 2006;64(3–4):99; with permission.)

integrity may not be straightforward. The authors concluded that low-demand patients with rheumatoid arthritis with severe deformity and bony erosion may still be good candidates for the Swanson silicone spacer implant as an alternative to wrist arthrodesis or TWA using the more complex, modern design prosthesis.

Second-generation Implants

Second-generation implants had separate radial and carpal components and relied on either a ball-and-socket design or hemispherical implants. In 1973, The Volz prosthesis was developed at Arizona Health Sciences Center as a semiconstrained cemented cobalt chrome alloy prosthesis.[15] The metacarpal component has a hemispherical surface with 2 different radii that allows for more wrist flexion and extension than radial and ulnar deviation, and minimizes radiocarpal rotation. The component fits through the capitate into the third metacarpal. The radial component has a polyethylene component with a concave surface that articulates with the metacarpal component. Volz reported on 25 cases in patients with rheumatoid arthritis and reported no infections, dislocations, implant loosening, or radioulnar imbalance.[16] Volz stressed the importance of soft tissue balance and musculotendinous forces across the radiocarpal joint. In a review of 30 Volz total wrist arthroplasties in patients with rheumatoid arthritis, Dennis and colleagues[17] reported 86% of patients had pain relief and satisfaction, but there were complications in 12 of 30 cases (40%) with a 24% rate of metacarpal component loosening. Gellman and associates[18] reviewed their series of 14 total wrist

arthroplasties with the Volz prosthesis with mean follow-up of 6.5 years. Migration of the radial component was seen in 2 patients with migration of the carpal component in 5 patients. Radiographic lucency was present in the radial component in 3 patients, the carpal component in 2 patients, and both components in 2 patients. There were 2 dislocations. The majority of the complications were related to technical problems with soft tissue balance and centering of the prosthesis and prosthetic design issues related to poor distal fixation.

Meuli introduced an unconstrained polyester ball-and-socket design in 1970 that used malleable metal forks to gain fixation in the second and third metacarpals. The rationale behind the ball joint was to allow for easier manufacturing, better range of motion in all planes, and to minimize unfavorable stresses and edge loading from impingement. The original Meuli prosthesis included a polyester ball that was replaced with an ultra-high-molecular-weight polyethylene with newer models. The newer prosthesis also incorporated eccentric prongs that allowed for more exact centering of the prosthesis.[19] Because the center of rotation of the radiocarpal joint is volar to the longitudinal axis of the radius, the malleable prongs allow the surgeon to adjust the component positioning intraoperatively (**Fig. 2**). Meuli described 41 implants of which 15 wrists required reoperation that were attributed mostly to technical errors and prosthesis centering, but ultimate satisfactory outcome was described in the majority of cases.[20] The Meuli implant has had a number of revisions, with the most recent MWP III Total Wrist Prosthesis, which uses a titanium alloy malleable design with a spherical head radial component that articulates with a polyethylene cup of the metacarpal component (Zimmer, Warsaw, IN).[9]

Vogelin and Nagy[21] reviewed 16 wrists that had complications with Meuli I, II, and III prostheses and found that a combination of both mechanical and soft tissue problems were causes for failures in 69% of the failures. Both loosening of the distal component and metacarpal perforation occurred in the majority of their reviewed failures. Cooney and colleagues[22] reviewed the Mayo Clinic experience with the Swanson silastic implant, the Volz prosthesis, and the Meuli prosthesis. Cooney attributed implant failure to 3 major factors: (1) centering of the prosthesis, (2) implant fixation, and (3) soft tissue balance. The Meuli prosthesis requires bending of the distal prongs to center the radiocarpal joint. The Volz prosthesis was modified with a dorsal offset on the metacarpal component to more accurately duplicate the

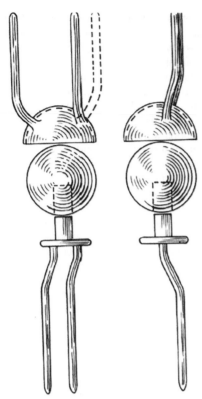

Fig. 2. The Meuli prosthesis required bending of the malleable forks to allow for better centering of the prosthesis. (*From* Beckenbaugh RD, Linscheid RL. Total wrist arthroplasty: a preliminary report. J Hand Surg 1977;2(5):339; with permission.)

center of rotation. In 140 Meuli arthroplasties at the Mayo Clinic there was reoperation rate of 33% for major complications including 8.6% dislocations, 2.9% prosthetic, 12.1% soft tissue deformity or contracture, and 6.4% tendon rupture. The authors recommended against the use of the Meuli prosthesis for clinical use despite the design changes based on the high complication rates.

Third-generation Implants

Third-generation implants include the Biaxial total wrist implant, the Trispherical prosthesis, and the Universal prosthesis. The third-generation prostheses were designed with the goal of minimizing bone resection, restoring the center of rotation of the wrist, and improving soft tissue balance and stability.

The Trispherical total wrist prosthesis has a radial component with a spherical head that articulates with a high-density polyethylene bearing on the metacarpal component to form a ball-and-socket joint.[23] There is an axle constraint to prevent dislocation. The metacarpal component

consists of a large third metacarpal stem and a smaller offset second metacarpal and scaphoid stem. The offset stem provides rotational stability. Figgie and colleagues[23] reviewed 35 cases of the Trispherical TWA with average follow-up of 9 years and reported no dislocations, implant fractures, or implant failures. However, the same group subsequently presented 8 failures out of 87 trispherical total wrist arthroplasties.[24] Two of the failures were from progressive wrist flexion contracture owing to loss of wrist extensor function. Mechanical failure occurred in 6 patients, with metacarpal loosening with dorsal perforation being the most common mode.

The Biaxial implant (Depuy Orthopedics, Inc, Warsaw, IN) is an unconstrained cemented cobalt chrome alloy implant with double-stemmed metacarpal component with an ellipsoidal head that articulates with a polyethylene-bearing surface that attaches to the radial component.[9] In addition to the long stem that inserts into the third metacarpal, there is a small stud that inserts to the trapezoid for added fixation and rotational stability. The shape of the ellipsoidal articular component is designed to reproduce the anatomic movements and stability in the native wrist.[9] In addition, the proximal radial component is offset ulnarly and palmarly to match the center of rotation. The stems have porous coated surfaces.

Cobb and Beckenbaugh[25] reviewed 57 cases of Biaxial TWA with mean follow-up of 6.5 years and found failures in 11 cases that included loosening of the distal implant in 8 cases (14%), as well as 1 case each of infection, dislocation, and progressive soft tissue imbalance. The authors felt that technical difficulties with poor intraoperative positioning contributed to failures in 5 of the cases. They suggested advising patients of a 20% failure rate at 6 years and consideration of long-stemmed multipronged implants, especially in revision cases and patients with poor bone stock (**Fig. 3**). Rizzo and Beckenbaugh[26] reviewed the Mayo Clinic experience with the long-stem biaxial prosthesis in 17 patients. There were no cases of prosthetic failures or revisions at a mean of 73.9 months. However, there were 2 cases of intraoperative metacarpal fractures. The authors caution that the longer metacarpal stem is more difficult to insert and potentially increases the risk of stress shielding. Takwale and colleagues[27] reviewed 76 biaxial total wrist implants and found no correlation between stem length in the third metacarpal component and loosening or terminal events. The probability of implant survival at 8 years was 83%. They found that uncemented fixation was predictive of future distal component loosening, and that the alignment of the distal

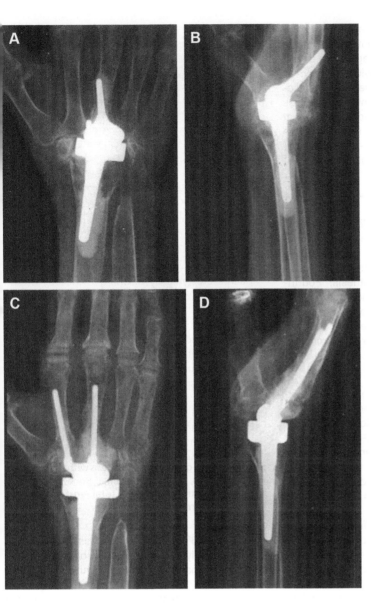

Fig. 3. Loosening and migration of distal component in a Biaxial total wrist arthroplasty (*A, B*) revised with a long-stem multipronged revision prosthesis (*C, D*). (*From* Cobb TK, Beckenbaugh RD. Biaxial long-stemmed multipronged distal components for revision/bone deficit total-wrist arthroplasty. J Hand Surg 1996;21A:768; with permission.)

component in extension predicted loosening and migration of the carpal component.

Menon's Universal I Total Wrist Implant (KMI Inc, San Diego, CA) is a nonconstrained implant with a Y-shaped radial component and a central carpal component that consists of a titanium plate holding a central capitate component with 2 screws on each side of that insert into the second and fourth metacarpal bones. A large, toroidal-shaped articular polyethylene-bearing surface attaches this plate to the cobalt chromium radial component, and the radial articular component has a 20° inclination similar to the native radial articular surface.[28,29] The large articular surface area was designed to resist instability and dislocation.[7]

Menon[29] reviewed this implant at average follow-up of 6.7 years and reported excellent pain relief in 88% of patients. However, he also reported a 32% complication rate with 5 volar dislocations in 37 wrists being the leading complication. Divelbiss and colleagues[30] also reviewed the Universal Total Wrist Implant and reported a 14% complication rate, all owing to instability in patients who were noted to have severe wrist laxity with advance rheumatoid arthritis.

Recently, Ward and colleagues[7] reviewed the 5- and 10-year outcomes of the Universal Total Wrist Implant in rheumatoid arthritis patients and reported a 50% revision rate at the latest follow-up at average 7.3 years. In 19 patients with a minimum 5-year follow-up, 9 prostheses had undergone revision surgery because of carpal component loosening. Only 1 patient had wrist instability that was ultimately managed with a wrist arthrodesis. At the time of revision surgery, all wrists had evidence of polyethylene wear, metallosis, and carpal component loosening. There was no evidence of loosening of the radial component in any of the wrists. All 10 prosthesis that were functioning at the time of follow-up had radiographic evidence of intercarpal fusion.

Fourth-generation Implants

Current generation implants were designed with the goal of improving the instability and fixation problems that plagued many of the earlier generation components. Loosening of the distal component remained the most difficulty challenge with the earlier generation prosthesis. Fourth-generation implants are mainly uncemented with porous titanium surfaces to allow for osseous integration. There are currently 3 designs that are approved by the US Food and Drug Administration[31] (**Fig. 4**).

Universal 2 Total Wrist System

With the goal of refining the instability of the Universal I implant, Adams established the Universal 2 Total Wrist System (Integra LifeSciences, Plainsboro, NJ) that featured an ultra-high-molecular weight polyethylene ellipsoidal articular surface rather than the toroidal surface of the original Universal implant. Grosland and colleagues[32] used both laboratory experiments and computer modeling to compare toroid- and ellipsoid-shaped TWA articulations and found that the ellipsoid articulation had improved centralization and greater contact through the total arc of motion, suggestive of a more stable design with less polyethylene wear. The Universal 2 system uses a beaded porous coating to the cobalt chromium radial and titanium carpal components to encourage osteointegration. The carpal baseplate has 2 variable angle screws and, similar to the Universal 1 design, has a central stem for capitate insertion.

Compared with both the original Universal 1 and other previous generation implants, stability data for the Universal 2 TWA have been promising. Anderson and Adams[33] described 25 patients with the Universal 2 TWA with pain relief reported in all patients and no dislocations at the time of publication. Van Winterswijk and Bakx[34] presented 17 Universal 2 TWAs with an average follow-up of 3.8 years and reported improved pain scores in all patients and only 1 prosthesis (6%) requiring removal owing to loosening of the carpal baseplate. These authors reported 1

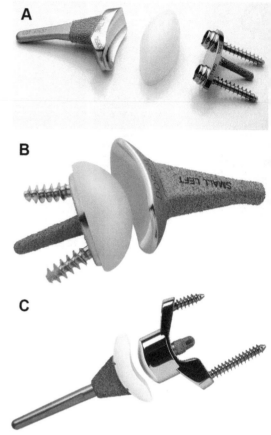

Fig. 4. Fourth-generation prosthesis with the Universal 2 (Integra) (*A*), RE-MOTION (Small Bone Innovations) (*B*), and Maestro (Biomet) (*C*) total wrist arthroplasty systems. (*Courtesy of* Arnold-Peter C. Weiss, MD.)

dislocation (6%) that was successfully managed nonoperatively. Ferreres and colleagues[35] reviewed 20 patients with the Universal 2 TWA implant and 2 patients with the original Universal TWA implant (the authors did not differentiate the results between the 2 prostheses) with an average follow-up of 5.5 years and reported 5 total complications, none of which were dislocations. They had 1 case of carpal subsidence and loosening of the carpal component and 2 patients with screw osteolysis in the index metacarpal. At the time of publication, no surgical component revisions were required. Morapudi and colleagues[36] reviewed 19 patients with Universal 2 TWA over a mean of 3.1 years and reported no dislocations or radiographic evidence of implant loosening. There were 3 superficial infections (16%), 2 patients with restricted range of motion requiring manipulation under anesthesia (11%), 1 patient requiring excision of a palmar bony bridge (5%), and 1 extensor pollicis longus rupture requiring tendon transfer (5%). Cooney and colleagues[37] retrospectively reviewed 46 wrist implants with the Biaxial, Universal 2, and RE-MOTION prostheses at a mean follow-up of 6 years. Of the 9 Universal 2 implants reviewed, 1 implant had instability and loosening and required wrist arthrodesis (11%), and the Disability of Arm Shoulder and Hand (DASH) questionnaire and Patient-rated Wrist Evaluation (PRWE) scores were the best among the Universal 2 patients, although this was not greater than the RE-MOTION wrist group.

RE-MOTION Total Wrist System

The RE-MOTION TWA (SBI, Morrisville, PA) uses an ultra-high-molecular weight polyethylene carpal ball that snaps to a rounded peg on the carpal plate for an ellipsoidal articulation with the radial component, but also uses a second articulation between the carpal plate and the ball to allow for 10° of additional rotation with the goal of both reducing distal torque stress and preserving more intricate motion.[31] The carpal plate has a central stem that inserts into the capitate and is surrounded on each side by 2 variable-angle screws for fixation into the hamate ulnarly, and the trapezoid and base of the second metacarpal radially. The radial component sits against the scaphoid and lunate fossa of the distal radius and allows for preservation of ligamentous attachments as well as preservation of the sigmoid notch and has a 10° palmar tilt approximating the native wrist. Cobalt chromium carpal and radial components are coated with porous titanium to promote osteointegration.

Herzberg[38] prospectively followed 20 wrists in both rheumatoid arthritis (13 wrists) patients and nonrheumatoid patients (7 wrists) treated with the RE-MOTION system. There were no dislocations or reoperations at an average follow-up of 2.6 years. There was 1 carpal loosening and 1 case of radial loosening, both of which occurred in rheumatoid patients and neither required surgical revision. The average visual analog scale with wrist flexion–extension improved from 7 preoperatively to 1 postoperatively in the rheumatoid group and improved from 7 preoperatively to 3 postoperatively in the nonrheumatoid group. Herzberg[39] then conducted a larger multicenter, prospective study using an Internet-based database with the RE-MOTION TWA that included 129 rheumatoid patients and 86 nonrheumatoid patients with a mean follow-up of 2 years. They found that 5% of the patients in the rheumatoid group and 6% of the nonrheumatoid group had complications that required surgical revision, and that both groups had an implant survival rate of 92% at maximum follow-up.

Using an Internet-based registry in which data are entered prospectively on the RE-MOTION TWA, Boeckstyns and colleagues[40] analyzed data from 7 centers performed between 2003 and 2007. Of the original 65 wrists included, 52 were available for follow-up and 5 revised cases were excluded. Of the excluded revisions, 4 were performed for loosening and 1 stiffened in an awkward position in a rheumatoid arthritis patient with almost no motion preoperatively. There were no infections or dislocations. In the 52 "surviving" implants, 6 showed signs of radiographic loosening but these were not treated surgically owing to the lack of severe pain. The overall implant survival was 90% at 5 to 9 years, which is a substantial improvement from previous generation implants.

Boeckstyns and Herzberg[41] analyzed 44 consecutive RE-MOTION TWA cases and found significant periprosthetic radiolucency (>2 mm in width) at the radial component side in 16 cases and at the carpal component side in 7 cases. Although they recommended continued close follow-up for patients with radiographic evidence of periprosthetic osteolysis, periprosthetic radiolucency was not necessarily related to implant loosening, and seemed to stabilize after 3 years.

Maestro Wrist Reconstruction System

The Maestro Wrist Reconstruction System (Biomet, Warsaw, IN) is the most recently Food and Drug Administration–approved TWA implant and features a concave polyethylene that locks into the proximal radial component and articulates with a convex carpal component. Distal fixation is achieved with a porous central titanium alloy capitate stem and 2 titanium alloy variable-angle radial and ulnar screws. The carpal and radial stems are treated with a titanium plasma coat to enhance fixation. This implant allows for use in both carpal hemiarthroplasty and TWA.

Dellacqua[42] presented 19 patients with the Maestro system with mean a follow-up of 2.25 years with pain relief and range of motion improvement in all patients. Nydick and colleagues[43] retrospectively reviewed 23 wrists in 22 patients treated with the Maestro TWA with an average follow-up of 2.33 years. Etiologies for TWA included posttraumatic arthritis (13 patients), rheumatoid arthritis (5 patients), primary osteoarthritis (2 patients), Kienbock disease (2 patients), and gout (1 patient). The mean pain visual analog scale improved from 8.0 preoperatively to 2.2 postoperatively, and pain was reported as none in 75% of the patients. They reported 7 complications (30%) with 4 cases of wrist contracture, 1 deep infection requiring wrist arthrodesis, 1 case

Table 1
Evolution of the total wrist arthroplasty implant designs

Implant	Design	Complications
Gluck, 1891	Ivory implant for tuberculosis of the wrist	Chronic draining fistula[3,8]
Swanson, 1972	Silicone spacer with flexible hinge for resection arthroplasty	Implant fracture, osteolysis, foreign body granuloma/giant cell synovitis, cystic changes to the wrist[10–14]
Volz, 1976	Cobalt chrome alloy third metacarpal and radial component that articulate via a semiconstrained hemispherical polyethylene bearing surface with 2 radii of curvature for flexion–extension and radial–ulnar deviation	Loosening of the metacarpal component, dislocation[9,18,50]
Meuli, 1980	Unconstrained polyester ball-and-socket articulation with malleable metal forks to gain fixation in the second and third metacarpal	Dislocation, imbalance[22]
Meuli MWP III Total Wrist Prosthesis, 1986	Unconstrained ball-and-socket design with a UHMWPE cup and titanium nitride coated head to improve wear characteristics	Component loosening, perforation[21,51,52]
Guepar, 1986	Radial polyethylene component that fits to a metal carpal component featuring 2 screws that fit into the second and third metacarpals	Radial component loosening, bone resorption at carpal component[53]
CFV wrist, 1988	Reverse polarity implant with an elliptical articular surface offset meant to facilitate balance	Infection, loosening of the distal component, imbalance[54]
Trispherical wrist, 1990	Cemented radial component and spherical head articulating the cemented carpal component via an axle-constrained articulation	Metacarpal loosening, metacarpal perforation[24]
Destot prosthesis, 1994	Unconstrained, metal-polyethylene condylar prosthesis with an extra empty polyethylene cylinder articulation in the metacarpal to increase wrist motion	Infection, metacarpal fracture[55]
Biaxial wrist, 1996	Ingrowth fixation into the radius and third metacarpal with an elongated distal stem; an ellipsoidal articulating shape to reproduce natural wrist motion	Loosening of the distal component, infection, dislocation, soft tissue imbalance[25,27]

Implant	Description	Complications
Universal I Total Wrist, 1998	A toroidal-shaped articular polyethylene-bearing surface attaches a carpal plate to the concave cobalt chromium radial component, and the radial articular component has a 20° inclination similar to the native radial articular surface	Dislocation, carpal component loosening, infection[7,29,30]
ATW/APH prosthesis, 1999	Radial component with an articular inclination of 10° toward the ulna and the carpal component has a mobile bearing surface with a radial inclination of 10°	Dislocation, infection[56]
Universal II Total Wrist, 2001	Modified the Universal I design with an ellipsoidal instead of toroid shape carpal plate, reduction in the radial component inclination, and beaded porous coating to the component surfaces	Carpal baseplate loosening, dislocation, screw osteolysis, superficial infections, palmar bony bridge, extensor pollicis longus rupture[34,35]
RWS Implant, 2003	Semiconstrained system with a radial articular surface is offset in a volar/ulnar direction allowing preservation of the radial styloid and the radioscaphocapitate ligament	Component loosening[57]
Total Modular Wrist Implant, 2004	Titanium radial component articulates with a carpal plate with an interposed polyethylene insert, and features an optional replacement of the distal radioulnar joint with a ball-and-socket articulation	Loosening, soft tissue infection, soft tissue imbalance[58]
Re-Motion, 2005	Features an UHMWPE carpal ball that snaps to a rounded peg on the carpal plate for an ellipsoidal articulation with the radial component, but also uses a second articulation between the carpal plate and the ball to allow for 10° of additional rotation for more intricate motion	Carpal and radial loosening, soft tissue complications and wound breakdown, periprosthetic osteolysis[38,40,59]
Maestro, 2005	Carpal and radial stems are treated with a titanium plasma coat to enhance fixation; modular implant allowing use in both carpal hemiarthroplasty and total wrist arthroplasty	Infection, synovitis related to a loose second[43] metacarpal, volar dislocation

Abbreviation: UHMWPE, ultra-high-molecular weight polyethylene.
Data from Refs.[3,7–14,18,21,22,24,25,27,29,30,34,35,38,40,43,50–59]

of synovitis related to a loose second metacarpal nonlocking screw, and 1 case of volar dislocation that occurred from a fall that was successfully closed reduced without recurrent instability.

CLINICAL OUTCOMES

Significant debate exists regarding arthroplasty and arthrodesis for management of wrist arthritis. Arthroplasty offers a motion-preserving alternative to wrist arthrodesis, which can be especially beneficial in patients with contralateral wrist fusions who will need motion in 1 wrist to retain function, or in patients with other ipsilateral upper extremity joint arthritis, such as in the shoulder, elbow, and hand. Patients who had a previous wrist arthrodesis, who then subsequently had an arthroplasty of the contralateral wrist, report improved function and preference toward arthroplasty.[35,44] To date, prospective randomized trials comparing wrist arthrodesis and arthroplasty have not been published, and many authors feel that to justify the higher cost of arthroplasty it should provide better function than traditional wrist arthrodesis.[45] However, the overall results of the newer fourth-generation implants have been very encouraging.

Cavaliere and Chung[46] conducted a systematic review using a MEDLINE database search comparing 20 total wrist arthrodesis studies (approximately 800 procedures) with 18 wrist arthroplasty studies (approximately 500 procedures) in rheumatoid arthritis patients and found that wrist fusion provided more reliable pain relief than arthroplasty, and that complication and revision rates were higher in the arthroplasty group. They found high satisfaction rates in both groups. They concluded that arthrodesis may provide better outcomes than TWA, and that their data did not support the widespread use of TWA for the rheumatoid wrist. However, most of the clinical series in their systematic review was based on earlier third generation implants.

Yeoh and Tourret[47] performed a systematic review of the clinical evidence on TWA from the last 5 years. They reviewed 8 articles on 405 prostheses from 7 different manufacturers that met the inclusion criteria. Rheumatoid arthritis was the most common indication, comprising 42% of the patients. These included third- and fourth-generation total wrist prosthesis. Implant survivorship ranged from 90% to 100% in the fourth-generation prosthesis with 100% survival at 3 to 5 years with the Universal 2 system. In a metaanalysis that included 18 published studies between 2003 and 2013, the overall survival rate was 92% at 4 years for the fourth-generation prostheses.[48] Of the published reports on fourth-generation prostheses, The Maestro had the best wrist flexion–extension arc of 90°, with mean wrist flexion of 43° and extension of 47°.[43]

Cooney and colleagues[37] performed a retrospective comparative study on outcomes of the Biaxial resectional arthroplasty with newer generation RE-MOTION and Universal 2 resurfacing implants. They included patients with rheumatoid arthritis and posttraumatic wrists with a mean follow-up of 6 years. They found a stable wrist with physiologic range of motion in 22 of 22 (100%) RE-MOTION wrists, 7 of 8 Universal 2 wrists (88%), and 8 of 16 (50%) Biaxial wrist implants. There were 9 total failures, and 8 of these were with the Biaxial implant (89%) and 1 with the Universal 2 implant (11%), with loosening of the distal component and instability being causes of failure. They concluded that TWA provided functional motion and pain relief in greater than 80% of all cases and in 97% of the current generation RE-MOTION and Universal 2 implants.

Several studies have also demonstrated the correlation between component malignment and implant failure.[22,24,49] Ocampos and colleagues[49] radiologically reviewed RE-MOTION arthroplasties on 14 cadaver wrists performed by 14 inexperienced surgeons (procedure performed for the first time). The authors found that none of the implants had satisfactory alignment, illustrating the difficulty in achieving proper component alignment in novice wrist arthroplasty surgeons.

SUMMARY

Although early generation implants had high complication and failure rates, improvement in implant design has contributed to the progress of TWA as an acceptable motion-preserving and pain-relieving surgical option for patients with debilitating wrist arthritis (**Table 1**). An understanding of the evolution of the development of total wrist prosthesis since the original Swanson implant in 1970 and the mode of failure in earlier generation implants are paramount to the improved clinical outcomes seen with modern surgical technique and the improvements in prosthesis design in fourth-generation implants. The newer prosthesis requires less bony resection, restores the center of rotation of the radiocarpal joint, provides more natural wrist motion and stability with the ellipsoidal articulating surface, and promotes osseous integration of the carpal components. We have also learned the importance of addressing soft tissue contractures and imbalance to minimize the risk of complications. Although current fourth-generation prostheses show clinical promise with 90% to 100% implant mid-term survivorship and good to excellent clinical outcomes, further long-term data and randomized prospective trials comparing wrist arthrodesis with TWA are necessary to establish what specific role both of these surgical interventions should play in the patient with advanced wrist arthritis.

REFERENCES

1. Palmer AK, Werner FW. Biomechanics of the distal radioulnar joint. Clin Orthop Relat Res 1984;(187): 26–35.
2. Ryu JY, Cooney WP, Askew LJ, et al. Functional ranges of motion of the wrist joint. J Hand Surg Am 1991;16(3):409–19.
3. Eynon-Lewis NJ, Ferry D, Pearse MF. Themistocles Gluck: an unrecognised genius. BMJ 1992;305: 1534–6.
4. Swanson AB. Flexible implant resection arthroplasty. Hand 1972;4:119–34.
5. Adams BD. Total wrist arthroplasty. Tech Hand Up Extrem Surg 2004;8(3):130–7.
6. Weiss AP, Kamal RN, Shultz P. Total wrist arthroplasty. J Am Acad Orthop Surg 2013;21:140–8.
7. Ward CM, Kuhl T, Adams BD. Five to ten-year outcomes of the universal total wrist arthroplasty in patients with rheumatoid arthritis. J Bone Joint Surg Am 2011;93:914–9.
8. Ritt MJPF, Stuart PR, Naggar L, et al. The early history of arthroplasty of the wrist. J Hand Surg 1994; 19B(6):778–82.
9. Shepherd DET, Johnstone AJ. Design considerations for wrist implant. Med Eng Phys 2002;24: 641–50.
10. Fatti JF, Palmer AK, Greenky S. Long-term results of Swanson interpositional wrist arthroplasty: part II. J Hand Surg 1991;16A:432–7.
11. Fatti JF, Palmer AK, Mosher JF. The long-term results of Swanson silicone rubber interpositional wrist arthroplasty. J Hand Surg 1986;11A:166–75.
12. Brase DW, Millender LHF. Failure of silicone-rubber wrist arthroplasty in rheumatoid arthritis. J Hand Surg Am 1986;11:175.
13. Jolly SL, Ferlic DC, Clayton ML, et al. Swanson silicone arthroplasty of the wrist in rheumatoid arthritis: a long-term follow-up. J Hand Surg 1992;17A:142–9.
14. Kistler U, Weiss APC, Simmen BR, et al. Long-term results of silicone wrist arthroplasty in patients with rheumatoid arthritis. J Hand Surg 2005;30A:1282–7.
15. Volz RG. The development of a total wrist arthroplasty. Clin Orthop Relat Res 1976;(116):209–14.
16. Volz RG. Total wrist arthroplasty. A clinical review. Clin Orthop Relat Res 1984;(187):112–20.
17. Dennis DA, Ferlic DC, Clayton ML. Volz total wrist arthroplasty in rheumatoid arthritis: a long-term review. J Hand Surg 1986;11A:483–90.
18. Gellman H, Hontas R, Brumield RH, et al. Total wrist arthroplasty in rheumatoid arthritis. A long-term clinical review. Clin Orthop Relat Res 1997;(342):71–6.
19. Meuli HC. Meuli total wrist arthroplasty. Clin Orthop Relat Res 1984;(187):107–11.
20. Meuli HC. Arthroplasty of the wrist. Clin Orthop Relat Res 1980;(149):118–25.
21. Vogelin E, Nagy L. Fate of failed Meuli total wrist arthroplasty. J Hand Surg 2003;28B:61–8.
22. Cooney WP, Beckenbaugh RD, Linscheid RL. Total wrist arthroplasty: problems with implant failures. Clin Orthop Relat Res 1984;(187):121–8.
23. Figgie MP, Ranawat CS, Inglis AE, et al. Trispherical total wrist arthroplasty in rheumatoid arthritis. J Hand Surg 1990;15A:217–23.
24. Lorei MP, Figgie MP, Ranawat CS, et al. Failed total wrist arthroplasty: analysis of failures and results of operative management. Clin Orthop Relat Res 1997;(342):84–93.
25. Cobb TK, Beckenbaugh RD. Biaxial total-wrist arthroplasty. J Hand Surg 1996;21A:1011–21.
26. Rizzo M, Beckenbaugh RD. Results of biaxial total wrist arthroplasty with a modified (long) metacarpal stem. J Hand Surg 2003;28A:577–84.
27. Takwale VJ, Nuttall D, Trail IA, et al. Biaxial total wrist replacement in patients with rheumatoid arthritis. J Bone Joint Surg Br 2002;84:692–9.
28. Stanley K. Arthroplasty and arthrodesis of the wrist. In: Green D, Wolfe S, editors. Green's operative hand surgery. 6th edition. Philadelphia: Elsevier; 2011. p. 454–60.
29. Menon J. Universal total wrist implant: experience with a carpal component fixed with three screws. J Arthroplasty 1998;13(5):515–23.
30. Divelbiss BJ, Sollerman C, Adams BD. Early results of the universal total wrist arthroplasty in rheumatoid arthritis. J Hand Surg 2002;27A:195–204.
31. Ogunro S, Ahmed I, Tan V. Current indications and outcomes of total wrist arthroplasty. Orthop Clin North Am 2013;44:371–9.
32. Grosland NM, Rogge RD, Adams BD. Influence of articular geometry on prosthetic wrist stability. Clin Orthop Relat Res 2004;(421):134–42.
33. Anderson MC, Adams BD. Total wrist arthroplasty. Hand Clin 2005;21:621–30.
34. Van Winterswijk PJ, Bakx PA. Promising clinical results of the universal total wrist prosthesis in rheumatoid arthritis. Open Orthop J 2010;4:67–70.
35. Ferreres A, Lluch A, del Valle M. Universal total wrist arthroplasty: midterm follow-up study. J Hand Surg 2011;36A:967–73.
36. Morapudi S, Marlow WJ, Withers D, et al. Total wrist arthroplasty using the universal 2 prosthesis. J Orthop Surg 2012;20(3):365–8.
37. Cooney W, Manuel J, Froelich J, et al. Total wrist replacement: a retrospective comparative study. J Wrist Surg 2012;1:165–72.

38. Herzberg G. Prospective study of a new total wrist arthroplasty: short term results. Chir Main 2011;30: 20–5.

39. Herzberg G. Promising preliminary results seen with last generation wrist arthroplasty implant. Orthopedics Today 2012;32(10):18.

40. Boeckstyns ME, Herzberg G, Merser S. Favorable results after total wrist arthroplasty: 65 wrists in 60 patients followed for 5-9 years. Acta Orthop 2013; 84(4):415–9.

41. Boeckstyns ME, Herzberg G. Periprosthetic osteolysis after total wrist arthroplasty. J Wrist Surg 2014; 3(2):101–6.

42. Dellacqua D. Total wrist arthroplasty. Tech Orthop 2009;24(1):49–57.

43. Nydick JA, Greenberg SM, Stone JD, et al. Clinical outcomes of total wrist arthroplasty. J Hand Surg 2012;37A:1580–4.

44. Goodman MJ, Millender LH, Nalebuff ED, et al. Arthroplasty of the rheumatoid wrist with silicone rubber: an early evaluation. J Hand Surg Am 1980; 5(2):114–21.

45. Murphy DM, Khoury JG, Imbriglia JE, et al. Comparison of arthroplasty and arthrodesis for the rheumatoid wrist. J Hand Surg 2003;28A:570–6.

46. Cavaliere CM, Chung KC. A systematic review of total wrist arthroplasty compared with total wrist arthrodesis for rheumatoid arthritis. Plast Reconstr Surg 2008;122:813–25.

47. Yeoh D, Tourret L. Total wrist arthroplasty: a systematic review of evidence from the last five years. J Hand Surg 2015;40(5):458–68.

48. Nair R. Review article: total wrist arthroplasty. J Orthop Surg 2014;22(3):399–405.

49. Ocampos M, Corella F, del Campo B, et al. Component alignment in total wrist arthroplasty: success rate of surgeons in their first cases. Acta Orthop Traumatol Turc 2014;48(3):259–61.

50. Costi J, Krishnan J, Pearcy M. Total wrist arthroplasty: a quantitative review of the last 30 years. J Rheumatol 1998;25:451–8.

51. Meuli HC, Fernandez DL. Uncemented total wrist arthroplasty. J Hand Surg Am 1995;20:115–22.

52. Meuli HC. Total wrist arthroplasty. Experience with a noncemented wrist prosthesis. Clin Orthop Relat Res 1997;342:77–83.

53. Fourastier K, Le Breton L, Alnot Y, et al. Guepar's total radio-carpal prosthesis in the surgery of the rheumatoid wrist. Apropos of 72 cases reviewed. Rev Chir Orthop Reparatrice Appar Mot 1996;82: 108–15.

54. Ferlic DC, Jolly SN, Clayton ML. Salvage for failed implant arthroplasty of the wrist. J Hand Surg Am 1992;17:917–23.

55. Levadoux M, Legre R. Total wrist arthroplasty with Destot prostheses in patients with posttraumatic arthritis. J Hand Surg 2003;28A:405–13.

56. Radmer S, Andresen R, Sparmann M. Wrist arthroplasty with a new generation of prostheses in patients with rheumatoid arthritis. J Hand Surg 1999; 24:935–43.

57. Rahimtoola ZO, Rozing PM. Preliminary results of total wrist arthroplasty using the RWS Prosthesis. J Hand Surg Br 2003;28:54–60.

58. Rahimtoola ZO, Hubach P. Total modular wrist prosthesis: a new design. Scand J Plast Reconstr Surg Hand Surg 2004;38:160–5.

59. Bidwai AS, Cashin F, Richards A, et al. Short to medium results using the Remotion total wrist replacement for rheumatoid arthritis. Hand Surg 2013;18(2):175–8.

Flexor Tendon Repair
Healing, Biomechanics, and Suture Configurations

Christopher Myer, MD, John R. Fowler, MD*

KEYWORDS

- Flexor tendon • Suture configuration • Biomechanics • Growth factors • Biological augmentation

KEY POINTS

- Tendon healing is a complex process that must coordinate healing within the tendon while limiting the amount of fibrosis in the surrounding tissues.
- The ultimate goal of surgical intervention has remained constant: to achieve enough strength to allow early motion, to prevent adhesions within the tendon sheath, and to restore the finger to normal range of motion and function.
- Although certain suture materials may have superior tensile properties, the number of strands crossing a repair site is the most important factor in the overall strength of the repair.
- Recent research has been focused on using pharmacologic agents to modify the healing environment to increase the healing response within the tendon while decreasing the adhesion formation between the tendon and its sheath.

INTRODUCTION

Before the 1960s, tendon repairs in the digits were rarely performed because of the universally poor outcomes, particularly in zone II, lending to the term "no man's land."[1] Sterling Bunnell is often credited as being one of the first to stress the necessity of gentle and precise surgical technique in the treatment of flexor tendon injuries.[2] Additional research has focused on different suture configurations or number of core sutures to maximize the strength of tendon repair and postoperative rehabilitation protocols to maximize function.[3,4] The ultimate goal of surgical intervention has remained constant: to achieve enough strength to allow early motion, to prevent adhesions within the tendon sheath, and to restore the finger to normal range of motion and function. In recent years, basic science research has focused on biological factors that will increase the tendon stability after surgical repair, increase intratendinous healing, and decrease extratendinous fibrosis in order to maximize clinical outcomes.[5,6] It is in this area that there is the potential for great advancement of our understanding of tendon healing.

The purpose of this article is to review the relevant tendon anatomy, biology of tendon healing, biomechanics of tendon healing, biological strategies to augment tendon healing, and suture configurations to maximize strength and motion.

TENDON ANATOMY

Tendons are collagen-based tissues that connect muscle to bone. Tendons are primarily composed of type I collagen, whereas the surrounding endotenon and epitenon are primarily composed of type III collagen. Collagen is synthesized and secreted by tenocytes present within the tendon.

Department of Orthopaedics, University of Pittsburgh, Suite 1010, Kaufmann Building, 3471 Fifth Avenue, Pittsburgh, PA 15213, USA
* Corresponding author.
E-mail address: johnfowler10@gmail.com

Orthop Clin N Am 47 (2016) 219–226
http://dx.doi.org/10.1016/j.ocl.2015.08.019
0030-5898/16/$ – see front matter © 2016 Elsevier Inc. All rights reserved.

Once secreted, the collagen fibers arrange into triple helices and undergo cross-linking to increase their strength and stability.[7] The surrounding extracellular matrix (ECM) is thought to help with gliding between collagen fibrils and to provide functional stability to the fibers.

The collagen fiber units are bound together by endotenon fascicles. These fascicles bind together within the epitenon to form the tendon (**Fig. 1**). Lymphatic, vascular, and neural elements are present within the endotenon to supply the fibroblasts. The epitenon contains the blood vessels and tracts for the lymphatics and nerves. The tendon sheath is covered with synovial cells that provide lubrication to aid in gliding of the tendon within the sheath. Outside of the hand, tendons are not typically enclosed within a sheath and are covered by a continuous paratenon that contains the vascular elements to supply the endotenon and epitenon.

Both the flexor digitorum profundus (FDP) and flexor digitorum superficialis (FDS) tendons in the digits receive dual nutritional supply from vascular perfusion and synovial diffusion.[8,9] The vascular supply is through vincula with each tendon having 2: a longus and a brevis. Proceeding from proximal to distal, the first vinculum encountered is the vinculum longus superficialis (VLS), arising just proximal to the decussation of the FDS and coming off the floor of the digital sheath of the proximal phalanx (**Fig. 2**). The vinculum brevis superficialis consists of small triangular mesenteries near the insertion of the FDS. The vinculum longus profundus arises from the superficialis at the level of the proximal

interphalangeal (PIP) joint. Finally, the vinculum brevis profundus arises near the insertion of the FDP. Each vinculum inserts on the dorsal aspect of the tendon, creating a richer blood supply on the dorsal side of the tendon. The vincula are important in the repair of injured tendons as they may hold the tendons out to length after injury, and one must be careful not to injure any maintained vincula while repairing an injured tendon, thereby decreasing the already tenuous blood supply.

The flexor tendons pass through the carpal canal and then enter a series of pulleys, creating the flexor tendon sheath in the digits. The flexor tendon sheath starts with the first annular pulley, or A1, overlying the metacarpal heads. There are a total of 5 annular pulleys (A1–A5) and 3 cruciate pulleys (C1–C3). The more stout annular pulleys help hold the tendon close to the phalanges, whereas the cruciate pulleys allow for some mobility of the sheath with finger flexion. The tendon sheath needs to be preserved, if at all possible, to maintain the normal function of the repaired tendon. The A1, A3, and A5 pulleys all arise from the volar plates of the metacarpophalangeal, PIP, and distal interphalangeal joints, respectively. These pulleys may be incised and used as windows through which to perform tendon repairs.[10] The A2 and A4 pulleys should be maintained to prevent bowstringing of the tendon after repair.

BIOLOGY OF TENDON HEALING

Tendon healing is a complex process that must coordinate healing within the tendon while limiting

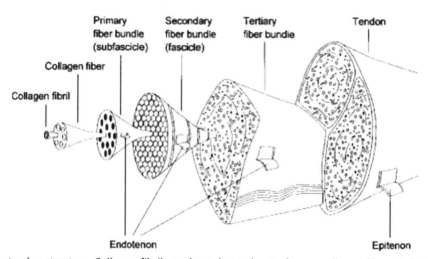

Fig. 1. Basic tendon structure. Collagen fibrils are bound together to form a collagen fiber. Multiple fibers are surrounded by endotenon in multiple stages to form a tertiary fiber bundle. Several tertiary fiber bundles are bound together by the epitenon to form the tendon. (*From* Kannus P. Structure of the tendon connective tissue. Scand J Med Sci Sports 2000;10:313; with permission.)

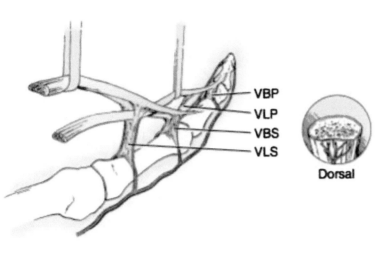

Fig. 2. The vascular supply to both flexor tendons is through vincula with each tendon having 2. The FDS receives its supply from the VLS and the vinculum brevis superficialis (VBS). The FDP receives its supply from the vinculum longus profundus (VLP) and the vinculum brevis profundus (VBP). The supply enters the tendons through the dorsal aspect of each tendon. (*From* Wolfe S, Hotchkiss R, Pederson W, et al. Flexor tendon injury. In: Wolfe S, Hotchkiss R, Pederson W, et al. Green's operative hand surgery. 6th edition. Philadelphia: Elsevier Churchill Livingstone; 2011; with permission.)

the amount of fibrosis in the surrounding tissues. The initial healing of flexor tendons consists of 3 separate stages: inflammatory, fibroblastic or reparative, and remodeling.[10,11]

Starting within the first week after injury, blood vessels within the tendon and tendon sheath form a clot at the injury site that is involved in the recruitment of vasodilators and proinflammatory cells.[11] These cells migrate to the injury site from both local tissues as well as from distant sites. They also help with removal of necrotic tissue, fibrin clot, and cellular debris through phagocytosis. Canine models have shown that angiogenic factors, such as vascular endothelial growth factor (VEGF), help initiate the vascular invasion to the site of injury.[12]

In the third week after injury, the tendon enters the fibroblastic stage. In this stage, the fibroblasts rapidly proliferate, synthesize immature collagen in an unorganized manner, and assist with the production of ECM. The initial collagen laid down is type III collagen, a weaker form of collagen than the type I collagen present in native tendons. The combination of type III collagen and previously initiated vascular network leads to scar formation within the tendon, initially decreasing its strength before entering into the final stage of healing.

The remodeling stage begins 6 to 8 weeks after injury. In this stage, type I collagen fibers are reoriented in a longitudinal manner along the long axis of the tendon and collagen fibrils begin cross-linking to one another, increasing the strength of the tendon complex. Unfortunately, the end result of the tissue repair never completely mimics the normal native tendon. It is during this stage that adhesions between the tendon and its sheath become more apparent.

Two separate models have been proposed to explain the overall mechanism of tendon healing. Extrinsic healing occurs when the fibroblasts and inflammatory cells move in from outside the tendon and invade the healing site. This process is thought to include the initial formation of adhesions. In contrast, intrinsic healing occurs through the migration of cells from the endotenon and epitenon. In most cases of tendon healing both types are present. Typically the extrinsic mechanism is activated earlier than the intrinsic mechanism and is thought to be responsible for the adhesion formation, whereas the intrinsic system is thought to help with collagen realignment and cross-linking.

BIOMECHANICS OF TENDON HEALING

Although primary tendon repair with current techniques maximizes tendon healing and decreases tendon adhesions, it is not currently possible to recreate the biomechanical properties of the normal tendon. Native tendons have a stress-strain curve that is not directly linear in nature. The collagen fibrils are aligned with one another but are not on full tension while at rest. On tensioning of the tendon, there is an initial toe region in which the tendon fibrils fully align with one another (**Fig. 3**). The curve then follows a linear progression as the tendon is increasingly tensioned. It maintains this linear slope until reaching the failure area of the curve. When tendons initially undergo surgical fixation, they have a decrease in their tension strength. It is not until the sixth to eighth week after repair when the strength of the tendon starts to increase as the collagen fibrils are realigning and the type I collagen begins to replace the initial type III collagen.

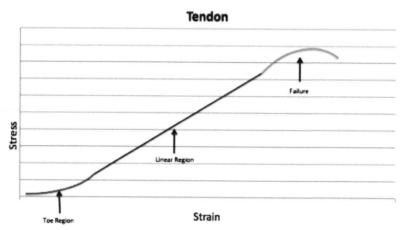

Fig. 3. The collagen fibrils are not fully aligned at rest; once tensioned, the tendon has an initial toe region in which the tendon fibrils fully align with one another. The curve then follows a linear progression as the tendon is increasingly tensioned until it reaches the failure area of the curve.

By starting controlled early active mobilization of the repaired digit, the stress across the repair site is increased. If done at levels below the load to failure of the repair, collagen deposition across the repair site is increased. This benefit, along with the decrease in adhesions between the tendon and its surrounding sheath, is the basis for early mobilization immediately after surgical repair of the tendon or tendons.

BIOLOGICAL STRATEGIES TO AUGMENT TENDON HEALING

Careful surgical technique and initiation of early motion after surgical repair of flexor tendon injuries have been the main strategies for decreasing tendon adhesions after surgical repair. However, there has been increased interest in using pharmacologic agents to modify the healing environment. Recent research has been focused on increasing the healing response within the tendon while decreasing the adhesion formation between the tendon and its sheath.

Chang[13] has performed extensive research into the biomolecular aspect of tendon repair and adhesion formation, studying a variety of growth factors in native tendons, injured tendons, and repaired tendons. The most promising of these growth factors include transforming growth factor β (TGF-B), nuclear factor kappa β (NF-kβ), and VEGF.[13]

Transforming Growth Factor β

TGF-β has 3 main isoforms (-β1, -β2, and -β3). It is produced throughout the body by nearly all cell lineages. Chang and colleagues[14] have shown that TGF-β1 is present in small amounts in native tendon and its surrounding sheath and shows a significant increase in production both within the tendon and its surrounding sheath after tendon transection and repair.[14] TGF-β1 also seems to be involved in fibrosis and is a focus of manipulation in order to decrease scarring. Shah and colleagues[15,16] were able to show that a neutralizing antibody to TFG-β was able to help control scarring in rat dermal wounds. Chang and colleagues[17] also demonstrated that the TGF-β neutralizing antibodies were able to increase the total range of motion after flexor tendon repair in a rabbit model.

Chang and his group[14] then studied the ability to separate 3 separate cell lines (fibroblasts, epitenon tenocytes, and intrinsic tenocytes) and the ability to influence each line separately. The addition of all 3 TGF-β isoforms to the cell cultures created an increase in collagen type I and III production in an in vitro rabbit model. Attempts are currently underway to isolate cells from the surrounding epitenon and selectively limit the expression of TGF-β from these cells after flexor tendon repair.[18]

Nuclear Factor Kappa β

NF-kβ is a transcription factor that is found in nearly every cell line, within the cytoplasm of the cells bound to an inhibiting factor. After activation, it releases from the inhibiting factor and passes into the nucleus where it can then bind to and act on the DNA. There are a variety of different ways to activate NF-kβ, including bacterial exposure, growth factors, and medications. NF-kβ expression is increased after tendon injury and repair, but its exact role in the tendon healing process is still under further investigation.[19]

Vascular Endothelial Growth Factor

VEGF was initially described as a substance that tumors secreted to increase vascular growth; however, it is now known that neutrophils, platelets, keratinocytes, tenocytes, and astrocytes also secrete VEGF.[20–22] Most cells produce several different isoforms at the same time, and each of the isoforms has similar end results on the target tissues. After binding to its target, VEGF induces the release of additional growth factors, ultimately causing vasodilation, expression of a-integrins, and the production of interstitial collagenase.[23,24]

VEGF is present in synovial fibroblasts. Pufe and colleagues[25] showed that VEGF was present at very low levels in native Achilles tendons, and its expression increased after injury. Others have shown increases in VEGF mRNA levels after flexor tendon injury and repair.[12] If investigators are able to harness the VEGF production and direct it where necessary, it may be possible to increase the vascular inflow to the tenuous blood supply that currently limits flexor tendon healing.

Nonsteroidal Antiinflammatory Medications

Nonsteroidal antiinflammatories (NSAIDs) are a class of medication that functions by inhibition of the cyclooxygenase (COX) enzyme, thereby inhibiting prostaglandin biosynthesis.[26] There are 2 distinct isoforms of the COX enzyme, COX-1 and COX-2. COX-1 is the constitutive form, and its activation leads to the production of prostacyclin. Prostacyclin is antithrombogenic and is cytoprotective when released by the gastric mucosa. COX-2 is an inducible isoform that is stimulated by other inflammatory stimuli and cytokines. A recent animal study has shown that ibuprofen is more effective than COX-2 inhibitors and placebo in decreasing adhesion formation. The investigators transected and then repaired tendons in rabbit forepaws and then treated the rabbits with placebo, ibuprofen, or rofecoxib. At 12 weeks, the rabbits treated with ibuprofen had significantly greater range of motion than both placebo and rofecoxib ($P = .009$).[27]

A human study has shown that ibuprofen seems to improve range of motion of the involved fingers after flexor tendon injury. Patients with zone II flexor tendon laceration repairs were randomized into either placebo or high-dose ibuprofen (2400 mg/d) for 1 month. Total active motion (TAM) at 4 weeks, TAM at 12 weeks, flexion contracture at 3 months, and disabilities of the arm, shoulder, and hand scores at 3 months were all significantly improved in patients taking ibuprofen.[28]

SUTURE CONFIGURATIONS TO MAXIMIZE STRENGTH AND MOTION

Although many different suture materials and configurations have been developed over the years, there are several core principles that need to be maintained in order to obtain stable fixation of the tendon ends. These principles include using a core suture that goes through the ends of the tendons combined with an epitendinous suture to prevent gapping at the repair site. The strength of the repair is directly proportional to the size of the suture as well as the number of passes across the repair site. More dorsal placement of the core suture provides greater strength to the construct when compared with a slightly more volar placement of the core suture.[29]

Increasing the size of the core suture leads to both increased strength of the repair as well as a decrease in gap formation. Barrie and colleagues[30] showed in a cadaveric study that 3-0 - sutures lead to a 2- to 3-fold increase in fatigue strength when compared with 4-0 sutures. In that same study, they compared variations of 2- and 4-strand flexor tendon repairs using nonlocked, simple locked, and cross-stitch locked patterns. The 3-0 four-strand cross-stitch locked repair had significantly greater fatigue strength than all other repairs tested. Additionally, all repairs using 4-0 sutures failed secondary to suture rupture, whereas repairs using 3-0 most commonly failed through suture pullout. In contrast, Osei and colleagues[31] demonstrated that even though the cross-sectional area of the 3-0 polyfilament caprolactam suture is 42% greater than that of the 4-0 polyfilament caprolactam, an 8-strand 4-0 suture repair was 43% stronger than a 4-strand 3-0 suture repair. A major conclusion from this study was that, although certain suture materials may have superior tensile properties, the number of strands crossing a repair site likely plays a larger role in the overall strength of the repair.

Lawrence and colleagues[32] demonstrated that changing the strength and stiffness of the suture material also affects gap formation. By using a stiffer and stronger material, such as Fiberwire (Arthrex) or stainless steel, the amount of gap formation at the repair site is decreased when comparing equal diameter suture. Fiberwire was shown to withstand greater ultimate forces and have a greater load to gap formation when compared with nylon, Prolene, (Ethicon) and Ethibond (Ethicon).[33] In addition, Scherman and colleagues[33] showed us that not all sutures are created equal. By taking cross-sectional areas of Fiberwire, Prolene, and Ticron (Covidien), of both 3-0 and 4-0 caliber, they were able to show that the 3-0 Fiberwire was larger in cross-sectional area than both 3-0 Prolene and 3-0 Ticron. They also were able to show that 4-0 Fiberwire was larger in cross-sectional area than 3-0 Prolene and 3-0 Ticron. The difference in true cross-sectional area of different sutures is something that most surgeons are not aware of and must be kept in mind when choosing sutures for flexor tendon repair.

The purchase of the core suture has also been extensively studied. Several in vitro animal studies have shown that the distance from the cut tendon end can significantly influence the strength of the repair. These studies have also shown that the optimal length for the purchase of the core suture is between 7 and 12 mm. With a purchase less than 7 mm, the strength decreases significantly, whereas the purchase greater than 12 mm adds little to no strength to the construct.[34,35]

The type of suture used, the size of the suture used, and the number of strands across the repair site are not the only factors associated with increased strength and decreased gapping at the repair site. Wu and colleagues[36] found that asymmetry in the repair can also increase the strength and decrease gapping. Creating a repair in which the purchase of 2 separate modified Kessler stitches, one with a purchase length of 8 mm on one side and 12 mm on the other and the second stitch is a mirror image reversing the sides for the 8- and 12-mm purchase, created a construct that was shown to have decreased gapping at initial loading as well as after cyclical loading when compared with symmetric repairs with a purchase length of 10 or 12 mm from the laceration.

Using an epitendinous suture increases the strength of the repair. Traditionally, either a 5-0 or 6-0 monofilament suture has been used. Several studies have shown that some form of cross-stitch or interlocking horizontal mattress decreases gliding resistance and increases the maximal strength of the repair construct.[37] In an attempt to increase the strength of the repair and improve surgical times, fibrin glue has been used to augment the repair. A direct comparison was performed between repairs that were augmented with an epitendinous suture and repairs augmented with fibrin glue. The linear stiffness, force to produce a 2-mm gap, and ultimate failure were similar between the two groups, whereas the fibrin glue repair had an increased gliding resistance when compared with the epitendinous repair.[38] Based on this information, an epitendinous suture adds strength, decreases gap formation, and improves the overall construct

created with the tendon repair and should be used whenever possible.

Hwang and colleagues[39] showed that repairing the FDP and both slips of the FDS increases the work of flexion by 51%, whereas repairing the FDP alone increased the work by 21%. Repairing only one slip of the FDS increased the work by an additional 9%. Because of this, one may feel comfortable with only repairing one slip of the FDS if it improves gliding of the flexor tendons through their flexor sheath without compromising the patients' outcomes.

SUMMARY

Flexor tendon healing is a complex collaboration between the tendons and their surrounding milieu. The goal is to increase the strength of the repair construct to allow for appropriate tendon healing while minimizing the scar formation to the surrounding tissues. By preserving the blood supply to the tendon through its vincula, we can maintain the nutrients needed for tendon healing. The first stage of tendon healing relies on an initial inflammatory response; with the possibility of increasing the effectiveness and decreasing the side effects of biological factors, such as TGF-β, NF-kβ, and VEGF, we may be able to tilt the balance of tendon healing and adhesion formation in our favor. The use of simple and safe medications, such as NSAIDs, may also help with the battle between healing and scar.

Using an appropriate construct when repairing an injured tendon aids in the ability to mobilize the digits, which also aids in decreasing adhesion formation. Using at least a 4-strand repair, of either a 3-0 or 4-0 suture with a purchase length of 7 to 12 mm, is necessary to allow for early active motion of the injured digits. By adding an epitendonous suture, we can both increase the strength of the repair as well as decrease the gliding resistance of the repair site. This construct allows for early passive motion while decreasing the chance of gap formation, which should allow for appropriate healing of the tendon while limiting the adhesion formation with the tendon sheath.

REFERENCES

1. Kleinert H, Kutz J, Ashbell T, et al. Primary repair of lacerated flexor tendons in "no man's land." J Bone Joint Surg Am 1967;49:577.
2. Wolfe S, Hotchkiss R, Pederson W, et al. Green's operative hand surgery. 6th edition. Philadelphia: Elsevier Churchill Livingstone; 2011.
3. Lister GD, Kleinert HE, Kutz JE, et al. Primary flexor tendon repair followed by immediate controlled mobilization. J Hand Surg Am 1977;2(6):441–51.

4. Duran RJ, Houser RG, Coleman CR, et al. A preliminary report in the use of controlled passive motion following flexor tendon repair in zones II and III. J Hand Surg Am 1976;1:79.

5. Strickland JW. Flexor tendon injuries, I: foundations of treatment. J Am Acad Orthop Surg 1995;3:44–54.

6. Strickland JW. Flexor tendon injuries, II: operative technique. J Am Acad Orthop Surg 1995;3:55–62.

7. Kuhn K. The structure of collagen. Essays Biochem 1969;5:59–87.

8. Ochiai N, Matsui T, Miyaji N, et al. Vascular anatomy of flexor tendons. I. Vincular system and blood supply of the profundus tendon in the digital sheath. J Hand Surg Am 1979;4(4):321–30.

9. Lundborg G, Rank F. Experimental intrinsic healing of flexor tendons based upon synovial fluid nutrition. J Hand Surg Am 1978;3(1):21–31.

10. Seiler JG. Flexor tendon repair. J Am Soc Surg Hand 2001;1(3):177–91.

11. Gelberman RH, Vandeberg JS, Manske PR, et al. The early stages of flexor tendon healing: a morphologic study of the first fourteen days. J Hand Surg Am 1985;10(6):776–84.

12. Bidder M, Towler DA, Gelberman RH, et al. Expression of mRNA for vascular endothelial growth factor at the repair site of healing canine flexor tendon. J Orthop Res 2000;18:247–52.

13. Chang J. Studies in flexor tendon reconstruction: biomolecular modulation of tendon repair and tissue engineering. J Hand Surg Am 2012;37:552–61.

14. Chang J, Most D, Stelnicki E, et al. Gene expression of transforming growth factor beta-1 in rabbit zone II flexor tendon wound healing: evidence for dual mechanisms of repair. Plast Reconstr Surg 1997;100(4):937–44.

15. Shah M, Foreman DM, Ferguson MWJ. Control of scarring in adult wounds by neutralising antibody to transforming growth factor beta. Lancet 1992;339:213–4.

16. Shah M, Foreman DM, Ferguson MWJ. Neutralisation of TGF-B1 and TGF-B2 or exogenous addition of TGF-B3 to cutaneous rat wounds reduces scarring. J Cell Sci 2005;108:985–1002.

17. Chang J, Thunder R, Most D, et al. Studies in flexor tendon wound healing: neutralizing antibody to TGF-B1 increases post-operative range of motion. Plast Reconstr Surg 2000;105:148–55.

18. Klein MB, Yalamanchi N, Pham H, et al. Flexor tendon healing in vitro: effects of TGF-beta on tendon cell collagen production. J Hand Surg Am 2002;27:615–20.

19. Tang JB, Xu X, Ding F, et al. Expression of genes for collagen production and NF-kB gene activation of in vivo healing flexor tendons. J Hand Surg Am 2004;29:564–70.

20. McCourt M, Wang JH, Sookhai S, et al. Proinflammatory mediators stimulate neutrophil-directed angiogenesis. Arch Surg 1999;134:1325–32.

21. Weltermann A, Wolzt M, Petersmann K, et al. Large amounts of vascular endothelial growth factor at the site of hemostatic plug formation in vivo. Arterioscler Thromb Vasc Biol 1999;19:1757–60.

22. Shweiki D, Itin A, Soffer D, et al. Vascular endothelial growth factor induced by hypoxia may mediate hypoxia-initiated angiogenesis. Nature 1992;359:843–5.

23. Unemori EN, Ferrara N, Bauer EA, et al. Vascular endothelial growth factor induces interstitial collagenase expression in human endothelial cells. J Cell Physiol 1992;153:557–62.

24. Dvorak HF. VPF/VEGF and the angiogenic response. Semin Perinatol 2000;24:75–8.

25. Pufe T, Petersen W, Tillmann B, et al. The angiogenic peptide vascular endothelial growth factor is expressed in foetal and ruptured tendons. Virchows Arch 2001;439:579–85.

26. Vane JR, Botting RM. Mechanism of action of nonsteroidal anti-inflammatory drugs. Am J Med 1998;104(3):2S–8S.

27. Tan V, Nourbakhsh A, Capo J, et al. Effects of nonsteroidal anti-inflammatory drugs on flexor tendon adhesion. J Hand Surg Am 2010;35:941–7.

28. Rouhani A, Tabrizi A, Ghavidel E. Effects of nonsteroidal anti-inflammatory drugs on flexor tendon rehabilitation after repair. Arch Bone Jt Surg 2013;1(1):28–30.

29. Soejima O, Diao E, Lotz JC, et al. Comparative mechanical analysis of dorsal versus palmar placement of core suture for flexor tendon repairs. J Hand Surg Am 1995;20:801–7.

30. Barrie KA, Tomak SL, Cholewicki J, et al. Effect of suture locking and suture caliber on fatigue strength of flexor tendon repairs. J Hand Surg Am 2001;26:340–6.

31. Osei DA, Stepan JG, Calfee RP, et al. The effect of suture caliber and number of core suture strands on zone ii flexor tendon repair: a study in human cadavers. J Hand Surg Am 2014;39(2):262–8.

32. Lawrence TM, Davis TRC. A biomechanical analysis of suture materials and their influence on a four-strand flexor tendon repair. J Hand Surg Am 2005;30:836–41.

33. Scherman P, Haddad R, Scougall P, et al. Cross-sectional area and strength differences of fiberwire, prolene, and ticron sutures. J Hand Surg Am 2010;35:780–4.

34. Cao Y, Zhu B, Xie RG, et al. Influence of core suture purchase length on strength of four-strand tendon repairs. J Hand Surg Am 2006;31(1):107–12.

35. Tang JB, Zhang Y, Cao Y, et al. Core suture purchase affects strength of tendon repairs. J Hand Surg Am 2005;30:1262–6.

36. Wu YF, Tang JB. The effect of asymmetric core suture purchase on gap resistance of tendon repair in linear cyclic loading. J Hand Surg Am 2014; 39(5):910–8.

37. Moriya T, Zhao C, An K-N, et al. The effect of epitendinous suture technique on gliding resistance during cyclic motion after flexor tendon repair: a cadaveric study. J Hand Surg Am 2010;35(4): 552–8.

38. Xu NM, Brown PJ, Plate JF, et al. Fibrin glue augmentation for flexor tendon repair increases friction compared with epitendinous suture. J Hand Surg Am 2013;38(12):2329–34.

39. Hwang MD, Pettrone S, Trumble TE. Work of flexion related to different suture materials after flexor digitorum profundus and flexor digitorum superficialis tendon repair in zone II: a biomechanical study. J Hand Surg Am 2009;34:700–4.

Scapholunate Advanced Collapse
Motion-Sparing Reconstructive Options

Kevin Kruse, MD, John R. Fowler, MD*

KEYWORDS

- Proximal row carpectomy • Four-corner arthrodesis • Scapholunate advanced collapse
- Wrist denervation • Motion-sparing surgical treatment

KEY POINTS

- Scapholunate advanced collapse (SLAC) occurs as a result of altered biomechanics after scapholunate dissociation.
- Proximal row carpectomy (PRC), scaphoid excision and four-corner arthrodesis (FCA), and wrist denervation are motion-sparing techniques designed to treat SLAC wrist.
- There are no Level I studies comparing PRC with FCA for treatment of SLAC wrist; however, systematic reviews and comparative studies suggest that there are minimal differences between PRC and FCA with respect to functional outcomes.
- Specific subgroups of patients may benefit from 1 procedure over the other. PRC may be preferred in smokers, and FCA may be preferred in patients younger than 35 years.

INTRODUCTION

Scapholunate advanced collapse (SLAC) is a predictable pattern of degenerative wrist arthritis that develops as a result of scapholunate dissociation. Watson and Ballet described the sequence of degenerative changes starting with narrowing at the radial styloid, progressing to the radioscaphoid joint, and terminating at the capitolunate articulation (**Fig. 1**).[1] The radiolunate articulation is commonly spared in SLAC. Total wrist arthrodesis is a reliable method for obtaining pain relief but has the disadvantage of sacrificing wrist motion. Motion-sparing procedures have been designed to relieve pain while maintaining some wrist range of motion. The purpose of this article is to review outcomes for the various motion-sparing surgical treatments for SLAC wrist (**Fig. 2**).

FOUR-CORNER ARTHRODESIS

Intercarpal arthrodesis as a treatment for painful degenerative conditions of the wrist was initially proposed by Watson and Ballet[1] when it was noted that many patients with congenital coalitions of the carpal bones had pain-free fully functioning wrists.[2] In their technique, k-wire fixation was used to hold the lunate, capitate, hamate, and triquetrum in position until arthrodesis occurred (**Fig. 3**). Watson and Ballet reviewed 16 patients treated with scaphoid excision and 4-corner fusion and noted 1 nonunion that was successfully treated with repeat bone grafting. All patients returned to work and had minimal pain at follow-up in this series. Other authors have obtained similarly good results with high union rates using k-wire fixation.[3,4] Krakauer and colleagues[3] had a 91% union rate (21/23) using mostly k-wires

Department of Orthopaedics, University of Pittsburgh, Suite 1010, Kaufmann Building, 3471 Fifth Avenue, Pittsburgh, PA 15213, USA
* Corresponding author.
E-mail address: fowlerjr@upmc.edu

Orthop Clin N Am 47 (2016) 227–233
http://dx.doi.org/10.1016/j.ocl.2015.08.002
0030-5898/16/$ – see front matter © 2016 Elsevier Inc. All rights reserved.

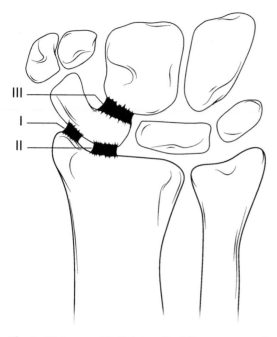

Fig. 1. Watson and Ballet described the sequence of degenerative changes starting with narrowing at the radial styloid (I), progressing to the radioscaphoid joint (II), and terminating at the capitolunate articulation (III).

for fixation (19/23). Patients obtained a mean flexion extension arc of 54°, and grip strength improved from 59% to 78.5% of the contralateral wrist. Cohen and Kozin[4] reported a union rate of 95% (18/19) and reported a mean flexion extension arc of 80° and grip strength of 79% of the contralateral side. The disadvantage of this technique is that the patient must return to the operating room, typically 8 to 10 weeks after the index procedure, to have the k-wires removed.

Although high union rates have been reported in the literature (>90%) with k-wire fixation, circular plate fixation was been introduced as alternative to theoretically improve union rates and avoid the need for k-wire removal. Despite the theoretic advantage of increased stability, the nonunion rates in several series have been surprisingly high (25%–63%).[5–7] Kendall and colleagues[5] reviewed the results of 4 surgeons using the circular plate for the first time. Only 3 of 8 patients who returned for final radiographs achieved union. Grip strength was 56% of the opposite wrist, and the mean flexion extension arc was 61°. Vance and colleagues[6] reviewed 58 patients who had undergone FCA with various techniques. Twenty-seven patients had plate fixation, and 31 patients had traditional fixation (k-wires, Herbert screws

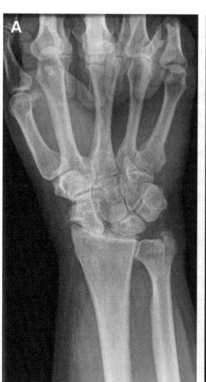

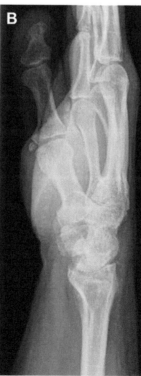

Fig. 2. AP (*A*) and lateral (*B*) radiographs of an SLAC wrist demonstrating scapholunate dissociation with radial styloid and radioscaphoid degenerative changes. The lateral radiographs show DISI of the lunate.

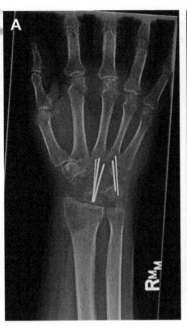
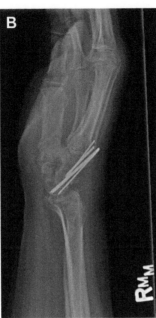

Fig. 3. Four-corner arthrodesis using K-wire fixation, AP (*A*) and lateral (*B*) radiographs.

staples). The traditional group had a nonunion rate of 3%, and the plate group had a nonunion rate of 26%. Grip strength and range of motion compared with the opposite side were 70% (plate)/79% (traditional) and 48% (plate)/50% (traditional), respectively. Shindle and colleagues reported on 16 patients undergoing 4-corner fusion with circular plate and had a 25% nonunion rate and a 56% overall complication rate. Circular plates have also been associated with decreased range of motion, compared with k-wires postoperatively. De Smet and colleagues[8] reported on 28 patients undergoing FCA and found that traditional methods had better postoperative flexion than the plate fixation group, 33° versus 23°, respectively. Despite the reports of high nonunion rates, other authors have published union rates as high as 100%.[9,10] Bedford and Yang[9] reported a 100% union rate on 15 patients undergoing 4-corner arthrodesis with a circular plate. Patients in this series achieved range of motion and grip strength of 71% and 78% of the opposite side, respectively. Merrell and colleagues[10] reported a 100% union rate for the capitolunate articulation in 28 patients using a circular plate. The mean flexion extension arc was 61°, and grip strength was 82% of the opposite side. These authors attributed the high union rate to using bone graft from the distal radius, placement of 2 screws in each bone, and thorough debridement of all chondral surfaces.

The primary goal of an FCA is the fusion of the capitolunate joint. The fusion of the triquetrum and hamate was added, because early reports of isolated capitolunate fusion had higher nonunion rates. Kirschenbaum reported a fusion rate of only 67% (12/18) in patients undergoing an isolated capitolunate fusion with a combination of staples and k-wires. The mean flexion extension arc was 50°, and grip strength was 67% of the opposite side.[11] Calandruccio and colleagues[12] reported on 14 patients who underwent isolated capitolunate fusion with a compression screw with scaphoid and triquetrum excision (**Fig. 4**). The authors reported a union rate of 86%, mean flexion extension arc of 53°, and grip strength 71% of the contralateral side. Gaston compared 16 patients who underwent capitolunate fusion with 18 patients who underwent traditional FCA. There was a slight increase in the mean flexion extension arc in the capitolunate group (58%) compared with the traditional FCA (48%). The capitolunate group had a 100% union rate, and there were no differences in any other outcome measures; however, 5 patients in the capitolunate group required screw removal for migration.[13] Overall clinical results of isolated capitolunate arthrodesis are similar those of FCA.

PROXIMAL ROW CARPECTOMY

Proximal row carpectomy (PRC) involves removal of the scaphoid, lunate, and triquetrum with creation of a new articulation between the capitate and radius (**Fig. 5**).[14] Imbriglia and colleagues[15] noted that the radius of the curvature of the capitate does not match the lunate fossa, resulting in a loose joint that disperses load on the lunate fossa despite increased contact area.[16–18] PRC

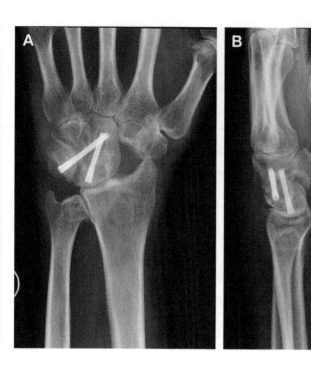

Fig. 4. Four-corner arthrodesis using headless compression screws, AP (*A*) and lateral (*B*) radiographs.

has been noted to be less technically demanding than 4-corner arthrodesis, and may allow earlier return to activity. Imbriglia and colleagues[15] reviewed 27 patients who underwent PRC at average follow-up of 4 years (range 2–8 years). Pain was relieved in 26 of 27 patients, and 24 of 27 patients returned to their previous level of activity. Grip strength improved to an average of 80% of the contralateral side. Culp and colleagues[19] retrospectively reviewed 20 patients, at average follow-up of 3.5 years (range 2–7 years), who underwent PRC. In nonrheumatoid

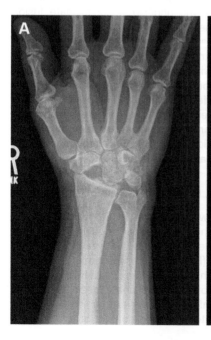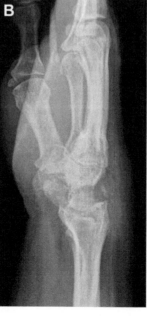

Fig. 5. AP (*A*) and lateral (*B*) radiographs after proximal row carpectomy.

patients, motion decreased to 52% of normal side and grip strength was 67% of normal side. Seventy-six percent of patients had little or no pain; 18% of patients had severe pain. Wrist scores showed 6% excellent, 35% good, 29% fair, and 30% poor results. Only 20% of laborers returned to work. The authors noted the radial styloidectomy improved radial deviation, but did not affect outcome scores. Tomaino and colleagues[20] reported on 23 patients who underwent PRC and found 20 of 23 patients were happy with their functional outcome and experienced pain relief. Two patients had persistent pain, and a third patient developed pain 3 years after surgery; all 3 patients required conversion to total wrist arthrodesis. Flexion and extension averaged 37° in each direction, for a mean arc of motion 61% of the contralateral side. Grip strength averaged 79% of the contralateral side. Twenty-one of 23 patients returned to work at an average of 5 months after surgery, including 9 of 13 heavy laborers in their original positions. Radiographs showed radiocapitate arthritis in 5 of 23 patients.

Several studies have reported long-term follow-up data at greater than 10 years. Jebson and colleagues[21] reported on 20 patients who underwent PRC, and 18 of 20 patients were evaluated at an average follow-up of 13.1 years (range 10–17 years). Persistent pain was present in 2 of 20 patients, and those patients underwent total wrist arthrodesis between 28 and 40 months after the index procedure. Average wrist range of motion (ROM) was 63%, and grip strength was 83%. Seventeen of 18 patients were satisfied with their outcome, and 16 of 18 patients returned to original work and activity level. Moderate or severe radiocapitate arthritis developed in 4 of 18 patients and did not correlate with pain or satisfaction. The authors felt that the translational movement described by Imbriglia led to less degeneration and that flattening of the capitate might be related to remodeling rather than arthritis. DiDonna and colleagues reviewed 22 wrists that underwent PRC for degenerative conditions and were followed for a mean of 14 years. Four of 22 (18%) wrists underwent wrist fusion at an average of 7 years and were deemed failures. All 4 failures occurred in patients who had the PRC when they were younger than 35 years of age. Average flexion–extension arc was 72°, and average grip strength was 91% of the contralateral side. The authors noted progression of radiocapitate narrowing as described by other authors,[15] but they concurred that this did not appear to correlate with clinical outcomes.[22]

STUDIES COMPARING PROXIMAL ROW CARPECTOMY AND FOUR-CORNER ARTHRODESIS

There are currently no Level I studies comparing PRC and FCA. However, there have been several studies that have compared cohorts of PRC and FCA.

Cohen and Cozen compared 2 groups of 19 patients that received either FCA or PRC at 2 different institutions. No difference was found between the groups in regards to flexion–extension (81° PRC and 80° FCA), pain, function, or grip strength (71% PRC and 79% FCA). The authors did note that the FCA group maintained better radial/ulnar deviation (31° PRC vs 53° FCA). There was no difference in complications between the groups.[4] Vanhove and colleagues[23] compared 15 patients with FCA and 15 patients with PRC in a retrospective study. The mean flexion extension arc was 70° in the FCA group and 80° in the PRC group. Grip strength was 71% of the opposite side in the FCA group and 77% in the PRC group. The PRC group returned to work in 9.8 weeks, and the FCA group returned in 38.6 weeks. Six patients in the FCA group had postoperative carpal tunnel syndrome requiring carpal tunnel release; 1 patient had a nonunion, and 3 patients had pin track infections. Overall, there was no significant difference in pain or function, but the authors found a higher complication rate and a later return to work in the 4-corner arthrodesis group. Krakauer and colleagues reported on 55 patients who underwent surgery for SLAC wrist using a variety of techniques (23 FCA, 8 capitolunate arthrodesis, 12 PRC, 5 radioscapholunate arthrodesis, 3 radioscaphoid arthrodesis, and 4 total wrist arthrodesis). Of the motion-sparing procedures, 6 of 51 procedures were converted to total wrist arthrodesis. The authors noted a mean arc of motion of 54° in the FCA group and 71° in the PRC group.

Mulford, in a systematic review of PRC versus FCA, found that grip strength, pain relief, and subjective outcomes were similar in both groups, although PRC lacked the complications of nonunion, hardware issues, and dorsal impingement. The author also noted a trend toward better range of motion in PRC, but the risk for early arthritis was higher.[24] Saltzman and colleagues[25] performed a systematic review of studies comparing FCA with PRC. The analysis included 240 patients and 242 wrists (119 FCA and 123 PRC) with a mean follow-up of 27 to 33 months. Proximal row carpectomy results in better postoperative wrist flexion and extension than FCA; however, FCA results in better radial deviation and grip strength. Postoperative flexion–extension arc was

62° in 4-corner fusion and 75° in PRC. Grip strength was slightly higher in FCA when compared with the contralateral side, 74% versus 67%. The overall complication rate of FCA was 29% versus 14% for PRC.

In a recent review of the literature, Kiefhaber found that 85% of patients report feeling good or better, regardless of the procedure performed. However, 25% of patients in each group still have residual pain, and approximately 5% are converted to total wrist arthrodesis. Range of motion in the flexion–extension arc is typically 75° to 80° (60%–70% of opposite side and 10° less than preoperatively) with either procedure, but average range of motion with 4-corner arthrodesis is about 10° less than with PRC. Grip strength returns to about 80% of the contralateral side in both PRC and FCA. Postoperative arthritis is more common with PRC, but this does not seem to affect the functional results. Based on a higher rate of conversion to total wrist arthrodesis in patients undergoing PRC under the age of 35, the author recommended that this subgroup be offered FCA.[26]

WRIST DENERVATION

In order to help alleviate the pain of SLAC wrist, denervation of the wrist joint has been described. This can be performed as a partial or complete denervation of the wrist. Silva reported on 49 patients who underwent a complete denervation of the carpus,[27] using 4 incisions about the wrist to denervate all nerves innervating the carpus. Patients in all groups reported 80% improvement in pain at 1 year, and grip strength improved from 43% opposite side preoperatively to 69% the opposite side postoperatively. Painful neuroma of the radial sensory nerve developed in 4 patients. Dellon reported on resection of the posterior interosseous nerve for various conditions and stressed the importance of a preoperative nerve block to assess the probability of a successful outcome of the procedure. In his series, all patients had pain relief with a preoperative block of the posterior interosseous nerve, and 90% of these patients had pain relief after posterior interosseous nerve neurectomy.[28] Not all authors have had as much success with wrist denervation. Radu and colleagues[29] studied 43 patients undergoing partial or complete wrist denervation, including SLAC and SNAC wrist diagnoses. Patients without arthritis experienced better pain relief than patients with arthritis. Only 53% of patients with arthritis and carpal instability were satisfied with the surgery. A total of 76% of all patients with a complete denervation and 57% of patients with a partial wrist denervation reported some pain reduction. The authors concluded that the results in patients with arthritic changes are unpredictable even with pain relief preoperatively with a nerve block, but still recommend the procedure in patients who would prefer to avoid wrist arthrodesis or PRC. There is currently no literature directly comparing the results of partial/complete wrist denervation with PRC/4-corner fusion.

SUMMARY

Scapholunate advanced collapse is a pattern of degenerative wrist arthritis that was traditionally treated with total wrist arthrodesis. Motion-sparing procedures such as FCA, PRC, and wrist denervation have successfully relieved pain and preserved motion in a majority of patients. Although no Level 1 evidence exists, systematic reviews and comparative studies suggest that there are minimal differences between PRC and FCA with respect to functional outcomes. Specific subgroups of patients may benefit from one procedure over the other. PRC may be preferred in smokers, and FCA may be preferred in patients younger than 35 years.

REFERENCES

1. Watson HK, Ballet FL. The SLAC wrist: scapholunate advanced collapse pattern of degenerative arthritis. J Hand Surg Am 1984;9(3):358–65.
2. Peterson HA, Lipscomb PR. Intercarpal arthrodesis. Arch Surg 1967;95(1):127–34.
3. Krakauer JD, Bishop AT, Cooney WP. Surgical treatment of scapholunate advanced collapse. J Hand Surg Am 1994;19(5):751–9.
4. Cohen MS, Kozin SH. Degenerative arthritis of the wrist: proximal row carpectomy versus scaphoid excision and four-corner arthrodesis. J Hand Surg Am 2001;26(1):94–104.
5. Kendall CB, Brown TR, Millon SJ, et al. Results of four-corner arthrodesis using dorsal circular plate fixation. J Hand Surg Am 2005;30(5):903–7.
6. Vance MC, Hernandez JD, DiDonna ML, et al. Complications and outcome of four-corner arthrodesis: circular plate fixation versus traditional techniques. J Hand Surg Am 2005;30(6):1122–7.
7. Shindle M, Burton K, Weiland A, et al. Complications of circular plate fixation for four-corner arthrodesis. J Hand Surg 2007;32(1):50–3.
8. De Smet L, Deprez P, Duerinckx J, et al. Outcome of four-corner arthrodesis for advanced carpal collapse: circular plate versus traditional techniques. Acta Orthop Belg 2009;75(3):323–7.
9. Bedford B, Yang SS. High fusion rates with circular plate fixation for four-corner arthrodesis of the wrist. Clin Orthop Relat Res 2010;468(1):163–8.

10. Merrell GA, McDermott EM, Weiss A-PC. Four-corner arthrodesis using a circular plate and distal radius bone grafting: a consecutive case series. J Hand Surg Am 2008;33(5):635–42.

11. Kirschenbaum D, Schneider LH, Kirkpatrick WH, et al. Scaphoid excision and capitolunate arthrodesis for radioscaphoid arthritis. J Hand Surg Am 1993;18(5):780–5.

12. Calandruccio JH, Gelberman RH, Duncan SF, et al. Capitolunate arthrodesis with scaphoid and triquetrum excision. J Hand Surg Am 2000;25(5):824–32.

13. Gaston RG, Greenberg JA, Baltera RM, et al. Clinical outcomes of scaphoid and triquetral excision with capitolunate arthrodesis versus scaphoid excision and four-corner arthrodesis. J Hand Surg Am 2009;34(8):1407–12.

14. Wall LB, Stern PJ. Proximal row carpectomy. Hand Clin 2013;29(1):69–78.

15. Imbriglia JE, Broudy AS, Hagberg WC, et al. Proximal row carpectomy: clinical evaluation. J Hand Surg Am 1990;15(3):426–30.

16. Zhu Y-L, Xu Y-Q, Ding J, et al. Biomechanics of the wrist after proximal row carpectomy in cadavers. J Hand Surg Eur Vol 2010;35(1):43–5.

17. Tang P, Gauvin J, Muriuki M, et al. Comparison of the "contact biomechanics" of the intact and proximal row carpectomy wrist. J Hand Surg Am 2009; 34(4):660–70.

18. Hogan CJ, McKay PL, Degnan GG. Changes in radiocarpal loading characteristics after proximal row carpectomy. J Hand Surg Am 2004;29(6):1109–13.

19. Culp RW, Bachoura A, Gelman SE, et al. Proximal row carpectomy combined with wrist hemiarthroplasty. J Wrist Surg 2012;1(1):39–46.

20. Tomaino MM, Delsignore J, Burton RI. Long-term results following proximal row carpectomy. J Hand Surg Am 1994;19(4):694–703.

21. Jebson PJ, Hayes EP, Engber WD. Proximal row carpectomy: a minimum 10-year follow-up study11 No benefits in any form have been received or will be received by a commercial party related directly or indirectly to the subject of this article. J Hand Surg Am 2003;28(4):561–9.

22. Stern PJ, Agabegi SS, Kiefhaber TR, et al. Proximal row carpectomy. J Bone Joint Surg Am 2005; 87(Suppl 1(Pt 2)):166–74.

23. Vanhove W, De Vil J, Van Seymortier P, et al. Proximal row carpectomy versus four-corner arthrodesis as a treatment for SLAC (scapholunate advanced collapse) wrist. J Hand Surg Eur Vol 2008;33(2): 118–25.

24. Stanley JK. Re: Mulford JS, Ceulemans LJ, Nam D, Axelrod TS. Proximal row carpectomy vs. four corner fusion for scapholunate (SLAC) or scaphoid nonunion advanced collapse (SNAC) wrists: a systematic review of outcomes. J Hand Surg Eur. 2009, 34: 256–63. J Hand Surg Eur Vol 2009;34(6): 819–20.

25. Saltzman BM, Frank JM, Slikker W, et al. Clinical outcomes of proximal row carpectomy versus four-corner arthrodesis for post-traumatic wrist arthropathy: a systematic review. J Hand Surg Eur Vol 2014;40(5):450–7.

26. Kiefhaber TR. Management of scapholunate advanced collapse pattern of degenerative arthritis of the wrist. J Hand Surg Am 2009;34(8):1527–30.

27. Jefferson BS, Roman JA, Padoin AV. Wrist denervation for painful conditions of the wrist. J Hand Surg Am 2011;36(6):961–6.

28. Dellon AL. Partial dorsal wrist denervation: resection of the distal posterior interosseous nerve. J Hand Surg Am 1985;10(4):527–33.

29. Radu CA, Schachner M, Tränkle M, et al. Functional results after wrist denervation. Handchir Mikrochir Plast Chir 2010;42(5):279–86.

Optimal Positioning for Volar Plate Fixation of a Distal Radius Fracture
Determining the Distal Dorsal Cortical Distance

Michael M. Vosbikian, MD[a],*,
Constantinos Ketonis, MD, PhD[b], Ronald Huang, MD[b],
Asif M. Ilyas, MD[c]

KEYWORDS

• Distal radius fracture • Loss of reduction • Screw position • Volar locked plate • Volar tilt

KEY POINTS

• Surgical treatment of distal radius fractures with volar locked plates can lead to satisfactory outcomes in most patients with the adequacy of the reduction and maintenance of this reduction leading to better outcomes.

• A number of radiographic parameters are used to assess adequate distal radius fracture reduction, including volar tilt, radial height, radial inclination, ulnar variance, and articular congruency. Among these, volar tilt has been shown to be most related to late fracture collapse and subsequent altered wrist kinematics.

• Loss of reduction is not uncommon after volar locked plate fixation of distal radius fractures, and is most closely related to subchondral screw position rather than plate position.

• The distal dorsal cortical distance (DDD), analogous to the "tip-apex" distance in the hip, may serve as a critical measurement that the surgeon can use intraoperatively to guide adequacy of subchondral screw position and fracture stability.

• We recommend a DDD of 6 mm as the maximum distance intraoperatively to avoid late fracture collapse.

INTRODUCTION

Fractures of the distal radius are among the most common injuries to the musculoskeletal system and typically result from a fall onto an outstretched arm.[1–8] The patients affected by this pathology tend to be distributed bimodally with a great variety of fracture patterns and clinical presentations. On one end of the spectrum, are the young high-energy trauma patients, and on the other end are the elderly patients with a low-energy mechanism of injury, typically a fall from standing height. With the prevalence of osteoporosis on

[a] Hand and Microvascular Surgery, Harvard–Beth Israel Deaconess Medical Center, 330 Brookline Avenue, Stoneman Building–10th Floor, Boston, MA 02215, USA; [b] Orthopaedic Surgery, Thomas Jefferson University Hospital, 1025 Walnut Street, College Building–Room 516, Philadelphia, PA 19107, USA; [c] The Rothman Institute at Thomas Jefferson University Hospital, 925 Chestnut Street, 5th Floor, Philadelphia, PA 19107, USA
* Corresponding author.
E-mail address: Michael.vosbikian@gmail.com

Orthop Clin N Am 47 (2016) 235–244
http://dx.doi.org/10.1016/j.ocl.2015.08.020
0030-5898/16/$ – see front matter © 2016 Elsevier Inc. All rights reserved.

the rise, and the aging population living longer and remaining more active, one can expect the incidence of these fractures to rise.[1,3,4,9]

When surgery is indicated to treat distal radius fractures, volar locked plates have recently become the treatment of choice. The literature is replete with studies examining the outcomes of this procedure, first introduced by Orbay and Fernandez in 2002.[2,5,7–14] The purported advantages of volar locked plates include a stable periarticular reduction affording earlier return to function, decreased need for postoperative immobilization, a consistent surgical approach, and a hardware complication profile relative to late tendon injury that can be minimized with thoughtful screw and plate positioning.

The goals of treatment for distal radius fractures are to achieve and maintain anatomic reduction relative to the radiographic parameters listed in this article.[2–4,7,8,10,15–19] The authors use the following values:

- Volar tilt (11° ± 5°)
- Radial height (14 ± 1 mm)
- Radial inclination (22° ± 3°)
- Ulnar variance (0.7 ± 1.5 mm)
- Articular step-off (≤2 mm) (**Fig. 1**).

INDICATIONS/CONTRAINDICATIONS FOR VOLAR LOCKED PLATING

The indications and contraindications are listed in **Table 1**.[10,18,20–22] However, they are intended to serve as a rough guideline, and may be titrated up or down based on individual patient characteristics, such as age, functional demands, and occupation.

The Concept of the Volar Locked Plate

The impetus for the development of volar locked plates came from the issues seen with previous fixation constructs. Nonlocking volar plates were limited by inadequate bicortical screw stability

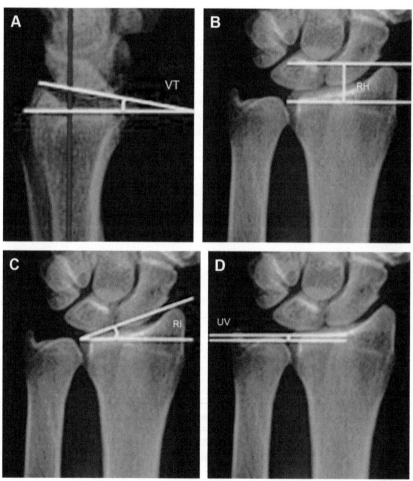

Fig. 1. Method of measuring the radiographic parameters of the distal radius fractures. (*A*) Volar tilt (VT). (*B*) Radial height (RH). (*C*) Radial inclination (RI). (*D*) Ulnar variance (UV).

Table 1 Indications/contraindications for volar locked plating	
Indications	**Contraindications**
Dorsal angulation ≥20°	Acceptable radiographic parameters after closed reduction and immobilization
Radial inclination ≤20°	Medical comorbidities precluding surgery
Ulnar variance ≥5 mm	Soft tissue condition precluding surgical approach
Articular step-off ≥2 mm	Dorsal shear fractures
Reduction loss on follow-up radiographs	—

Data from Refs.[10,18,20–22]

due to the presence of dorsal comminution. Dorsal plates also suffered from fracture displacement but also soft tissue complications, such as complex regional pain syndrome and extensor tendon irritation or rupture[13,23,24] (**Fig. 2**). The volar locked plate was intended to serve as a fixed-angle buttressing construct for the subchondral surface of the distal radius using a more generous soft tissue envelope provided by the volar side of the distal

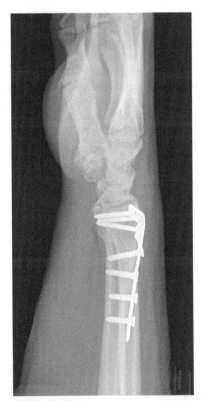

Fig. 2. Dorsal plates have been shown to be effective in managing dorsally displaced distal radius fractures; however, they can result in late soft tissue complications due to their intimate contact with the extensor tendons.

forearm.[13] The critical nuances of this technique and device are to achieve an appropriate reduction and proper plate placement proximal to the watershed line. As the initial implants were all fixed-angle constructs, the trajectory of the screw or pegs were predicated on a near anatomic reduction (**Fig. 3**). Initial designs included only 4 screws or pegs in the distal row, which were designed to capture the radial styloid, the central articular surface, and the volar-ulnar corner of the distal radius.[13]

With the advent of variable-angle locking screws, there is potentially more latitude with plate placement and articular fracture fixation (**Fig. 4**). Hart and colleagues[25] demonstrated that with the standard variable-angle locking plates, there was a 3-mm zone of forgiveness relative to the watershed line provided with these designs without compromising stability. However, the advantages afforded by variable-angle constructs have been called into question in other series.[26,27]

Achievement and Maintenance of Reduction

One of the principal tenets of fracture surgery is both restoring and maintaining normal anatomy. Surgical techniques and implants have evolved over time to better achieve these goals, and the distal radius is no exception. However, both achieving and subsequently maintaining fracture reduction can be challenging and highly variable, resulting in potentially disparate outcomes.

In a retrospective review of 185 distal radius fractures treated with a single implant performed by Mignemi and colleagues[10] in 2013, the investigators attempted to determine the ability of the volar locked plate to provide durable results with the maintenance of radiographic parameters. In their series, the volar tilt, radial inclination, ulnar variance, radial height, and articular step-off were measured immediately postoperatively and at final follow-up. They found that in most cases,

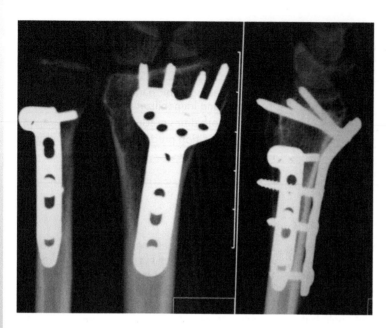

Fig. 3. Appropriate positioning of a fixed-angle volar plate is critical to optimize screw positioning and fracture fixation. Note a case of a volar fixed-angle locking plate applied in a suboptimal position. Consequently, note the prominence of the plate volarly, potentially injuring flexor tendons, imbalanced subchondral screw support, and prominent screws dorsally potentially injuring extensor tendons.

the articular step-off was less than 2 mm at all points in the postoperative course. However, this series demonstrated that there was a change in reduction over time with the volar tilt, radial inclination, and ulnar variance having changed but still within normal parameters in roughly 50% of the cases, but radial height in only 12% of cases. The loss of reduction was correlated to initial fracture severity.

Other studies have shown that radiographic parameters are typically maintained postoperatively.[3,4,6,10–12] However, on closer examination

of the results, there are nuances worth noting. In a review by Stevenson and colleagues[6] from 2009, the investigators conclude that the volar locking plate is a good technique for restoring and maintaining radiographic parameters of these fractures postoperatively. However, volar tilt was restored to an average of 1°, the range of values reported in their series ranged from 7.3° to 3.7° of undercorrection and overcorrection, respectively, yielding an 11° range. In the same series, radial inclination ranged from 10° undercorrected to overcorrection of 8.4°, with a mean of 1.9° of

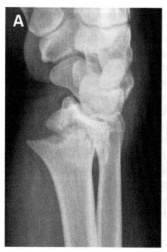
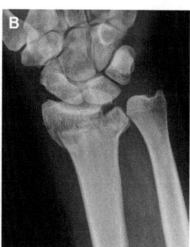
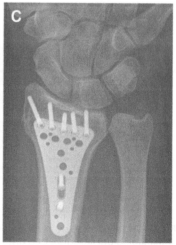

Fig. 4. Variable-angle locked plates afford more flexibility in both plate positioning as well as subchondral screw positioning. (*A*) Preoperative lateral view. (*B*) Preoperative posterior-anterior (PA) view. (*C*) Postoperative PA view.

undercorrection. The ulnar variance showed a tighter measurement range with an absolute measurement of −2 mm to +3.5 mm. Figl and colleagues[3,4] showed similar ranges of measurements in 2 other series. In a series from 2009 examining reduction in distal radius fractures treated with volar locked plates, there was a 22° range for radial inclination, and an 18° range for the volar tilt.[3] In their 2010 study, which focused on fractures in the elderly, there was similarly a 17° and 13° range in measurements for the radial inclination and volar tilt, respectively.[4]

The Importance of Maintaining Reduction

When normal anatomy is not restored, numerous adverse consequences have been noted. In particular, persistent radial shortening and/or distal radioulnar joint (DRUJ) incongruency has been shown to be a troublesome problem.[2] Common sequelae include altered carpal kinematics, Kïenbock disease, scapholunate instability, triangular fibrocartilage complex (TFCC) tears, and ulnar impaction.[1,10,16,18,20–22,28–30]

In a biomechanical cadaveric study by Nishiwaki and colleagues,[31] the effects of dorsal angulation of the distal radius on the kinematics of the DRUJ with and without an intact TFCC were evaluated. The impact of simulated malunions of 10°, 20°, and 30° of dorsal angulation on ulnar displacement in supination was shown to progressively adversely impact the kinematics of the DRUJ. Significant displacement of the ulna in the volar, ulnar, and distal directions was noted in all simulated malunions, with an increase in the volar translation in specimens with the TFCC sectioned. These changes were noted with as little as 10° loss of volar tilt, which is deemed an acceptable reduction by many investigators. This series has been echoed in other biomechanical studies that show an adverse effect on the DRUJ with dorsally angulated malunions.[32,33] An additional concern with altered kinematics with distal radius fractures is the high incidence of primary and secondary TFCC tears, which have been reported to be as high as 45% to 57% after a distal radius fracture.[34,35]

McQueen and Caspers[28] studied the final function of patients with varying anatomic reductions in distal radius fractures. In this series, a reduction in grip strength was noted in many patients. This was attributed to pain as well as the shortening of the radius, which decreases the power and mechanical advantage of the flexor tendons when compared with an uninjured wrist. The investigators go on to propose that increasing dorsal tilt will shift the axis of rotation of the wrist, leading

to compromise of the flexion-extension arc of the radiocarpal joint.

Focusing on secondary fracture displacement, when treated nonoperatively, Altissimi and colleagues[21] noted that with increased settling, patients had more functional deficits and were more predisposed to radiocarpal arthrosis. In this study, dorsal tilt of 1° to 15° resulted in 8% of patients having fair to poor results and in patients with 15° or greater, fair to poor outcomes were reported in 50% of patients. Although this is not a typical postoperative finding, there are patients in other series who fall into these ranges with fracture settling and may be experiencing underappreciated functional deficits.

Potential Factors Influencing Reduction Maintenance

Once surgical fracture reduction is achieved, maintaining the reduction with internal fixation presents the next challenge to the surgeon. Previous investigators have studied various parameters to be considered to maximize stable internal fixation with locked volar plates in distal radius fractures. In an osteoporotic biomechanical model, Wall and colleagues[36] studied the effect of screw length on stability in distal radius fracture volar locked plate constructs. Their work showed that a screw length greater than 75% of the bicortical distance provides excellent stability and minimizes the chance for extensor tendon rupture by obviating the need for bicortical drilling and eliminating the possibility of dorsal screw prominence, while still maintaining adequate subchondral screw support. With respect to the use of screws versus pegs for fixation, Weninger and colleagues[8] found that screws proved to be biomechanically superior, particularly when loaded in torsion, then compared with smooth pegs, which demonstrated a 17% reduction in stiffness. Crosby and colleagues,[37] in a biomechanical model using 24 sawbone specimens, sought to determine if the amount of screws in the distal fragment of the fracture had any impact on stability in extra-articular fragments. Their results supported the fact that the number of screws in the distal row did not show a significant influence on the stiffness or stability of the final construct.

The placement and position of the volar locked plate also has been a topic of a number of studies. Some investigators have recommended that the plate be placed as distal as possible without crossing the watershed line to place the screws as close as possible to the subchondral bone.[2,13] However, this requires diligence to avoid placing

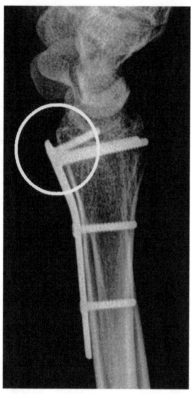

Fig. 5. Placement of volar locked plate too distally with residual dorsal angulation leading to potential flexor tendon irritation and injury.

the plate too distal and causing plate prominence and potential risk of flexor tendon ruptures. This risk is increased in cases with fractures healing in residual dorsal angulation[38–40] (**Fig. 5**).

On a larger scale, one can deduce that despite these advances and the evolution of techniques and practice that has come from these studies, there remain unanswered questions about the parameters needed for successful maintenance of reduction with distal radius fracture fixation. We posit that this demands a return to the principles initially proposed by Orbay and Fernandez,[13] who suggested that the buttress effect of the volar locked plate is the critical biomechanical advantage to this technique when compared with more traditional methods of fixation. The work of Crosby's group[37] supports this theory in that the buttress exists in a static location regardless of the number of screws in the distal row.[37] This implies that it is the position of these screws, and not the number or the length of the screws that dictates the capability of the construct to reproducibly maintain the reduction of the distal radial articular surface. In addition, with the advent of variable-angle locking screw and peg technology, the plate placement, as long as not too distal, is less important, as the screws are what provide the distal aspect of the buttress. Furthermore, the variable-angle screws can provide up to 3 mm of forgiveness with plate placement.[25]

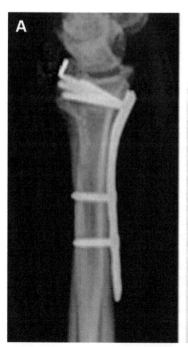

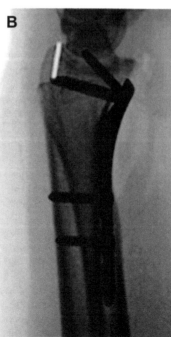

Fig. 6. (*A, B*) The DDD is measured (in mm) from the tip of the most distal screw to the dorsal rim of the distal radius, taken on a 20° inclined lateral view intraoperatively.

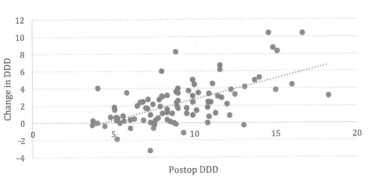

Fig. 7. Linear regression demonstrating the relationship between the change in DDD relative to the initial postoperative (postop) DDD ($P<.001$).

This implies that there should be a primary focus on an optimal distance for the screws in relation to the proximal aspect of the subchondral bone of the distal radius and not necessarily a focus on the position of the plate with respect to the watershed line. The work of Orbay and Fernandez,[13] as well as a study by Drobetz and colleagues,[2] suggest that placing these screws as close to the subchondral bone as possible is critical.[13] However, there is no consensus as to the optimal distance of the screws relative to the subchondral bone.

THE DISTAL DORSAL CORTICAL DISTANCE

In seeking a reproducible and reliable measurement that can serve as a valuable intraoperative tool to determine the optimal distance between the subchondral screws and the articular surface, we turn to the work of Baumgaertner and colleagues[41] and the "tip-apex" distance in the treatment of peritrochanteric fractures of the hip. In this series of 198 fractures in 193 patients, they found that there was a critical distance for the implant from a fixed point in the subchondral bone on

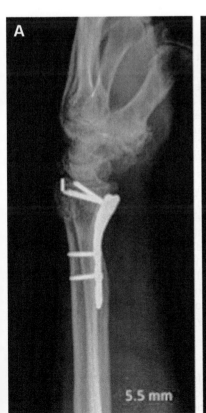
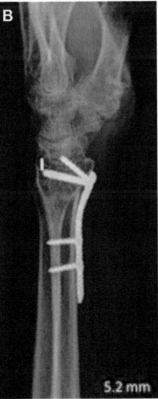

Fig. 8. Case of a DDD placed within the optimal distance. (*A*) Immediate postoperative lateral radiographic view demonstrating an initial DDD of 5.5 mm. (*B*) One-year follow-up lateral demonstrating a DDD of 5.2 mm, showing 0.3 mm of settling, and a concordant 0.84° loss of volar tilt.

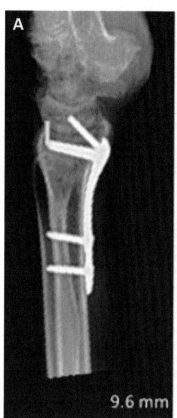
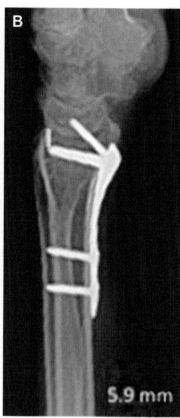

9.6 mm   5.9 mm

Fig. 9. Case of a DDD placed outside the optimal distance. (*A*) Immediate postoperative lateral radiographic view demonstrating an initial DDD of 9.6 mm. (*B*) One-year follow-up lateral demonstrating a DDD of 5.9 mm, showing 3.7 mm of settling, and a concordant 8° loss of volar tilt.

standardized radiographs that correlated with improved ability to maintain fracture reduction until union. We similarly propose a novel measurement that can be taken intraoperatively with fixed points of measurement that is reproducible and correlates to the amount of settling that can be predicted with respect to the articular surface and volar tilt, so as to avoid late altered wrist kinematics.[21,28,31–33] We have coined this the "distal dorsal cortical distance" (DDD). This tool can allow the surgeon to make intraoperative adjustments based on a fluoroscopic 20° true lateral view that allows visualization of the most distal screw and the dorsal rim of the radius in profile.

In our preliminary experience with this concept, a retrospective review of 95 closed extra-articular distal radius fractures repaired with a locked volar plate was performed at our tertiary care referral institution. There were 75 female patients and 20 male patients. All surgeries were performed by 5 fellowship-trained orthopedic hand surgeons. Postoperative radiographs were reviewed at a minimum of 1-year follow-up. Patients were excluded if the fracture was intra-articular or supplemental fixation was used. On the preliminary and final postoperative radiograph, the DDD was measured from the tip of the most distal screw in the construct to the edge of the dorsal rim of the distal radius (**Fig. 6**). Based on these numbers, the difference in the DDD with time was measured to reflect the amount of settling.

In our series, the initial postoperative radiograph DDD was found to be 9.01 mm, with a range of values from 3.68 mm to 18.26 mm. The mean difference in the DDD from initial to final radiographs at 1 year was 2.27 mm, with a range of −3.23 mm to 10.43 mm. Using a linear regression analysis, the change in DDD at final follow-up from the initial postoperative DDD, a significant correlation was found to exist, showing that the greater the initial DDD the greater chance of fracture settling to union ($P<.001$) (**Fig. 7**). The conclusion was that a DDD of less than 6 mm was found to be the critical value for maintaining fracture reduction and avoiding loss of volar tilt, radial shortening, and DRUJ incongruency (**Figs. 8 and 9**).

SUMMARY

Distal radius fractures are common injuries treated by orthopedic surgeons. Despite improvement in fracture fixation devices, the risk of late loss of fracture reduction persists. Many investigators have helped to provide guidelines for screw length, plate position, and other technical factors; yet, there is still a need for future research and improvement in surgical techniques. We propose utilization of the "DDD" measurement to serve as a simple, reliable, and reproducible measurement that can be readily determined intraoperatively to optimize subchondral screw position and fracture reduction. Based on our findings, the DDD should be kept less than 6 mm to optimize hardware placement and minimize the risk of losing fracture reduction.

REFERENCES

1. Chen NC, Jupiter JB. Management of distal radial fractures. J Bone Joint Surg Am 2007; 89(9):2051–62.
2. Drobetz H, Bryant AL, Pokorny T, et al. Volar fixed-angle plating of distal radius extension fractures: influence of plate position on secondary loss of reduction–a biomechanic study in a cadaveric model. J Hand Surg Am 2006;31(4):615–22.
3. Figl M, Weninger P, Liska M, et al. Volar fixed-angle plate osteosynthesis of unstable distal radius fractures: 12 months results. Arch Orthop Trauma Surg 2009;129(5):661–9.
4. Figl M, Weninger P, Jurkowitsch J, et al. Unstable distal radius fractures in the elderly patient: volar fixed-angle plate osteosynthesis prevents secondary loss of reduction. J Trauma 2010;68(4):992–8.
5. Rozental TD, Blazar PE, Franko OI, et al. Functional outcomes for unstable distal radial fractures treated with open reduction and internal fixation or closed reduction and percutaneous fixation. A prospective randomized trial. J Bone Joint Surg Am 2009;91(8): 1837–46.
6. Stevenson I, Carnegie CA, Christie EM, et al. Displaced distal radial fractures treated using volar locking plates: maintenance of normal anatomy. J Trauma 2009;67(3):612–6.
7. Weninger P, Schueller M, Drobetz H, et al. Influence of an additional locking screw on fracture reduction after volar fixed-angle plating—introduction of the "protection screw" in an extra-articular distal radius fracture model. J Trauma 2009;67(4):746–51.
8. Weninger P, Dall'Ara E, Leixnering M, et al. Volar fixed-angle plating of extra-articular distal radius fractures: a biomechanical analysis comparing threaded screws and smooth pegs. J Trauma 2010;69(5):E46–55.
9. Sokol SC, Amanatullah DF, Curtiss S, et al. Biomechanical properties of volar hybrid and locked plate fixation in distal radius fractures. J Hand Surg Am 2011;36(4):591–7.
10. Mignemi ME, Byram IR, Wolfe CC, et al. Radiographic outcomes of volar locked plating for distal radius fractures. J Hand Surg Am 2013; 38(1):40–8.
11. Minegishi H, Dohi O, An S, et al. Treatment of unstable distal radius fractures with the volar locking plate. Ups J Med Sci 2011;116(4):280–4.
12. Musgrave DS, Idler RS. Volar fixation of dorsally displaced distal radius fractures using the 2.4-mm locking compression plates. J Hand Surg Am 2005;30(4):743–9.
13. Orbay JL, Fernandez DL. Volar fixation for dorsally displaced fractures of the distal radius: a preliminary report. J Hand Surg Am 2002;27(2):205–15.
14. Williksen JH, Frihagen F, Hellund JC, et al. Volar locking plates versus external fixation and adjuvant pin fixation in unstable distal radius fractures: a randomized, controlled study. J Hand Surg Am 2013; 38(8):1469–76.
15. Bradway JK, Amadio PC, Cooney WP. Open reduction and internal fixation of displaced, comminuted intra-articular fractures of the distal end of the radius. J Bone Joint Surg Am 1989;71(6):839–47.
16. Jupiter JB. Fractures of the distal end of the radius. J Bone Joint Surg Am 1991;73(3):461–9.
17. Trumble TE, Schmitt SR, Vedder NB. Factors affecting functional outcome of displaced intra-articular distal radius fractures. J Hand Surg Am 1994;19(2):325–40.
18. Knirk JL, Jupiter JB. Intra-articular fractures of the distal end of the radius in young adults. J Bone Joint Surg Am 1986;68(5):647–59.
19. Medoff RJ. Essential radiographic evaluation for distal radius fractures. Hand Clin 2005;21(3): 279–88.
20. Mann FA, Wilson AJ, Gilula LA. Radiographic evaluation of the wrist: what does the hand surgeon want to know? Radiology 1992;184(1):15–24.
21. Altissimi M, Antenucci R, Fiacca C, et al. Long-term results of conservative treatment of fractures of the distal radius. Clin Orthop Relat Res 1986;(206): 202–10.
22. Porter M, Stockley I. Fractures of the distal radius. Intermediate and end results in relation to radiologic parameters. Clin Orthop Relat Res 1987;(220):241–52.
23. Rein S, Schikore H, Schneiders W, et al. Results of dorsal or volar plate fixation of AO type C3 distal radius fractures: a retrospective study. J Hand Surg Am 2007;32(7):954–61.
24. Yu YR, Makhni MC, Tabrizi S, et al. Complications of low-profile dorsal versus volar locking plates in the distal radius: a comparative study. J Hand Surg Am 2011;36(7):1135–41.
25. Hart A, Collins M, Chhatwal D, et al. Can the use of variable-angle volar locking plates compensate for suboptimal plate positioning in unstable distal radius

fractures? A biomechanical study. J Orthop Trauma 2015;29(1):e1–6.

26. Drobetz H, Weninger P, Grant C, et al. More is not necessarily better. A biomechanical study on distal screw numbers in volar locking distal radius plates. Injury 2013;44(4):535–9.

27. Hoffmeier KL, Hofmann GO, Mückley T. The strength of polyaxial locking interfaces of distal radius plates. Clin Biomech (Bristol, Avon) 2009;24(8):637–41.

28. McQueen M, Caspers J. Colles fracture: does the anatomical result affect the final function? J Bone Joint Surg Br 1988;70-B(4):649–51.

29. Lindau T, Hagberg L, Adlercreutz C, et al. Distal radioulnar instability is an independent worsening factor in distal radial fractures. Clin Orthop Relat Res 2000;(376):229–35.

30. Steyers CM, Blair WF. Measuring ulnar variance: a comparison of techniques. J Hand Surg Am 1989; 14(4):607–12.

31. Nishiwaki M, Welsh M, Gammon B, et al. Distal radioulnar joint kinematics in simulated dorsally angulated distal radius fractures. J Hand Surg Am 2014; 39(4):656–63.

32. Adams BD. Effects of radial deformity on distal radioulnar joint mechanics. J Hand Surg Am 1993; 18(3):492–8.

33. Kihara H, Palmer AK, Werner FW, et al. The effect of dorsally angulated distal radius fractures on distal radioulnar joint congruency and forearm rotation. J Hand Surg Am 1996;21(1):40–7.

34. Bombaci H, Polat A, Deniz G, et al. The value of plain X-rays in predicting TFCC injury after distal radial fractures. J Hand Surg Eur 2008;33(3): 322–6.

35. Hohendorff B, Eck M, Mühldorfer M, et al. Palmar wrist arthroscopy for evaluation of concomitant carpal lesions in operative treatment of distal intraarticular radius fractures. Handchir Mikrochir Plast Chir 2009;41(5):295–9 [in German].

36. Wall LB, Brodt MD, Silva MJ, et al. The effects of screw length on stability of simulated osteoporotic distal radius fractures fixed with volar locking plates. J Hand Surg Am 2012;37(3):446–53.

37. Crosby SN, Fletcher ND, Yap ER, et al. The mechanical stability of extra-articular distal radius fractures with respect to the number of screws securing the distal fragment. J Hand Surg Am 2013;38(6):1097–105.

38. Agnew SP, Ljungquist KL, Huang JI. Danger zones for flexor tendons in volar plating of distal radius fractures. J Hand Surg Am 2015;40(6):1102–5.

39. Soong M, Earp BE, Bishop G, et al. Volar locking plate implant prominence and flexor tendon rupture. J Bone Joint Surg Am 2011;93(4):328–35.

40. Tanaka Y, Aoki M, Izumi T, et al. Effect of distal radius volar plate position on contact pressure between the flexor pollicis longus tendon and the distal plate edge. J Hand Surg Am 2011;36(11):1790–7.

41. Baumgaertner MR, Curtin SL, Lindskog DM, et al. The value of the tip-apex distance in predicting failure of fixation of peritrochanteric fractures of the hip. J Bone Joint Surg Am 1995;77(7):1058–64.

Open Fractures of the Hand

Review of Pathogenesis and Introduction of a New Classification System

Jacob E. Tulipan, MD*, Asif M. Ilyas, MD

KEYWORDS

- Open fractures • Hand • Pathogenesis • Classification system • Infection • Treatment

KEY POINTS

- Open fractures of the hand are commonly encountered, and vary widely in mechanism, location, and severity.
- Current evidence shows that antibiotic use and the extent of contamination are predictive of infection risk, but time to debridement is not.
- Open fractures of the hand are less susceptible to infection than other open fractures.
- The different regions of the hand are unique with regard to the osseous anatomy, blood supply, and soft tissue coverage, all of which factor into the risk of infection after an open fracture.
- Current classification schemas for open fractures are insufficient to describe and indicate treatment of fractures of the hand. A specialized classification is introduced that may better take into account risk factors for infection specific to the hand when determining best treatment of open fractures of the hand.

INTRODUCTION

Fractures of the finger, hand, and wrist constitute a significant disease burden, estimated to comprise up to 1.5% of emergency department visits and constituting 1.4 million cases in 1998 alone.[1] Like all fractures, distal upper extremity fractures range in severity based on several factors, including mechanism of injury, fracture location, fracture pattern, and associated soft tissue injury.

Open fractures of the hand are a common occurrence. A database study in 2001 estimated that 5% of hand fractures are open.[1] Like all open fractures, open hand and finger fractures are at increased risk for infection compared with their closed counterparts. Beginning with anecdotal observations that these fractures were less likely than other open fractures of the body to become infected, several studies have attempted to stratify these injuries by infection risk.

AVAILABLE EVIDENCE ON OPEN HAND FRACTURES

A study by McLain and colleagues[2] examined 208 consecutive patients with open fractures of the hand. Overall, the cohort showed an 11% infection rate. This study had limited subject retention (143 of 208 patients) and excluded both farm injuries and human bite wounds. All injuries were irrigated and debrided in the operating room and received cephalosporin plus/minus penicillin and an aminoglycoside preoperatively.

A similar retrospective analysis of factors correlating with infection in open hand fractures was performed by Swanson and colleagues.[3] These

Department of Orthopaedic Surgery, Thomas Jefferson University, 925 Chestnut Street, Philadelphia, PA 19107, USA
* Corresponding author. 1025 Walnut Street, Room 516 College, Philadelphia, PA 19107.
E-mail address: jacob.tulipan@gmail.com

Orthop Clin N Am 47 (2016) 245–251
http://dx.doi.org/10.1016/j.ocl.2015.08.021

orthopedic.theclinics.com

investigators showed a 6% incidence of infection in a series of 154 patients, with 35 lost to follow-up. As in the prior study, all patients were treated with prompt intravenous antibiotics and bedside or operative irrigation and debridement.

An in-depth analysis of functional recovery following open fractures in 75 patients performed by Duncan and colleagues[4] showed an infection rate of 6 per 171 fractures (3.5%), all in Gustilo-Anderson type III injuries. This group also underwent standard treatment with antibiotics and urgent irrigation and debridement.

More recent retrospective reviews have varied in the reported incidence of infection in open hand fracture. A 2011 review of 145 cases by Capo and colleagues[5] showed a 1.4% infection rate, even in a series with a high proportion (91 out of 145) of Gustilo-Anderson type III injuries. Similarly, a 2006 review of bone grafting for open fractures of the hand found a 0% infection rate even in more severe fractures.[6] Moreover, a 2010 retrospective review of 432 metacarpal and phalanx fractures requiring internal fixation found no significant difference in infection rates between the open (133 fractures) and closed (299 fractures) injury groups.[7]

These infection rates are significantly lower than that identified in a 2012 meta-analysis of all open fractures, not only hand open fractures, by Schenker and colleagues.[8] That review found an 8% infection rate in Gustilo-Anderson class I and II fractures, and a 12.7% rate in class III fractures. This finding supports the traditional wisdom that the hand is more resilient and less prone to infection after an open fracture than other open fractures of the body.

VARIABLES AFFECTING INFECTION RISK FOLLOWING AN OPEN FRACTURE OF THE HAND

There are several potential variables that may cause an open fracture to be more or less prone to developing an infection. These variables include the local osseous and soft tissue anatomy, the extent of contamination, the integrity of the soft tissue envelope, and the vascularity of the extremity.

Anatomy

Within the hand, distal to the radius and ulna, there are 27 bones that are prone to injury and an open fracture. Each has its unique anatomy, blood supply, and soft tissue coverage. Divided broadly, they can be separated into 3 regions: the phalanges, the metacarpals, and the carpal bones.

The soft tissue coverage of the phalanges consists of skin, tendon, ligament, areolar connective tissue, and nail. The 14 phalanges of each hand are devoid of muscle. As a result, the digits are prone to open injury with minimal amounts of trauma or fracture displacement, especially in the dorsal surface where the fascial layers lack the robustness of the palmar side. Furthermore, these structures do not possess the bulk or vascularity of muscle, potentially limiting their ability to fight infection.

The metacarpals share some morphologic features with the phalanges. Among these are palmar layers of tough fascia and alveolar connective tissue, and a dorsal surface with a thin covering of skin, tendon, and fascia. However, the metacarpals also benefit from the presence of interosseous, thenar, and hypothenar musculature, providing bulky coverage and blood supply. As a result, the metacarpals are vulnerable to dorsal open injuries and wounds but benefit from a robust blood supply.

The carpal bones possess the most dense soft tissue coverage of the osseous regions of the hand. However, they have the most fragile blood supply because of their absence of muscular coverage and otherwise extensive articular nature. Subsequently their blood supply is derived from their ligamentous and capsular attachments, structures that can be readily compromised with trauma. However, these soft tissue attachments, combined with the deep position of the carpus and its highly congruent and strong intercarpal attachments, provide resistance to open fractures in this region.

Vascular Supply

The digits receive most of their blood supply via the palmar digital arteries, with contribution from the dorsal digital arteries. Distally, these palmar arteries anastomose to form the blood supply to the digital pulp.[9] The palmar digital arteries run superficial to the digital nerves and lie directly deep to the skin. As a result of their position, these vessels are easily injured during digital trauma, compromising blood supply and increasing infection risk of the digit. This effect can be mitigated by the arterial anastomoses in the digit, which provide redundant blood supply in case of injury. Degloving, ring avulsion, and other circumferential injuries are a particular risk for dysvascularity, and loss of both radial and ulnar digital arteries can result in an avascular digit.

More proximally, the hand benefits from a robust and redundant vascularity. The vascular supply of the hand is provided by the palmar arches and variable dorsal arches, anastomotic networks composed of contributions from radial and ulnar circulation. These networks provide multiple perforators supplying both the metacarpal bones and the soft tissues surrounding them. The intrinsic muscles of the hand also possess multiple points of vascular supply, and provide a vascular bed that can supply the metacarpals. This region of the hand is more resistant to devascularization from trauma, although extensive soft tissue damage can still compromise its blood supply.

Proximal devascularization in hand injuries does not guarantee loss of blood supply distal to the injury. Although certain sites in the hand and wrist (eg, the proximal scaphoid) have tenuous vascular supply, the extensive network of anastomoses means that blood flow often has many alternate paths to reach distal structures. This supply is especially relevant to the carpus.

Because of the extensive articulations of the carpal bones, many have a limited, tenuous blood supply. A landmark study examining 75 cadaver limbs showed that the scaphoid received most of its blood supply via distal, dorsal nutrient vessels, with no intraosseous anastomosis to the palmar circulation. In 70% of capitates examined, most of the blood supply was dorsally based and did not anastomose with the palmar circulation. Likewise, in 8% of the lunate specimens examined, the vascular supply of the bone arose from a single vessel.[10]

Although the other carpal bones possess more redundant blood supply, all are vulnerable to disruption from high-energy injuries. In the case of the scaphoid and the capitate, in particular, small soft tissue disruptions may result in avascular bone stock, increasing the risk of infection and nonunion.

Severe vascular injuries of the hand may require emergent revascularization, regardless of the level of contamination of the wound. Although the literature is limited with regard to thrombosis and infection rate of revascularized hands in open fractures, inadequate perfusion necessitates emergent surgical intervention. Primary repair or grafting of damaged vessels prevents ischemic injury to distal structures, and must be performed if collateral circulation is not adequate. Poor blood supply is clearly a risk factor for subsequent infection.[11] However, the hand differs to some extent from other sites of open fracture in its extensive network of collateral circulation. Gustilo-Anderson type IIIc lower-limb fractures carry an infection risk as high as 39% according to one series.[12] However, there are limited data on infection rates in open hand injuries with vascular compromise.

Soft Tissue Envelope

The hand has a unique soft tissue envelope, both protective and potentially injurious in the setting of open hand fractures. The palmar surface of the hand benefits from a robust skin and dense subcutaneous tissue via its glabrous skin and deep fascial connections and muscular subcompartments. Significant trauma is required to result in open fractures on the palmar side. In contrast, the dorsal hand has only a thin layer of skin with minimal alveolar subcutaneous tissue, leaving the osseous and tendinous structures prone to ready exposure even with minor trauma.

When soft tissue loss is present, the hand poses a unique challenge in coverage. Securing adequate coverage in hand trauma is necessary to protect the deep osseous and soft tissue structures such as the many nerves, vessels, and tendons. However, many soft tissue coverage options exist that are indicated based on the nature of the injury and surgeon preference, including primary closure, secondary closure, acellular dermal substitutes, local rotational or advancement flaps, pedicled flaps, and free flaps. Each option has its own unique characteristics and risks and benefits for infection that must be taken into account in the setting of an open fracture.

Contamination

Frank contamination of an open fracture intuitively increases the risk for infection. Contamination of wounds often occurs as a result of injury mechanism, because debris is deposited into the wound site. These contaminant particles provide a nidus for bacterial growth, as well as serving as a source of bacterial bioburden. Certain types of contamination warrant specific consideration. Among these are soil contamination, which carries a high risk of anaerobic infection[13]; fecal contamination, which carries a risk of polymicrobial and gram-negative infection[14]; and bite wounds, which may be contaminated by organisms including *Eikenella* and *Pasteurella* species.[15] A 1978 study performed by Lawrence and colleagues[16] analyzed bacterial cultures of open fractures at time of presentation, and found that infections developed in a small proportion of patients (3 of 95 fractures), and only in those with high levels of contamination, providing evidence that initial degree of contamination affects infection risk.

Tscherne and Oestern[17] attempted to quantify this risk with their classification of open fractures. This classification takes into account the severity of associated soft tissue disruption, ranging from grade I (small puncture wound, negligible contamination, low-energy fracture) to grade III (heavy contamination, extensive soft tissue damage, associated neurovascular injury) and grade IV (traumatic amputation).[17] A 2015 retrospective review of 122 patients by Matos and colleagues[18] found that Tscherne II and III fractures were associated with a significantly higher rate of infection (48% and 26% respectively). Although this study examined both upper-limb and lower-limb injuries, it did not differentiate hand injuries specifically.

PREDICTIVE FACTORS IN OPEN HAND FRACTURES

A recent meta-analysis of 12 studies on open hand fractures meeting the inclusion criteria were reviewed to assess factors related to infection risk.[19] These factors included antibiotic administration and timing of debridement. Use of antibiotics varied between studies in the meta-analysis, but all studies using antibiotics used either a cephalosporin or a penicillin derivative. With all patients pooled, antibiotic use was significantly ($P = .0057$) associated with lower risk of infection, with a 4.4% infection rate in the antibiotic-treated group versus a 9.4% rate in the control group. Alternatively, timing to debridement was specifically examined in 2 of the studies used in the meta-analysis.[2,20] Neither study was able to show correlation between timing to debridement and infection rate, and nor did the pooled results.

Although not specific to the hand, several other studies have also examined open fractures of the distal radius and forearm, and studied different associated variables relative to infection risk.

A 2009 study by Glueck and colleagues[14] retrospectively reviewed 42 open distal radius fractures to determine infection risk. Three fractures ultimately became infected, of which 2 were grossly contaminated with fecal matter at the time of injury. Although the study found a statistically significant correlation between contamination and risk for infection, it failed to find any significant association between infection and either fixation method or time to debridement. All 3 infections occurred in Gustilo-Anderson type II or III injuries. These findings were mirrored in a 2011 study by Kurylo and colleagues,[21] which retrospectively identified 32 open radius fractures. This study failed to show any infections in the cohort, regardless of time to debridement or method of fixation. This study did not report degree of contamination.

A 2014 study by Zumsteg and colleagues[22] reviewed 200 open forearm fractures, and found a 5% infection rate. Deep infection risk was correlated with injury severity as measured by the Gustilo-Anderson classification, but was not associated with either time to debridement or

time to antibiotics. This study did not include information on the degree of contamination in these injuries.

The correlation between gross contamination and infection in the first study discussed earlier provides an indication that this is a significant contributor to infection risk. Although the distal radius differs from the hand in soft tissue coverage and vascularity, this association of injury characteristics and infection risk can be assumed to be analogous.

INAPPLICABILITY OF THE GUSTILO-ANDERSON CLASSIFICATION TO OPEN HAND FRACTURES

The Gustilo-Anderson classification[11,23] (Table 1), initially developed for use in long bones, is not optimal in classifying hand fractures. Specifically, the variables used to classify fractures in the Gustilo-Anderson system, particularly wound size, and the different nuances of soft tissue coverage and dysvascularity unique to the hand, make it less applicable to open hand fractures. For example, the laceration size cutoffs for Gustilo-Anderson types (1 cm and 10 cm) are not realistic for a limb as small as the hand and its fingers. In addition, the indications and options for soft tissue coverage of open long bone fractures (ie, Gustilo-Anderson type IIIB injuries) are very different in the hand. Furthermore, there are multiple common mechanisms for open fractures of the hand. The first is direct laceration or penetrating injury. In these cases, a sharp object (eg, a saw) cuts through

| Table 1 |
| The Gustilo-Anderson classification of open fractures |

Type	Description
I	Wound <1 cm
II	Wound >1 cm
IIIa	Extensive soft tissue laceration, wound >10 cm, adequate bone coverage, segmental fractures
IIIb	Inadequate soft tissue coverage over bone
IIIc	Arterial injury requiring repair

Data from Gustilo RB, Anderson JT. Prevention of infection in the treatment of one thousand and twenty-five open fractures of long bones: retrospective and prospective analyses. J Bone Joint Surg Am 1976;58(4):453–8; and Gustilo RB, Mendoza RM, Williams DN. Problems in the management of type III (severe) open fractures: a new classification of type III open fractures. J Trauma 1984;24(8):742–6.

Table 2
Proposed classification scheme for open fractures of the hand and fingers

Type	Location	Modifiers
I	Phalanges	a: Primary soft tissue
II	Metacarpals	coverage not possible **(Fig. 1)**
III	Carpus	b: Frank contamination **(Fig. 2)**
		c: Dysvascularity requiring revascularization **(Fig. 3)**

skin and then the underlying soft tissues and bone. In the second mechanism, a crush injury tears skin while fracturing the bone below. In the third, shear forces avulse skin and break underlying bone. In addition, direct blows or falls can result in a bone spike being forcibly pushed through the skin. Each of these injuries can result in similar skin defects (and thus similar Gustilo-Anderson classes) while causing vastly different amounts of damage to the soft tissues and underlying bone.

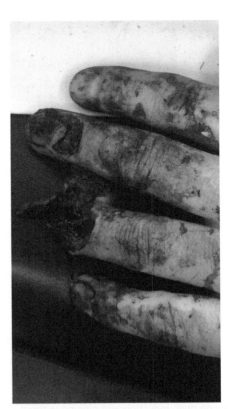

Fig. 2. A fracture showing frank contamination with soil. This fracture is classified as type Ib by the proposed classification scheme.

NEW CLASSIFICATION OF OPEN HAND FRACTURES

Given the current uncertainty with regard to risk factors for infection and appropriate timing to debridement of open fractures of the hand, we recommend the development of a new classification system to predict infection risk based on established risk factors for infection specifically after an open hand fracture. Subsequently, the classification system we are proposing (**Table 2**) deemphasizes wound size as the primary variable, and instead takes into account fracture location, extent of contamination, integrity of the soft tissue coverage, and viability of the vascularity.

By taking into account both anatomic and injury-specific factors, this classification can serve as a more effective tool for guiding treatment by providing insight for early infection risk stratification and long-term prognosis. We recommend using the classification in the following manner:

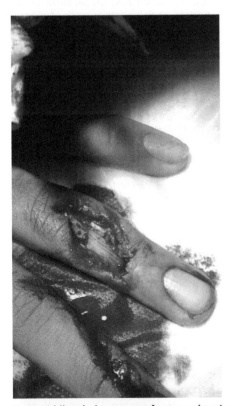

Fig. 1. A middle phalanx open fracture showing a soft tissue defect that cannot be closed primarily. This fracture is classified as type Ia by the proposed classification scheme.

- Any open fracture type (I–III) without a modifier does not require emergent surgical treatment and can be managed with antibiotics and

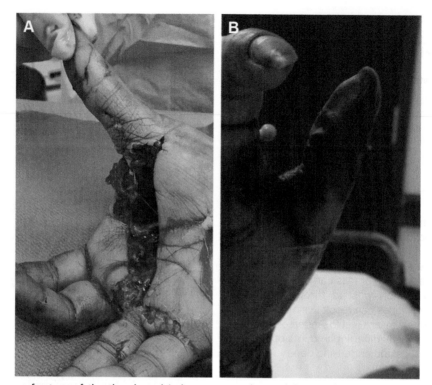

Fig. 3. An open fracture of the thumb and index metacarpal seen (*A*) immediately on presentation and (*B*) following open reduction and pinning without primary revascularization, showing late necrosis of avascular tissue. Although no direct vascular transection was evident, the traction and degloving nature of the injury resulted in late vascular compromise and subsequent infection. This fracture is classified as type IIc based on the proposed classification system and would have potentially benefited from early revascularization.

emergency room washout alone, followed by standard fracture management.

- Any open fracture type with the modifier "a" requires immediate antibiotics with emergency room washout alone, followed by semi-elective surgical soft tissue coverage and standard fracture management.
- Any open fracture type with the modifier "b" requires immediate antibiotics and urgent surgical debridement, followed by early versus delayed fracture management.
- Any open fracture type with the modifier "c" requires immediate antibiotics and emergent surgical revascularization and fracture management.

Using this system and algorithm has resulted in promising and consistent results in our patients. It is our expectation that with future research this open hand fracture–specific classification will be validated as a tool to help guide early treatment and prognose long-term outcome and infection risk more effectively than the currently used, nonspecific to hand, open fracture classifications.

REFERENCES

1. Chung KC, Spilson SV. The frequency and epidemiology of hand and forearm fractures in the United States. J Hand Surg 2001;26(5):908–15.
2. McLain RF, Steyers C, Stoddard M. Infections in open fractures of the hand. J Hand Surg 1991; 16(1):108–12.
3. Swanson TV, Szabo RM, Anderson DD. Open hand fractures: prognosis and classification. J Hand Surg 1991;16(1):101–7.
4. Duncan RW, Freeland AE, Jabaley ME, et al. Open hand fractures: an analysis of the recovery of active motion and of complications. J Hand Surg 1993; 18(3):387–94.
5. Capo JT, Hall M, Nourbakhsh A, et al. Initial management of open hand fractures in an emergency department. Am J Orthop 2011;40(12):E243–8.
6. Saint-Cyr M, Gupta A. Primary internal fixation and bone grafting for open fractures of the hand. Hand Clin 2006;22(3):317–27.
7. Bannasch H, Heermann AK, Iblher N, et al. Ten years stable internal fixation of metacarpal and phalangeal hand fractures-risk factor and outcome analysis show no increase of complications in the

treatment of open compared with closed fractures. J Trauma 2010;68(3):624–8.

8. Schenker ML, Yannascoli S, Baldwin KD, et al. Does timing to operative debridement affect infectious complications in open long-bone fractures? A systematic review. J Bone Joint Surg Am 2012;94(12): 1057–64.

9. Park HC, Bahar-Moni AS, Cho SH, et al. Classification of distal fingertip amputation based on the arterial system for replantation. J Hand Microsurg 2013; 5(1):4–8.

10. Gelberman RH, Gross MS. The vascularity of the wrist. Identification of arterial patterns at risk. Clin Orthop Relat Res 1986;(202):40–9.

11. Gustilo RB, Anderson JT. Prevention of infection in the treatment of one thousand and twenty-five open fractures of long bones: retrospective and prospective analyses. J Bone Joint Surg Am 1976; 58(4):453–8.

12. Soni A, Tzafetta K, Knight S, et al. Gustilo IIIC fractures in the lower limb: our 15-year experience. J Bone Joint Surg Br 2012;94(5):698–703.

13. Templeman DC, Gulli B, Tsukayama DT, et al. Update on the management of open fractures of the tibial shaft. Clin Orthop Relat Res 1998;(350): 18–25.

14. Glueck DA, Charoglu CP, Lawton JN. Factors associated with infection following open distal radius fractures. Hand 2009;4(3):330–4.

15. Kennedy SA, Stoll LE, Lauder AS. Human and other mammalian bite injuries of the hand: evaluation and management. J Am Acad Orthop Surg 2015;23(1): 47–57.

16. Lawrence RM, Hoeprich PD, Huston AC, et al. Quantitative microbiology of traumatic orthopedic wounds. J Clin Microbiol 1978;8(6):673–5.

17. Tscherne H, Oestern HJ. A new classification of soft-tissue damage in open and closed fractures (author's transl). Unfallheilkunde 1982;85(3):111–5 [in German].

18. Matos MA, Lima LG, de Oliveira LA. Predisposing factors for early infection in patients with open fractures and proposal for a risk score. J Orthop Traumatol 2015;16(3):195–201.

19. Dwyer J, Ilyas A, Ketonis C. Timing of debridement and infection rates in open fractures of the hand: a systematic review. Journal of Hand Surgery 2014;39(9):e44.

20. Ng T, Unadkat J, Bilonick RA, et al. The importance of early operative treatment in open fractures of the fingers. Ann Plast Surg 2014;72(4):408–10.

21. Kurylo JC, Axelrad TW, Tornetta P III, et al. Open Fractures of the Distal Radius: The Effects of Delayed Debridement and Immediate Internal Fixation on Infection Rates and the Need for Secondary Procedures. Journal of Hand Surgery 2011;36(7):1131–4.

22. Zumsteg JW, Molina CS, Lee DH, et al. Factors influencing infection rates after open fractures of the radius and/or ulna. J Hand Surg 2014;39(5):956–61.

23. Gustilo RB, Mendoza RM, Williams DN. Problems in the management of type III (severe) open fractures: a new classification of type III open fractures. J Trauma 1984;24(8):742–6.

Oncology

Preface

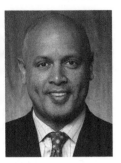

Felasfa M. Wodajo, MD
Editor

In the Oncology section of this issue of *Orthopedic Clinics of North America*, we proudly present three terrific reviews exploring the cutting edge of orthopedic oncology. In "Innovations in Intraoperative Tumor Visualization," Drs Visgauss, Eward, and Brigman shine a light onto one of today's most exciting avenues in oncologic research–technologies that allow us to detect tumor cells in real time during surgery. This group at Duke University is in fact leading some of the ground-breaking research in this field. In "Reconstruction After Tumor Resection in the Growing Child," Drs Groundland and Binitie from the Moffitt Cancer Center in Tampa, FL explore the modern surgical options available to the preadolescent and adolescent patient facing resection of a lower extremity bone sarcoma. Finally, in "Update on Survival in Osteosarcoma," Dr Megan Anderson from Boston Children's Hospital brings to our readers the state of the art in osteosarcoma chemotherapy, and how we might reasonably counsel our patients and families facing this cancer.

This issue also marks the conclusion of my editorship of the Oncology section as the series heads into a new direction without specialty-specific sections in each issue. To see the scope of what we have covered, below are some of the reviews published in this section over the last two years.

- Malignant Soft Tissue Tumors in Children, Mihir M. Thacker, Alfred I. DuPont Hospital for Children, Wilmington, DE
- How Intraoperative Navigation Is Changing Musculoskeletal Tumor Surgery, Robert L. Satcher Jr, MD Anderson Cancer Center, Houston, TX
- Management of Open Wounds: Lessons from Orthopedic Oncology, Herrick J. Siegel, University of Alabama, Birmingham, AL
- The Practicing Orthopedic Surgeon's Guide to Managing Long Bone Metastases, Felix H. Cheung, Marshall University, Huntington, WV
- The Principles and Applications of Fresh Frozen Allografts to Bone and Joint Reconstruction, Luis A. Aponte-Tinao and colleagues, Buenos Aires, Argentina
- Nonneoplastic Soft Tissue Masses That Mimic Sarcoma, Matthew W. Colman and colleagues, Massachusetts General Hospital, Boston, MA
- Use of Bisphosphonates in Orthopedic Surgery: Pearls and Pitfalls, Santiago A. Lozano-Calderon and colleagues, Massachusetts General Hospital, Boston, MA
- Five Polyostotic Conditions That General Orthopedic Surgeons Should Recognize (or Should Not Miss), Saravanaraja Muthusamy and colleagues, University of Miami, Miami, FL
- Novel Applications of Osseointegration in Orthopedic Limb Salvage Surgery, R. Lor Randall and colleagues, University of Utah, Salt Lake City, UT
- Top Five Lesions That Do Not Need Referral to Orthopedic Oncology, Felasfa Wodajo, Virginia Commonwealth University, Fairfax, VA
- PET Imaging in Sarcoma, Drs Becher and Oskouei, Emory University, Atlanta, GA
- Soft Tissue Masses for the General Orthopedic Surgeon, Drs. Jernigan and Esther, UNC, Chapel Hill, NC

Orthop Clin N Am 47 (2016) xxvii–xxviii
http://dx.doi.org/10.1016/j.ocl.2015.10.008
0030-5898/16/$ – see front matter © 2016 Published by Elsevier Inc.

- Paget Disease of Bone, Mamun Al-Rashid and colleagues, Massachusetts General Hospital, Boston, MA
- Targeted Chemotherapy in Bone and Soft Tissue Sarcoma, Joel Mayerson and colleagues, The Ohio State University, Columbus, OH

It has been truly an honor and a privilege to solicit and to edit reviews from some of the thought-leaders in our specialty. I want to thank the *Orthopedic Clinics of North America* for the opportunity to contribute to our field. But, most importantly, I want to offer my deepest thanks to the authors who worked hard, surely into many late nights, to assemble their manuscripts, to consider my suggestions, and then to submit them again, often within tight deadlines.

Felasfa M. Wodajo, MD
Musculoskeletal Tumor Surgery
Inova Fairfax Hospital
VCU School of Medicine
Inova Campus
Georgetown University Hospital
8503 Arlington Boulevard
Suite 400
Fairfax, VA 22031, USA

E-mail address:
wodajo@sarcoma.md

Innovations in Intraoperative Tumor Visualization

Julia D. Visgauss, MD, William C. Eward, DVM, MD, Brian E. Brigman, MD, PhD*

KEYWORDS

- Intraoperative tumor imaging • Surgical margin assessment • Optical imaging
- Near-infrared fluorescent imaging • Targeted fluorescent probes

KEY POINTS

- Intraoperative tumor visualization has the potential to significantly improve surgical cancer care by improving adequacy of resection, decreasing resection of normal tissue and structures, and directing adjuvant therapy.
- Various techniques for intraoperative tumor imaging exist, including optical fluorescent imaging, high-frequency ultrasound, optical coherence tomography, optoacoustic imaging, confocal microscopy, elastic scattering spectroscopy, Raman spectroscopy, and radiofrequency spectroscopy; however, no single technique has yet been perfected.
- Optical fluorescence imaging has been further refined with the use of near-infrared techniques and selective probes, improving the sensitivity and accuracy of intraoperative images.

INTRODUCTION

The surgical oncologist is tasked with a great responsibility, with little margin for error. One must localize the tumor and resect it, preferably en bloc, with as little morbidity and contamination to surrounding tissues as possible. Adequacy of resection has implications on local recurrence[1] and survival for many tumor types. Incorrect estimation of tumor resection margins may result in incomplete excision of disease, or increased morbidity with resection of excess normal tissue. Various methods of intraoperative tumor visualization have been, and are being, developed to aid in the real-time assessment of tumor extent and adequacy of resection. Better understanding of the resection margins has implications for adjuvant treatment as well. Knowledge of an increased or decreased risk of local recurrence may inform decisions about adjuvant therapies, such as radiation.

Assessment of the margins of resected tumor is a surrogate measure for the ultimate question: whether or not tumor remains in the patient. Analysis is performed via gross and histologic evaluation of the resected tissue, and is a lengthy and imperfect process. The standard and most widely used method of intraoperative identification of tumor margin is frozen section pathologic analysis. Although it is an accurate way of identifying tumor in the sampled tissue,[2,3] only a small percentage of the margin of resected tissue is actually analyzed. Thus, there is great potential for sampling error both from random sampling of the resected tissue, as well as heterogeneity of the tumor itself. Furthermore, the process is time-consuming and correlation of orientation/localization between the tumor and tumor bed are distorted after excision.[4] Final histologic analysis of complete tumor margins can take up to 5 to 7 days. If margins are found to be positive, the patient may be subjected to reoperation, adjuvant treatments, or both.

Department of Orthopaedic Surgery, Duke University, Box 3312 DUMC, Durham, NC 27710, USA
* Corresponding author.
E-mail address: brian.brigman@dm.duke.edu

Orthop Clin N Am 47 (2016) 253–264
http://dx.doi.org/10.1016/j.ocl.2015.08.023

Multiple methods for intraoperative tumor visualization have been developed and continue to be refined. Many of these advances have been driven by brain and head and neck cancers due to the morbidity associated with tissue resection, as well as breast cancers with the increase in breast-conserving surgical techniques. However, a mature technique for intraoperative tumor visualization would benefit surgeons and their patients across all disciplines, guiding accuracy of biopsies, increasing adequacy of resections, and in some instances even providing diagnostic information.

TRADITIONAL IMAGING TECHNIQUES

Traditional imaging techniques, such as MRI and ultrasound. have been studied in brain tumor resection and breast-conserving surgery, respectively. Studies have shown increased rates of complete tumor resection without increased neurologic deficits, and improved survival rates with intraoperative MRI-guided resection of gliomas.[5–7] Although safe and effective, there are disadvantages to this technique. For one, it requires the surgeon to interpret the imaging and correlate the location of the lesion from the image to the tumor bed. Second, previously treated areas may have treatment effects or postoperative changes that affect the MRI image and decrease the accuracy of this technique. Third, obtaining an MRI can be time-consuming, resulting in significant surgical disruptions and prolonged operative time. Finally, there is considerable investment required to create operative suites with the ability to accommodate the logistical needs of the MRI magnet. Ultrasound has fewer logistical pitfalls

than MRI, and has been used to localize the tumor, guide resection, and confirm completeness of excision. Studies show ultrasound-guided resection of breast lesions to have improved resection margins and decreased excision volumes than traditional techniques, such as palpation guided, wire localization, or quantitative radionucleotide-guided localization.[8–11] However, the resolution of ultrasound is poor, and similar to other structural imaging modalities, the accuracy is affected by previously treated surgical fields.

Computer-assisted navigation using fiducial markers that are calibrated to the patient's anatomy and cross-sectional (computed tomography [CT] or MRI) imaging can be used for indirect tumor imaging. Calibrated pointers, or surgical instruments (ie, osteotome, burr, cautery) can localize the instrument within the patient's cross-sectional images on a monitor in real time. This can be used to correlate to the planned resection margin, to the tumor, or to other vital anatomic structures. Computer-assisted navigation systems have gained popularity in pelvic resections for technically demanding, complex multiplanar osteotomies, and joint-preserving excisions.[12,13] They have been shown to improve excision accuracy[14] with adequate resection margins (**Fig. 1**). However, accuracy with navigation of soft tissue tumors is poor because of inability to place a stable fiducial, and disruption of the localizers may result in misguided navigation.

OPTICAL FLUORESCENT IMAGING

Optical imaging is based on fluorescence variation between normal and tumor tissue, which may be driven by intrinsic tissue properties or exogenously

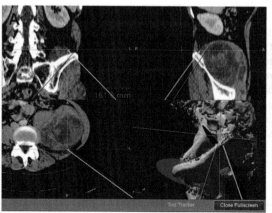
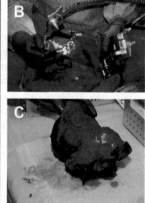

Fig. 1. Computer navigated resection of a large pelvic tumor. (*A*) CT cross-sectional and 3D reformatted images with lines representing anatomic correlate of instruments within the patient. (*B*) Calibrated localizer on an osteotome displays location and trajectory of bone cuts in real time on the patient's cross-sectional imaging. (*C*) Resected pelvic tumor en bloc. (*Courtesy of* Stryker Inc. Kalamazoo, MI, USA; with permission.)

infiltrated optical agents. It requires 3 basic components: a fluorophore agent that will emit light when excited (may be endogenous to tissues or administered exogenously), a light source (at a wavelength that will excite the fluorophore), and a camera system (that will capture the fluorescence emitted from the excited fluorophore). There are many different variations of optical imaging techniques that will be discussed in more detail, but the basic method is described as follows[15]:

1. A light source emits light at a specific wavelength known to excite the chosen fluorophore.
2. The fluorophore may be endogenous to tissues (autofluorescence) or administered to the patient (fluorescent probe). Exogenous probes can be administered preoperatively via intravenous (IV) or local infiltration, or applied topically onto the tumor bed or resected tissue intraoperatively.
3. This light wavelength (photon) travels into the tissue and is absorbed by the fluorophore. It is subjected to reflection, refraction, and scattering as it penetrates the tissues.
4. The fluorophore enters a state of excitation for a fraction of a second (depending on the lifetime of the fluorophore).
5. When the fluorophore returns to its ground state, it emits the photon at another given wavelength of light.
6. This light wavelength travels out of the tissue (again subjected to reflection, refraction, and scattering) and is captured and recorded by the camera system.

Autofluorescence

This technique uses a light source in the UV to visible range, and exploits differences in the inherent optical properties between normal and pathologic tissue, resulting in differences in light scatter and autofluorescence. One such technique, described by Wilke and colleagues,[16] is based on the premise that tumor tissue has a different profile of β-carotene and hemoglobin from surrounding normal tissue. Evaluation of the margins of resected tissue correctly identify 79% of histologically positive margins by this technique. Autofluorescence also has been used to assess the margins of surgical beds during resection of oral cavity cancers. In this method, the destruction of collagen matrix and increased vascularity within the tumors resulted in a decrease in autofluorescence recorded by a handheld camera device.[4]

Advantages

- Real-time, intraoperative visualization of tumor
- Takes advantage of tissue property differences without administration of exogenous fluorophores
- Can image tumor or tumor bed
- Wide field imaging
- Can be used to both localize tumor and assess tumor bed for residual disease, or assess excised tissue for status of margins

Disadvantages

- Relatively low tumor-to-background signal ratio
- Blood pooling and cauterized tissue in the surgical field increases the scattering/absorption of light, and may falsely decrease the fluorescent signal
- Tissue optical properties may be altered by neoadjuvant cancer therapies
- Changes in tissue morphology after resection may alter the evaluation of margins in excised tissue
- Shallow depth of penetration (~2 mm)

Near-Infrared Fluorescent Imaging

The light source chosen for optical imaging techniques may be in the visible (400–800 nm) or the near-infrared (NIR; 700–900 nm) spectrum, based on the excitation properties of the given fluorophore. Compared with visible light, NIR light has many advantages. First, it has better penetration of soft tissues (on the order of centimeters compared with the millimeters of penetration by visible light). Second, NIR fluorescence techniques can use an exogenous fluorescent probe that localizes to tumor cells to increase the fluorescent signal produced by tumor tissue. NIR light generates minimal autofluorescence by the surrounding tissues in the background, resulting in increased tumor "signal"-to-background "noise" ratio with use of exogenous fluorescent probes.[4,17,18] This increases the sensitivity of NIR compared with visual spectrum fluorescence in tumor detection. NIR systems can be free-standing, adapted into intraoperative microscopes, laparoscopes, and robots, or small handheld probes (Fig. 2). Fluorescence molecular tomography uses complex mathematical formulas to derive 3-dimensional images from optical fluorescent techniques. These fluorescent renditions can be superimposed onto CT or MRI images to create an anatomic reference with high sensitivity and resolution.[19,20]

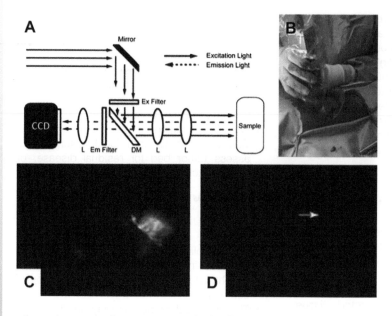

Fig. 2. (*A*) A diagram illustrates the optical layout of the intraoperative imaging device. Light enters the device through the fiber bundle where it is reflected through an excitation filter (ex filter) and reflected with a dichronic mirror (DM) onto the tumor sample/tumor bed where emitted light returns through the emission filter (em filter) to the detector. Several lenses (L) are used to relay the fluorescence image at no magnification into a charge-coupled device (CCD) where the fluorescence emission of the individual cancer cells is mapped into 2 to 4 pixels. (*B*) A photograph shows the device in use in a dog with a chest wall soft tissue sarcoma. (*C, D*) Representative intraoperative NIR fluorescence imaging after removal of a canine mast cell tumor. Images display fluorescence from the (*C*) tumor as well as (*D*) fluorescence (*arrow*) from small foci of residual tumor in the tumor bed. (*Adapted from* Eward WC, Mito JK, Eward CA, et al. A novel imaging system permits real-time in vivo tumor bed assessment after resection of naturally occurring sarcomas in dogs. Clin Orthop Relat Res 2013;471(3):837–38; with permission.)

Advantages

- Greater depth of field
- Decreased scattering/reflectance, and use exogenous fluorescent probes increase the fluorescent "signal"
- Decreased autofluorescence reduces the background "noise"
- Decreased absorption by hemoglobin and lipid improves optimal use in surgical field

Disadvantages

- Not visible with the naked eye: requires a camera system able to capture light and translate onto an imaging screen; however, newer hand-held systems have greatly improved the convenience of use

Nontargeted Fluorescent Probes

Optical imaging can be performed with fluorescent probes that are administered to the patient and preferentially infiltrate into the tumor tissue. Nontargeted probes are based on the enhanced permeability and retention (EPR) effect. EPR exploits properties of the tumor, such as increased vascularity, leaky capillary membranes, and abnormal lymphatic drainage, which result in increased delivery and retention of the exogenous fluorophores to the target tissue.[21] These non–tumor specific agents include fluorescein, indocyanine green dye (ICG), cresyl violet, toluidine blue, Lugol iodine, and acridine orange.[17] These can be administered intravenously, applied topically, or injected in or near the tumor. Local injection, termed diffusion molecular retention, typically uses pegylated probes to further enhance interstitial diffusion and tumor uptake.[22] This results in slowed uptake and clearance by vascular channels, prolonging interstitial diffusion and further decreasing systemic circulation.

Advantages

- ICG, the predominant fluorophore used in NIR fluorescence, is rapidly cleared by the liver and has low rates of toxicity
- Camera devices used in NIR techniques are designed to capture ICG fluorescence, but also are able to image other fluorophores with similar excitation and emission profiles as newer tumor specific agents become approved for clinical use

Disadvantages

- Contrast allergy is a relative contraindication to ICG use[4]
- Time sensitive due to the rapid clearance of ICG
- Relatively low signal-to-background ratio

Targeted Fluorescent Probes

Recent advancements have led to the development of probes linking a fluorescent agent to a tumor-specific target, many of which are based on existing cancer-targeted therapies.[17] These targets, as outlined in **Table 1**, are based on the premise that gene dysregulation of tumor cells leads to increased angiogenesis, metabolism, and expression of growth signal receptors that can be exploited as biomarker targets for tumor-specific probes.[17,23]

The Target Selection Criteria (TASC) is a scoring system that has been developed to choose biomarker targets for a given tumor to enable optimal pharmacokinetics and bio-distribution with minimal toxicity, high signal-to-noise ratio, and homogeneous distribution within the tumor[17,24] (**Table 2**).

Probes that exploit increased metabolism in tumor cells include 5-aminolevulinic acid (5-ALA) and folate conjugated with fluorescein isothiocyanate (folate-FITC). The 5-ALA is involved in hemoglobin synthesis and when given in excess doses results in accumulation of protoporphyrin IX, which absorbs blue light and fluoresces in the visible red light range. Folate-FITC binds to the folate receptor and also fluoresces in the visible light range. The 5-ALA has been shown to improve tumor

Table 2
Target selection criteria scoring system

Biomarker Characteristic	Score
Extracellular localization of protein	
Bound to cell surface (ie, receptor)	5
Close proximity to tumor cell	3
Diffuse upregulation throughout tumor tissue	4
Percentage of upregulation	
>90	6
70–90	5
50–69	3
10–49	0
Tumor/Normal cell ratio >10	3
Prior success with in vivo imaging	2
Enzymatic activity	1
Internalization	1
Total Maximum	22

Score ≥18 has potential for imaging target (21–22 with high potential).

Data from van Oosten M, Crane LM, Bart J, et al. Selecting potential targetable biomarkers for imaging purposes in colorectal cancer using TArget Selection Criteria (TASC): a novel target identification tool. Transl Oncol 2011;4(2):71–2.

Table 1
Targeted probes for fluorescent imaging

Unique Tumor Property	Target	Example
Unlimited replication potential	Increased metabolism	IRDye800CW 2-deoxyglucose (Li-Cor Bioscience, Lincoln, NE, USA)
Increased angiogenesis	Increased hemoglobin concentration	Spectroscopy
	VEGF receptor	NIRF-labeled bevacizumab (Genentech, Inc., San Francisco, CA, USA)
	Avβ3-Integrin	IRDye800CW RGD, IntegriSense (PerkinElmer, Waltham, MA, USA)
	Increased vascular permeability	IRDye800CW PEG, AngioSense (PerkinElmer)
Tissue invasion and metastasis	Matrix metalloproteinases	MMPSense (PerkinElmer, Waltham, MA, USA)
	Cathepsins	ProSense (PerkinElmer)
Upregulation of growth signals	EGF receptor	IRDye800CW EGF, NIRF-labeled cetuximab (ImClone LLC, Branchburg, NJ, USA), NIRF-labeled trastuzumab (Genentech, Inc.)

Abbreviations: EGF, epithelial growth factor; MMP, matrix metalloproteinase; NIRF, near-infrared fluorescence; PEG, polyethylene glycol; VEGF, vascular epithelial growth factor.

Data from de Boer E, Harlaar NJ, Taruttis A, et al. Optical innovations in surgery. Br J Surg 2015;102(2):e56–72; and Keereweer S, Kerrebijn JD, van Driel PB, et al. Optical image-guided surgery: where do we stand? Mol Imaging Biol 2011;13(2):199–7.

resection and progression-free survival rates in patients with glioma,[25,26] and folate-FITC has shown improved detection of intraperitoneal metastases in patients with ovarian cancer.[27]

Other probes target growth factors, growth factor receptors, and integrins. Existing biologics, such as bevacizumab (an anti–vascular endothelial growth factor monoclonal antibody), trastuzumab, and cetuximab (anti–epithelial growth factor receptor monoclonal antibodies) have been conjugated to a fluorescent dye (IRDye800) for use with NIR techniques.[28] These types of probes have shown encouraging results for tumor resection in mouse models,[29] and clinical trials for use in humans are currently under way in Europe[4] (Clinicaltrials.gov, NCT01508572). In a mouse model with human breast tumor xenograft, fluorescence-guided resection using an $\alpha v \beta 3$-integrin receptor-targeted fluorescent probe, was successful in detecting tumor and improving resection margins, and correlated with high specificity to histologic analysis.[30]

Activated probes take advantage of the upregulation of certain proteolytic enzymes in tumor cells. These probes are injected in an inactive state, but fluoresce after cleavage by specific proteases, such as cathepsins and matrix metalloproteinases (MMPs).[31] Prosense 680 (PerkinElmer, Inc., Waltham, MA, USA) and VM249 (Visen Medical/PerkinElmer Inc., Waltham, MA, USA) are examples of cathepsin-activated fluorescent probes, which have shown to improve sarcoma resection margins, and local control in mice.[32] **Fig. 3** shows the correlation between tumor bed fluorescence and tissue histology, as well as a survival curve showing improved disease-free survival with complete resection margins, as measured by a lack of residual fluorescence in the tumor bed. When used

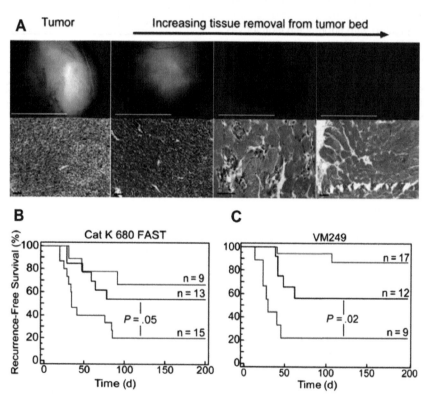

Fig. 3. Intraoperative detection and removal of microscopic residual sarcoma using wide-field imaging. Intraoperative, image-guided surgery improves local control. (A) Representative histology is shown from the removal of tumor using the imaging device. The top row corresponds to fluorescence images of the tumor (*first column*) and the tumor bed after 1, 2, and 3 resections (scale bars = 5 mm). The bottom row shows the corresponding histology from a biopsy of the tumor bed at each step in the surgery (scale bars = 50 μm). The removal of residual fluorescence from the tumor bed improves local control with either (B) the cathepsin K-specific Cat K 680 FAST probe or (C) the multicathepsin imaging agent VM249 (hazard ratio, 2.5 [P = .05] and 3.4 [P = .02], respectively). Blue lines represent single resections with no residual NIR fluorescence; red lines, single resections with residual NIR fluorescence; black lines, multiple resections to a tumor bed free of residual NIR fluorescence. Numbers of mice in each cohort are noted above each line. (*From* Mito JK, Ferrer JM, Brigman BE, et al. Intraoperative detection and removal of microscopic residual sarcoma using wide-field imaging. Cancer 2012;118(21):5328; with permission.)

to aid sarcoma resection in dogs, our laboratory has demonstrated an excellent correlation between intraoperative imaging of the tumor bed and histopathologic analysis of the resected tissue margins.[33,34] Clinical trials using a cathepsin-activated fluorescent probe, LUM015 (Lumicell Diagnostics, Inc., Waltham, MA, USA), in humans are currently under way (Clinicaltrials.gov, NCT01626066). Tumor Paint BLZ-100 (Blaze Bioscience, Inc., Seattle, WA) is another activated probe with great potential. Found in scorpion venom, the peptide chlorotoxin is conjugated to ICG, and fluoresces on cleavage by MMP-2 in tumor cells. Preclinical studies ·in mouse models have confirmed the ability to differentiate tumor tissue from surrounding normal tissue, as well as identify small foci of metastasis for various cancer types, including malignant glioma, medulloblastoma, prostate cancer, intestinal cancer, and sarcoma.[35,36] Safety and phase I studies using BLZ-100 in humans are under way (Clinicaltrials.gov, NCT02234297, NCT02097875).

Advantages

- Tumor-specific probes exploit molecular differences between normal and tumor tissue
- Ability to use existing biologic cancer therapies as targeting agents for fluorescent-linked probes
- Tumor-specific targets improve accuracy
- Good penetration with NIR techniques
- Improved signal-to-noise ratio

Disadvantages

- Requires exogenous fluorescent agent given to patient
- Targeted probes still in preclinical and clinical trials

High-frequency Ultrasound

The propagation of ultrasound waves through tissues is dependent on its cellular density, tissue heterogeneity, tissue structure, and cellular structure variables that are affected by neoplastic processes. The speed, amplitude, and spectral frequencies of high-frequency ultrasound wavelengths (20–80 MHz) as they travel through tissue can be recorded using both through-transmission and pulsed-echo techniques. Although no single variable has been shown to be predictive of tissue type, multivariate spectral analysis using attenuation coefficients and peak densities have demonstrated ability to differentiate among normal, benign, and malignant conditions, of excised breast tissue.[37]

Advantages

- Minimally invasive
- Resolution <1 mm
- Does not require preoperative administration of fluorescent agent

Disadvantages

- Sensitivity and specificity vary based on tissue pathology
- Multivariate algorithm varies among tissue types and would need to be redefined for each tumor type

Optical Coherence Tomography

The premise of optical coherence tomography (OCT) is similar to that of ultrasound, but using light instead of sound. It takes advantage of the native optical properties of tissues, and measures the time delay and intensity of backscattered/reflected light. This is measured along multiple locations and collected to form a cross-sectional image.[38] OCT is a powerful imaging technique with resolution capabilities to the cellular level. It can detect morphologic changes in tissue architecture characteristic of neoplasia, such as changes in epithelial thickness and integrity of the basement membrane.[39] Although trained personnel can interpret the OCT images with good accuracy for highly contrasted tissue types, other tissues are hard to differentiate (ie, normal fibrous vs fibrous tumor). Therefore, complex computer algorithms, using multiple variables based on the optical properties of the backscattered/reflected light, have been created to produce automated interpretation of tissue type (eg, fatty, fibrous, tumor)[40] or tumor margins (homogeneous normal tissue, homogeneous tumor tissue, heterogeneous tumor margin).[41] Recent data show successful delineation, with high resolution, of tumor margins using OCT imaging and automated interpretation of OCT with histologic comparison in breast cancer[42,43] and soft tissue sarcoma[41] (**Fig. 4**).

Advantages

- Does not require exogenous fluorescent probes
- High resolution ($\sim$ 10–15 μm) allows visualization of tissue architecture and cellular morphology similar to that of histopathology; greater than high-frequency ultrasound
- Can be handheld, or can integrate with existing surgical instrumentation, such as microscopes

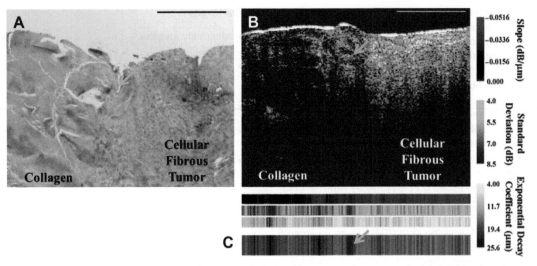

Fig. 4. Vertical tumor margin between collagen and cellular fibrous tumor presented with (*A*) histology image, (*B*) OCT image, and (*C*) color-coded plot combining the parameters of the A-line slope, the SD of the slope-removed A-line, and the exponential decay coefficient of its spatial frequency spectrum. The arrows point at the estimated position of the vertical tumor margin. The scale bars represent 0.5 mm. (*From* Wang S, Liu CH, Zakharov VP, et al. Three-dimensional computational analysis of optical coherence tomography images for the detection of soft tissue sarcomas. J Biomed Opt 2014;19(2):21102; with permission.)

- Small fiberoptic components facilitate use with small instrumentation for endoscopic or needle biopsy techniques
- Imaging techniques require experienced interpretation, but development of computational algorithms allow fast, automated interpretation

Disadvantages

- Shallow depth of field (~2 mm); less than high-frequency ultrasound
- Tumor heterogeneity in the setting of small field of view/depth of field may lead to sampling and type 2 errors

Optoacoustic imaging

In contrast to other optical imaging, this technique can produce high-resolution imaging with depth of field up to several centimeters. A short pulse of light is directed to the tissue and the resulting acoustic ultrasound waves produced by the tissues are recorded. Multispectral optoacoustic tomography (MSOT) is a process of computerized subtraction algorithms to differentiate the optoacoustic wavelengths produced by the exogenous fluorescent dyes or endogenous chromophores (ie, hemoglobin in vascular-rich tumors, or melanin in primary or metastatic melanoma) from the background tissue signal.[17,44,45] Although more work is needed to bring it to clinical application, technological advances have increased the feasibility and interest in research and development of optoacoustic imaging techniques.

Advantages

- Rapid technique
- High resolution with improved depth of field

Confocal Microscopy

Confocal microscopy is a microscopic technique with ability to visualize in vivo tissue at the cellular, histologic level. It depends on multiple flexible optical fibers that are ideal for endoscopic environments, and particularly has shown diagnostic potential during colonoscopies.[46] It has capabilities for fluorescent imaging as well as dynamic observations.

Advantages

- Resolution on the order of microns
- Real-time high-resolution (on the order of microns) imaging

Disadvantages

- Very small field of view
- Requires histologic interpretation of imaging

Elastic Scattering Spectroscopy (Diffuse Reflectance Spectroscopy)

Elastic scattering spectroscopy (ESS), otherwise referred to as diffuse reflectance spectroscopy, is similar to OCT, in that it is based on the differences in the reflection and scattering profiles of light through tissue. A light source (typically with wavelengths in the 300–900 nm, near UV-visible range) is directed to the target tissue, and the scattered and reflected light is recorded. Properties of the detected light wavelengths are analyzed using pattern recognition schemes to then determine tissue morphology and pathology. Certain configurations are sensitive enough to depict changes in subcellular components (eg, nucleus, mitochondria) affected by malignant transformation of tissue.[47] ESS has been shown to accurately differentiate malignant from nonmalignant tissue in breast tissues as well as colonic polyps using endoscopic techniques[48] (**Fig. 5**).

Advantages

- Small fiberoptic components facilitate use with small instrumentation for endoscopic or needle biopsy techniques
- Hardware includes small handheld probes and foot petals for easy control and use by the operator
- Rapid data acquisition and display time (less than 1 second for each measurement)
- No exogenous fluorescent probes required
- Strong optical signal (100 times stronger than fluorescence and 1000 times stronger than Ramen)[49]

Disadvantages

- Results affected by blood (hemoglobin) on the probe and in the operative field
- Despite background to noise subtraction techniques, the system can be overwhelmed by high-intensity operative lighting if not dimmed/shielded

- Small devices coupling the light source and light detector with close proximity have shorter depth of field compared with devices with greater offset

Raman Spectroscopy

Raman spectroscopy analyzes the inelastic scattering of light as it interacts with tissues. The Raman effect is the frequency/wavelength shift noted between the energy emitted to and the energy recorded from various tissues. However, although light is often the source of energy emission to the target tissue, Raman spectroscopy is based on the measurement of energy shifts in the form of molecular vibrations. This method is briefly outlined as follows:

1. Light energy of a given wavelength/frequency is directed toward the tissues (as in other techniques described previously).
2. Photons are absorbed by the molecules in tissues, which then enter an excited state.
3. The molecule then emits the photon as it enters a "less-excited state"; however, this is not necessarily the same ground state in which it started.
4. Therefore, the emitted photon is either at a higher or lower energy state than initial emission and interaction with the tissue.
5. This "Raman spectra" is recorded as a function of the frequency shifts of the emitted and recorded photons.

A spectroscopic model can be derived, and the cellular and molecular composition of a given tissue is represented by their fit coefficients (FCs). In one

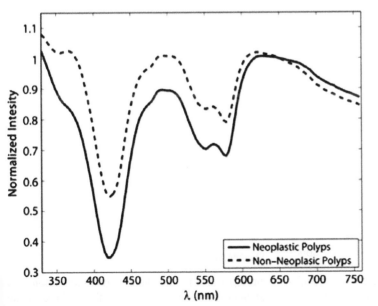

Fig. 5. Representative ESS spectra for neoplastic polyps (*solid line*) and non-neoplastic polyps (*dashed line*). (*From* Rodriguez-Diaz E, Huang Q, Cerda SR, et al. Endoscopic assessment of colonic polyps by using elastic scattering spectroscopy. Gastrointest Endosc 2015; 81(3):541; with permission.)

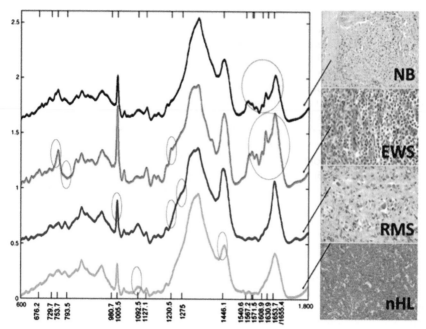

Fig. 6. Mean spectra of neuroblastoma (NB), Ewing sarcoma (EWS), rhabdomyosarcoma (RMS), and non-Hodgkin lymphoma (nHL) (Burkitt lymphoma) are shown. The 18 diagnostic peaks are marked with tick marks along the top and bottom of the graph with areas of specific interest circled on each spectrum. (*From* Kast R, Rabah R, Wills H, et al. Differentiation of small round blue cell tumors using Raman spectroscopy. J Pediatr Surg 2010;45(6):1112; with permission.)

technique, the FCs of fat and collagen were the distinguishing variables in an algorithm to differentiate normal, benign, and malignant breast tissue.[50,51] Spatially offset Raman spectroscopy probes have increased the depth of field with this technique to 2 mm, with successful qualitative analysis of breast cancer margins (positive or negative).[52] Raman spectroscopy is not only able to qualify the presence of tumor, but can also classify different tissue and tumor types, as shown in a study of various small round blue cell tumor types[53] (**Fig. 6**).

Advantages

- Depth of field up to 2 mm
- Can distinguish both tissue/tumor type as well as marginal status

Disadvantages

- Results affected by blood (hemoglobin) or cauterized tissues
- Although data analysis takes 1 to 2 minutes, data acquisition can take up to 30 minutes

Radiofrequency Spectroscopy

Similar to Raman and ESS, radiofrequency spectroscopy (RFS) is based on the differences between normal and tumor tissue's penetration of and interaction with radiofrequency energy, due to derangements of cellular and extracellular composition in tumor cells (eg, cellular organization, size, morphology, membrane structure, extracellular composition). RFS records conductivity (ability to move electric charges) and permittivity (ability to store electric charges) of electromagnetic waves in tissues, and is able to detect small differences consistent with tumor tissue at or near the margins of resected tissue.[54] RFS has been shown to differentiate between benign and malignant tissues of breast and prostate.[54–56]

Advantages

- Does not require fluorescent probes
- Immediate data collection and computed reporting (1–3 seconds)
- Simple handheld device

Disadvantages

- Small field of view (<1 cm)
- Very shallow depth of field (0.1–0.2 mm) is not ideal for evaluation of tumor bed, and ensures very narrow margin of resection when evaluating tumor resection

SUMMARY

Intraoperative tumor visualization has the potential to significantly improve surgical cancer care by improving adequacy of resection, decreasing resection of normal tissue and structures, and directing adjuvant therapy. This is an exciting, new, and rapidly evolving area of research that addresses a critical unmet need. We have outlined a variety of methods here, some of which have not been attempted in human patients, most of which are investigational and not currently approved by the Food and Drug Administration. Although the need for real-time, intraoperative assessment of an oncologic resection drives this research forward, data on important clinical outcomes, such as local recurrence and survival, remain years away.

REFERENCES

1. Simon MA, Enneking WF. The management of soft-tissue sarcomas of the extremities. J Bone Joint Surg Am 1976;58(3):317–27.
2. Ashford RU, McCarthy SW, Scolyer RA, et al. Surgical biopsy with intra-operative frozen section. An accurate and cost-effective method for diagnosis of musculoskeletal sarcomas. J Bone Joint Surg Br 2006;88(9):1207–11.
3. Howanitz PJ, Hoffman GG, Zarbo RJ. The accuracy of frozen-section diagnoses in 34 hospitals. Arch Pathol Lab Med 1990;114(4):355–9.
4. Rosenthal EL, Warram JM, Bland KI, et al. The status of contemporary image-guided modalities in oncologic surgery. Ann Surg 2015;261(1):46–55.
5. Senft C, Bink A, Franz K, et al. Intraoperative MRI guidance and extent of resection in glioma surgery: a randomised, controlled trial. Lancet Oncol 2011; 12(11):997–1003.
6. Claus EB, Horlacher A, Hsu L, et al. Survival rates in patients with low-grade glioma after intraoperative magnetic resonance image guidance. Cancer 2005;103(6):1227–33.
7. Kuhnt D, Becker A, Ganslandt O, et al. Correlation of the extent of tumor volume resection and patient survival in surgery of glioblastoma multiforme with high-field intraoperative MRI guidance. Neuro Oncol 2011;13(12):1339–48.
8. Krekel NM, Zonderhuis BM, Schreurs HW, et al. Ultrasound-guided breast-sparing surgery to improve cosmetic outcomes and quality of life. A prospective multicentre randomised controlled clinical trial comparing ultrasound-guided surgery to traditional palpation-guided surgery (COBALT trial). BMC Surg 2011;11:8.
9. Krekel NM, Zonderhuis BM, Stockmann HB, et al. A comparison of three methods for nonpalpable breast cancer excision. Eur J Surg Oncol 2011;37(2):109–15.
10. Krekel NM, Haloua MH, Lopes Cardozo AM, et al. Intraoperative ultrasound guidance for palpable breast cancer excision (COBALT trial): a multicentre, randomised controlled trial. Lancet Oncol 2013;14(1):48–54.
11. Yu CC, Chiang KC, Kuo WL, et al. Low re-excision rate for positive margins in patients treated with ultrasound-guided breast-conserving surgery. Breast 2013;22(5):698–702.
12. Krettek C, Geerling J, Bastian L, et al. Computer aided tumor resection in the pelvis. Injury 2004; 35(Suppl 1):S-A79–83.
13. Wong KC, Kumta SM. Use of computer navigation in orthopedic oncology. Curr Surg Rep 2014;2:47.
14. Cartiaux O, Banse X, Paul L, et al. Computer-assisted planning and navigation improves cutting accuracy during simulated bone tumor surgery of the pelvis. Comput Aided Surg 2013;18(1–2):19–26.
15. Keereweer S, Van Driel PB, Snoeks TJ, et al. Optical image-guided cancer surgery: challenges and limitations. Clin Cancer Res 2013;19(14):3745–54.
16. Wilke LG, Brown JQ, Bydlon TM, et al. Rapid noninvasive optical imaging of tissue composition in breast tumor margins. Am J Surg 2009;198(4):566–74.
17. de Boer E, Harlaar NJ, Taruttis A, et al. Optical innovations in surgery. Br J Surg 2015;102(2):e56–72.
18. Vahrmeijer AL, Hutteman M, van der Vorst JR, et al. Image-guided cancer surgery using near-infrared fluorescence. Nat Rev Clin Oncol 2013;10(9):507–18.
19. Stuker F, Ripoll J, Rudin M. Fluorescence molecular tomography: principles and potential for pharmaceutical research. Pharmaceutics 2011;3(2):229–74.
20. Ntziachristos V. Fluorescence molecular imaging. Annu Rev Biomed Eng 2006;8:1–33.
21. Bertrand N, Wu J, Xu X, et al. Cancer nanotechnology: the impact of passive and active targeting in the era of modern cancer biology. Adv Drug Deliv Rev 2014;66:2–25.
22. Guo Y, Yuan H, Cho H, et al. High-efficiency diffusion molecular retention tumor targeting. PLoS One 2013; 8(3):e58290.
23. Keereweer S, Kerrebijn JD, van Driel PB, et al. Optical image-guided surgery–where do we stand? Mol Imaging Biol 2011;13(2):199–207.
24. van Oosten M, Crane LM, Bart J, et al. Selecting potential targetable biomarkers for imaging purposes in colorectal cancer using TArget Selection Criteria (TASC): a novel target identification tool. Transl Oncol 2011;4(2):71–82.
25. Widhalm G, Kiesel B, Woehrer A, et al. 5-Aminolevulinic acid induced fluorescence is a powerful intraoperative marker for precise histopathological grading of gliomas with non-significant contrast-enhancement. PLoS One 2013;8(10):e76988.
26. Stummer W, Pichlmeier U, Meinel T, et al, ALA-Glioma Study Group. Fluorescence-guided surgery with 5-aminolevulinic acid for resection of malignant glioma: a randomised controlled multicentre phase III trial. Lancet Oncol 2006;7(5):392–401.
27. van Dam GM, Themelis G, Crane LM, et al. Intraoperative tumor-specific fluorescence imaging in

ovarian cancer by folate receptor-α targeting: first in-human results. Nat Med 2011;17(10):1315–9.

28. Warram JM, de Boer E, Sorace AG, et al. Antibody-based imaging strategies for cancer. Cancer Metastasis Rev 2014;33(2–3):809–22.

29. Terwisscha van Scheltinga AG, van Dam GM, Nagengast WB, et al. Intraoperative near-infrared fluorescence tumor imaging with vascular endothelial growth factor and human epidermal growth factor receptor 2 targeting antibodies. J Nucl Med 2011;52(11):1778–85.

30. Themelis G, Harlaar NJ, Kelder W, et al. Enhancing surgical vision by using real-time imaging of αvβ3-integrin targeted near-infrared fluorescent agent. Ann Surg Oncol 2011;18(12):3506–13.

31. Savariar EN, Felsen CN, Nashi N, et al. Real-time in vivo molecular detection of primary tumors and metastases with ratiometric activatable cell-penetrating peptides. Cancer Res 2013;73(2):855–64.

32. Mito JK, Ferrer JM, Brigman BE, et al. Intraoperative detection and removal of microscopic residual sarcoma using wide-field imaging. Cancer 2012;118(21):5320–30.

33. Eward WC, Mito JK, Eward CA, et al. A novel imaging system permits real-time in vivo tumor bed assessment after resection of naturally occurring sarcomas in dogs. Clin Orthop Relat Res 2013;471(3):834–42.

34. Troyan SL, Kianzad V, Gibbs-Strauss SL, et al. The FLARE intraoperative near-infrared fluorescence imaging system: a first-in-human clinical trial in breast cancer sentinel lymph node mapping. Ann Surg Oncol 2009;16(10):2943–52.

35. Butte PV, Mamelak A, Parrish-Novak J, et al. Near-infrared imaging of brain tumors using the tumor paint BLZ-100 to achieve near-complete resection of brain tumors. Neurosurg Focus 2014;36(2):E1.

36. Veiseh M, Gabikian P, Bahrami SB, et al. Tumor paint: a chlorotoxin:Cy5.5 bioconjugate for intraoperative visualization of cancer foci. Cancer Res 2007;67(14):6882–8.

37. Doyle TE, Factor RE, Ellefson CL, et al. High-frequency ultrasound for intraoperative margin assessments in breast conservation surgery: a feasibility study. BMC Cancer 2011;11:444.

38. Fujimoto JG, Pitris C, Boppart SA, et al. Optical coherence tomography: an emerging technology for biomedical imaging and optical biopsy. Neoplasia 2000;2(1–2):9–25.

39. Pitris C, Goodman A, Boppart SA, et al. High-resolution imaging of gynecologic neoplasms using optical coherence tomography. Obstet Gynecol 1999;93(1):135–9.

40. Mujat M, Ferguson RD, Hammer DX, et al. Automated algorithm for breast tissue differentiation in optical coherence tomography. J Biomed Opt 2009;14(3):034040.

41. Wang S, Liu CH, Zakharov VP, et al. Three-dimensional computational analysis of optical coherence tomography images for the detection of soft tissue sarcomas. J Biomed Opt 2014;19(2):21102.

42. Savastru D, Chang EW, Miclos S, et al. Detection of breast surgical margins with optical coherence tomography imaging: a concept evaluation study. J Biomed Opt 2014;19(5):056001.

43. Nguyen FT, Zysk AM, Chaney EJ, et al. Intraoperative evaluation of breast tumor margins with optical coherence tomography. Cancer Res 2009;69(22):8790–6.

44. Buehler A, Herzog E, Ale A, et al. High resolution tumor targeting in living mice by means of multispectral optoacoustic tomography. EJNMMI Res 2012;2:14.

45. Ntziachristos V, Razansky D. Molecular imaging by means of multispectral optoacoustic tomography (MSOT) [review]. Chem Rev 2010;110(5):2783–94.

46. Kiesslich R, Burg J, Vieth M, et al. Confocal laser endoscopy for diagnosing intraepithelial neoplasias and colorectal cancer in vivo. Gastroenterology 2004;127(3):706–13.

47. Bigio IJ, Bown SG, Briggs G, et al. Diagnosis of breast cancer using elastic-scattering spectroscopy: preliminary clinical results. J Biomed Opt 2000;5(2):221–8.

48. Rodriguez-Diaz E, Huang Q, Cerda SR, et al. Endoscopic histological assessment of colonic polyps by using elastic scattering spectroscopy. Gastrointest Endosc 2015;81(3):539–47.

49. Dhar A, Johnson KS, Novelli MR, et al. Elastic scattering spectroscopy for the diagnosis of colonic lesions: initial results of a novel optical biopsy technique. Gastrointest Endosc 2006;63(2):257–61.

50. Haka AS, Volynskaya Z, Gardecki JA, et al. In vivo margin assessment during partial mastectomy breast surgery using Raman spectroscopy. Cancer Res 2006;66(6):3317–22.

51. Haka AS, Shafer-Peltier KE, Fitzmaurice M, et al. Diagnosing breast cancer by using Raman spectroscopy. Proc Natl Acad Sci U S A 2005;102(35):12371–6.

52. Keller MD, Vargis E, de Matos Granja N, et al. Development of a spatially offset Raman spectroscopy probe for breast tumor surgical margin evaluation. J Biomed Opt 2011;16(7):077006.

53. Kast R, Rabah R, Wills H, et al. Differentiation of small round blue cell tumors using Raman spectroscopy. J Pediatr Surg 2010;45(6):1110–4.

54. Dotan ZA, Fridman E, Lindner A, et al. Detection of prostate cancer by radio-frequency near-field spectroscopy in radical prostatectomy ex vivo specimens. Prostate Cancer Prostatic Dis 2013;16(1):73–8.

55. Allweis TM, Kaufman Z, Lelcuk S, et al. A prospective, randomized, controlled, multicenter study of a real-time, intraoperative probe for positive margin detection in breast-conserving surgery. Am J Surg 2008;196(4):483–9.

56. Karni T, Pappo I, Sandbank J, et al. A device for real-time, intraoperative margin assessment in breast-conservation surgery. Am J Surg 2007;194(4):467–73.

Reconstruction After Tumor Resection in the Growing Child

John S. Groundland, MD[a], Odion Binitie, MD[a,b],*

KEYWORDS

- Pediatric limb salvage • Tumor • Endoprosthesis • Allograft • Allograft-prosthetic composite

KEY POINTS

- Limb salvage may be a viable alternative to amputation in even the youngest of pediatric patients with an extremity bone tumor.
- Expandable metallic endoprosthesis can achieve meaningful growth, resulting in little to no limb length discrepancy for skeletally immature patients by the end of their growth.
- Many case series have been presented in the literature, but there is no evidence graded level II or higher, limiting the ability to identify 1 construct as superior to another.
- Failure rates in the pediatric population of the 3 main forms of limb salvage constructs (metallic endoprosthesis, allograft, allograft-prosthetic composite) are high, but comparable with failure rates reported in adults.
- Function after limb salvage for bone tumor in the growing child has been inadequately reported in the literature.

HISTORICAL BACKGROUND

The prognosis of bone sarcoma of the extremities in the pediatric patient was historically described as poor, hopeless, or grave.[1–3] In the first half of the twentieth century, the only curative procedure was amputation, which provided a reported 5-year survival of 12% to 23%.[3–5] Amputation was not available for all patients; rather, it was reserved for patients who met appropriate criteria, which included no evidence of metastatic disease. With such a bleak prognosis, the idea of limb salvage seemed implausible.

In 1975, several studies were published that changed the landscape in the treatment of extremity sarcoma.[6–8] Chemotherapy and radiation began to have an impact on the course of the disease, improving 5-year survival outcomes from 20% to 65%.[9–13] As late as 1979, Copeland and Sutow[14] noted that "following diagnostic biopsy, amputation of the extremities remains the treatment of choice. In selected cases, limb-saving radical en bloc resection may surface." However, by 1986, Simon and colleagues[15] reported on their results in 227 patients younger than 30 years with osteosarcoma; they reported no survival difference in 5-year follow-up between those patients who underwent amputation versus limb salvage. With this improvement in survival afforded by chemotherapy and radiation, the

Disclosure: No benefits in any form have been received or will be received from a commercial party related directly or indirectly to the subject of this article; neither author is a paid consultant, or receives royalties, from any manufacturer or supplier of medical commercial interests.

[a] Department of Orthopedics and Sports Medicine, University of South Florida, 13220 USF Laurel Drive, Tampa, FL 33612, USA; [b] Department of Sarcoma, H. Lee Moffitt Cancer Center, 12902 Magnolia Drive, Tampa, FL 33612, USA

* Corresponding author. Sarcoma Department, Moffitt Cancer Center, FOB-1, 12902 Magnolia Drive, Tampa, FL 33612.

E-mail address: Odion.Binitie@moffitt.org

treatment paradigm shifted from radical amputation to en bloc resection and reconstruction of the resultant defect. Limb salvage is the prevailing treatment of most sarcomas of the extremities, with 90% to 95% of skeletally mature patients with primary bone tumors receiving some fashion of limb salvage surgery.[16–19]

Although the overall trend in orthopedic oncology moved from amputation to limb salvage, the treatment of the pediatric patient with primary bone tumor remained controversial.[20–22] This is partly because of the generally high complication rates after tumor resection and subsequent reconstruction and partly because of the unique issues related to pediatric patients when compared with their adult counterparts. With the rate of failure requiring operative revision nearing 25% in adults, some orthopedic oncologists have questioned the appropriateness of subjecting children with bone sarcoma to a lifetime of surgical complications and revisions. In addition, surgical resection of tumor in the skeletally immature patient is often complicated by the loss of a physis, with a resultant potential for clinically relevant leg length discrepancy. For these reasons, some tumor surgeons maintained that children with a malignant bone tumor of the lower extremity, especially those far from skeletal maturity, might be best served by a single amputation surgery with subsequent prosthesis fitting. From this point of view, amputation would provide the most consistent outcome with the least amount of surgeries and complications.[23] In a review article published in *Journal of the American Academy of Orthopedic Surgery* in 2003, DiCaprio and Freidlaender[24] list "immature skeletal age with a predicted leg length discrepancy greater than 8 cm" as a relative contraindication to limb salvage.

However, an increasing body of literature has reported limb salvage techniques for the skeletally immature, including patients younger than 5 years. Expandable prostheses have been developed and modified to address the issue of leg length discrepancy, and both surgical and functional outcome studies have been performed that suggest that limb salvage might be a preferable alternative to amputation in the skeletally immature patient with a primary bone tumor.[25–40]

STATE OF THE LITERATURE

There are several features inherent to pediatric orthopedic oncology that hamper the development of a robust literature. First, the relative rarity of pediatric bone tumor limits the amount of patients any single treatment center may see over the course of a reasonable timespan. When segregated for anatomic location of the tumor, the

number of patients can become even more limited. For example, in a 10-year span, many large regional cancer centers may have only a few pediatric patients with a distal femur tumor that was treated with en bloc resection and a specific limb salvage option, such as endoprosthesis, allograft, or allograft-prosthetic composite (APC). By the time a sufficient number of patients have been accumulated, the interventions may have been modified and no longer be comparable. Second, tumor resections are not homogenous. Outcomes also depend on soft tissue maintenance, nerve function, and health of the patient. However, these factors cannot be randomized or controlled, because they are subject to the specifics of the tumor and the patient; strict exclusion criteria for study would only lead to further restriction on patient number, often to the point of reporting on patients on a case-by-case basis.[41]

In a recent review of the literature,[41] an attempt was made to investigate the surgical and functional outcomes in pediatric patients after en bloc bone sarcoma excision followed by limb salvage reconstruction with an endoprosthesis, an allograft, or an allograft-prosthesis reconstruction. The study segregated each limb salvage type by anatomic location, reporting on the proximal femur, total femur, distal femur, and the proximal tibia individually. The state of the literature was noted to be limited. No study rose above level IV evidence. In total, 62 articles were found that clearly reported on the surgical and functional outcomes of pediatric patients after limb salvage surgery for bone tumor at a specific anatomic location. No study had more than 40 patients, and 82% of the studies had 10 or fewer patients. Twenty-six of the 62 studies (42%), reported on 1 subject per described anatomic region. One hundred and seventy-five papers were excluded because of overinclusion and inability to reliably parse the data. That is, most studies combined pediatric patients with adult and elderly patients or combined hip, knee, and shoulder patients together as 1 group. Future research studies are needed that segregate pediatric patients from adults; more specifically, they should distinguish between those far from skeletal maturity versus patients in their peak of growth versus those patients nearing physeal closure. In addition, anatomically specific reporting should become the standard, because each region has unique challenges and surgical considerations.[41]

CURRENT ALTERNATIVES TO LIMB SALVAGE
Amputation

Even in an era of expanding indications for limb salvage, amputation as the primary surgical modality in the treatment of pediatric extremity bone tumor remains a common intervention.[42] Schrager and colleagues[43] analyzed the registry data from the National Cancer Institute's SEER (Surveillance Epidemiology and End Results) Program from 1988 to 2007. These investigators compared the incidence of amputation versus limb salvage in 890 patients with osteosarcoma younger than 20 years. They found that 66.3% of the reported sample underwent limb salvage, whereas 33.7% had amputation. A study using the same database[44] noted that patients with an age of 5 years or less were more likely to undergo amputation than their 6-year-old to 19-year-old counterparts, with the former receiving amputation in 55% of cases versus 27% for the latter. This finding suggests that young age continues to be an exclusion criterion for many surgeons when considering limb salvage. This situation may be because of the clinically significant longitudinal and cross-sectional growth remaining in the child and the understanding that limb salvage means multiple surgeries throughout adolescence, even if a growing prosthesis was successfully used.

In addition to young age, traditional indications for amputation include patients with tumors whose resections would necessitate sacrifice of a major neurovascular bundle; tumors of the distal tibia; and patients in areas of the world that lack the economic resources to provide a complex implant.[42] Although these indications are being challenged by an increasing body of literature showing alternatives to amputation, amputation remains a major tool for many orthopedic oncologists, as shown by the percentages noted earlier.

Rotationplasty

Because most of the primary bone tumors occur about the hip and knee, amputation often requires an above-knee amputation or hip disarticulation. This option imparts a significant increase in oxygen demand while walking when compared with a below-knee amputation and has been linked to less favorable psychosocial outcomes. For cases in which an above-knee amputation would be required to achieve tumor resection, rotationplasty is available as a means to effectively convert an above-knee amputation to a below-knee amputation.

First described by Borggreve in the 1930s and expanded by Van Nes in the 1950s to treat proximal focal femoral deficiency, rotationplasty involves the resection of the distal femur and proximal tibia, with subsequent tibiofemoral osteosynthesis, after rotating the distal tibia and foot 180°.[45–47] This technique allows the residual

distal tibia to augment the length of the foreshortened femur and uses the reversed but functional ankle to operate as a knee. The prosthesis fits on the foot and the patient functions as a below-knee amputee.

When considered for the growing child, rotationplasty offers a form of a growing reconstruction. The preserved proximal femoral physis remains and the distal tibial physis is preserved as well, providing potential growth at both ends of the newly fashioned femorotibial composite. Although the transferred distal tibial physis does not have the same growth potential as the contralateral distal femoral physis, the growth potential that is preserved allows procedures such as contralateral epiphysiodesis to be reasonably considered. The literature on rotationplasty is understandably limited to small case series, but reports of interventions in patients as young as 14 months old show the potential of this surgical alternative.[48]

Surgical complications include the standard orthopedic oncology issues, such as infection, local recurrence, and pathologic fracture. Rotationplasty also may be subject to malrotation as well as failure of the vascular anastomosis. In a series of 25 pediatric patients receiving rotationplasty for tumor, Sawamura and colleagues[49] reported 3 (12%) vascular complications requiring subsequent amputation. Six additional patients (24%) required subsequent surgical intervention for complications, including sciatic nerve palsy because of hematoma, distal tibia fracture, nonunion of the osteosynthesis, slipped capital femoral epiphysis, and wound complications.

When considering rotationplasty for the pediatric patient with a complex sarcoma about the knee, parents and surgeons must consider more than just the reconstruction and surgical complications. Amputation is a disfigurement in itself, and rotationplasty potentially magnifies this effect by altering the morphology of the extremity, beyond mere ablation.[50] Forni and colleagues[51] studied the emotional acceptance of children who underwent this procedure. These investigators found relational and emotion difficulty in adolescence after rotationplasty, which abated as the patient grew into adulthood. On the other hand, in a case series comparing rotationplasty with endoprosthetic reconstruction for treatment of tumors about the knee, Hillmann and colleagues[52] reported equivalent functional scores between the groups, as measured by the Musculoskeletal Tumor Society (MSTS) questionnaire; moreover, significantly fewer of the rotationplasty patients required assistive walking devices, fewer had limiting pain, and more rotationplasty patients resumed hobbies and sports than their endoprosthesis-treated counterparts.

Because of the limitations of the literature, secondary to the rare nature of sarcoma and the even more limited number of rotationplasties, the outcomes of rotationplasty remain incompletely described. However, given the moderate support in the literature, rotationplasty remains a viable option in select cases, pending a thorough and frank discussion between the patient's family and the surgeon.

LIMB SALVAGE: GENERAL PRINCIPLES FOR THE SKELETALLY IMMATURE

Initial efforts in limb salvage surgery for bone tumors were sporadic, controversial, and varied. Early attempts that were described included endoprostheses made of vitallium, ceramic, polyethylene, and cobalt-chrome.[53–55] Alternatively, cadaveric allograft and autogenous cortical bone grafting were used. Some surgeons spanned the affected joint with a fusion construct, hoping to maintain length of the limb to preserve distal function, whereas more ambitious surgeons sought to restore joint function in addition to saving the limb. However, application of these preliminary techniques to the pediatric population was largely avoided.[56,57] In 1976, Scales[58] broke with this tradition, describing an expandable prosthesis designed specifically for the pediatric patient. Developed at the Division of Biomedical Engineering in Stanmore, England, the extendible endoprosthesis sought to reconstruct the posttumor resection defect and also to address the issue of anticipated limb length discrepancy after physis excision. Over the ensuing 40 years, the literature has come to reflect the increasing acceptance of limb salvage after bone tumor resection in the pediatric population, although considerable variation in reconstruction design persists.

Selecting a Prosthesis

Age-related concerns for the lower extremity
When considering the options for reconstruction after bone tumor resection in the lower extremity of a growing child, 3 distinct subpopulations based on age and skeletal maturity must be appreciated. The first subpopulation contains those patients nearing skeletal maturity, typically in the age ranges of 14 to 17 years. If the remaining anticipated growth of the resected physis is 2 cm or less, an adult implant may be used. The limb length discrepancy of this amount may be well tolerated without need to augment the limb with an external shoe lift. Alternatively, the adult implant can be selected such that the operated limb is lengthened intraoperatively to the expected adult length, allowing the contralateral side to catch up

over time. The amount of overcorrection tolerated depends on the starting size of the limb and is limited by the potential to induce sciatic neuropraxia or loss of motion at the knee, secondary to the acute length change.

The second group of patients based on age is the skeletally immature with roughly 2 to 6 cm of growth remaining at the resected physis. This intermediate group may be addressed from various perspectives. Although the anticipated leg length discrepancy would be too great to simply overcorrect the affected side with a long implant, a combination of ipsilateral overcorrection with contralateral epiphysiodesis may result in acceptable limb length equality. The benefit of this approach lies in the fact that an adult implant is placed during the index procedure, forgoing the need to transition from a growing prosthesis to an adult implant once skeletal maturity is achieved. Alternatively, a growing prosthesis may be used. This option has several potential advantages over initial placement of an adult implant. An expandable prosthesis, if it functions properly, can be used to match the growth of the contralateral side. Although growth prediction provides a reasonable expectation of ultimate limb length, it is only an estimate and prone to error, especially in the face of chemotherapy and local radiation, which may affect physeal growth.[59–61] Also, a growing prosthesis permits the greatest potential final patient height, as a result of preclusion of contralateral epiphysiodesis, which may be a concern in some cases.

The third and final subpopulation to consider in regards to age is the group far from skeletal maturity. Ranging from 2 to 8 years old, the only reliable option these patients have for limb salvage is a growing endoprosthesis. Showing the potential of limb salvage, reports have been published describing a proximal femur replacement in a 3-year-old,[62] a total femur in a 2-year-old,[63] distal femur replacement in a 5-year-old,[38] and a proximal tibia replacement in a 4-year-old.[64] At this extreme of young age, not only must longitudinal growth be considered but cross-sectional growth must also be taken into account. For the patient younger than 8 years to have successful limb salvage surgery, taking them to skeletal maturity with limb length equality and a functional limb, more than 1 growing prosthesis is likely required. With additional surgery for final conversion to an adult implant, limb salvage in this subpopulation requires a major commitment among the patient, the family, and the surgeon.

Age-related concerns for the upper extremity
Tolerance for limb length inequality is a major concern in the lower extremity, as a consequence

of bipedal human ambulation, but limb length inequality in the upper extremity is not without its considerations. Moderate amount of limb length inequality is well tolerated in the upper extremity, and the patient can easily accept several centimeters of difference. This situation allows the surgeon to choose a final prosthesis based on the structural needs of the patient, whether that entails a metallic endoprosthesis (ME), allograft, or APC.

However, when performing a resection in the very young, a growing prosthesis in the humerus may be appropriate, to provide an upper limb that is morphologically similar to the contralateral side. However, these reconstructions are rare, because of the limited occurrence of sarcoma in general, and the even more restricted occurrence in the very young and in the upper extremity. Case reports have been published, but no substantial case series has been presented.[65]

Metal Endoprostheses: Historical Background

Growing prosthesis

By 1992, Unwin and Walker[66] were able to report on the outcomes of 168 skeletally immature patients who had bone tumors treated with en bloc resection and reconstruction with an extendible Stanmore custom ME. During the period reported, from 1976 to 1992, these investigators noted 4 distinct designs in the growing mechanism. The initial design used a worm-drive screw to extend the telescoping titanium components. That design was switched to a ball-bearing mechanism in 1982, because of reported mechanical failure of the device, attributed to difficulties associated with the manufacturing process. The ball-bearing mechanism was replaced in 1988 by a C-collar mechanism, in which expansion required open dissection to the area of the telescoped components, manual longitudinal traction, and the subsequent interposition of the C-collar spacer to maintain the gained length between the 2 components. This design was then replaced in 1992 with a minimally invasive device that used a mechanism similar to the original worm-screw design. An Allen wrench could be percutaneously inserted to turn the drive that engaged the screw mechanism. This history reflects the overall trend in expandable endoprosthetic design and use. The original attempts were limited by manufacturing capabilities and required invasive, open surgical procedures for every lengthening. As manufacturing techniques improved, the design could return to the screw mechanism and minimally invasive techniques could be used.[67]

In 2006, Gupta and colleagues[68] reported on the next step of development from the Stanmore group: the noninvasive growing prosthesis (Stanmore, Elstree, United Kingdom). This latest generation endoprosthesis, first used in 2002, houses a rare-earth magnetic disk within the endoprosthesis, which connects to a gearbox, which is in turn connected to a power screw. Expansion of the prosthesis is achieved when the extremity is placed in the core of a circular external drive unit. This external drive unit induces a rotating magnetic field that acts on the magnetic disk mechanism noninvasively within the endoprosthesis. The rotating magnetic field pulls the magnetic disks within the prosthesis, engaging the gearbox, which rotates the power screw, leading to the predictable lengthening of the prosthesis. The amount of potential expansion is determined by the size of the telescoping mechanism. Three lengths are available for the proximal femur, distal femur, and proximal tibia endoprosthesis, which provide 50 mm, 70 mm, or 90 mm of available growth, determined by the remaining growth of the child and the length of resection. The advantages of this latest generation of expandable prosthesis include reduced risk of infection because of noninvasive expansions, outpatient expansion without need for anesthesia, and precise and reversible lengthening. The specific disadvantages relative to other endoprostheses include high cost and limited availability in nonspecialized centers. **Figs. 1–4** show a distal femur implant, the magnetic expansion device, and radiographic progression of expansion in an implanted total femur Stanmore device.

Alternatives to the Stanmore design have been developed and used. The Repiphysis expandable prosthesis is an example (**Figs. 5** and **6**). Originally marketed as the Phenix prosthesis, the Repiphysis is a noninvasively expandable titanium endoprosthesis (Wright Medical, Arlington, TX). The expansion mechanism is housed within the tubular portion of the prosthesis and works by releasing

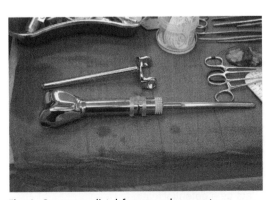

Fig. 1. Stanmore distal femur replacement.

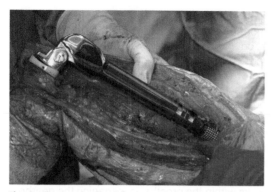

Fig. 2. Stanmore distal femur expandable implant.

stored energy from compressed springs within the mechanism. The spring is held compressed by 2 tubes, made of polyether ethylketone. When expansion is desired, the tubes are heated under the guidance of fluoroscopy by induction from an external magnetic coil; the heat melts the polymer and the coiled spring is released, creating the force to expand the tubular insert.[69] However, general acceptance of the Repiphysis system has been limited because of concerns regarding the high rate of complications. Although limb salvage in general is plagued with failure rates in the 25% to 33% range, the Repiphysis system has been noted to have failure rates in excess of 50%. The group from Rush University reported, over the course of 2 studies,[70,71] a failure rate of 58% (15 of 26 patients), with associated bone loss around the prosthesis often limiting revision options. Likewise, Staals and colleagues[72] reported that 9 of the 10 patients they treated with Repiphysis reconstruction at the distal femur required revision surgery: 8 for implant breakage and 1 for aseptic loosening. In addition, these investigators noted that expansion lengthening was erratic and unpredictable. They cautioned against use of the device.

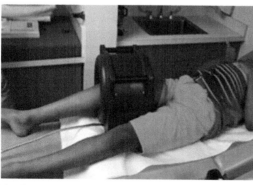

Fig. 3. Stanmore magnet.

As an example of the innovative nature of endoprosthesis design in response to documented complications, Webber and Seidel combined the Compress compliant prestress device (Biomet, Warsaw, IN) with the Repiphysis endoprosthesis.[73] Although these investigators presented only a single case report, and this has not been adopted or documented in any substantial number, this modification shows the ongoing adaptation occurring in pediatric limb salvage surgery. This will unlikely solve the high rate of complications associated with the Repiphysis, but the lesson in understanding and addressing the modes of failure of a device is worthy of note.

The MUTARS (Modular Universal Tumour and Revision System) shows additional innovation in expansion technology. In their Xpand prosthesis line, growth may be achieved through both mechanical as well as biological means. The mechanical device uses a high-frequency transmitter to activate the internal actuator within the prosthesis; to achieve biological growth, the stem of the prosthesis can be replaced with a growing intramedullary rod system that lengthens the host bone through distraction osteogenesis.

Although not exhaustive by any means, the synopsis given earlier reflects the early trials and subsequent innovations made in expandable prosthesis design. There are certainly other prostheses that should be considered in a complete history, such as the Lewis expandable adjustable prosthesis, which was the first widely used expandable device used in the United States. In addition to the noninvasive models noted earlier, minimally invasive expansion designs by Stryker and Biomet are available for use (**Figs. 7** and **8**). A list of the current expandable MEs is presented in **Table 1**.

LIMB SALVAGE SURGERY: CURRENT PRACTICES

No database study has been published that details the relative use of the various types of reconstruction after bone tumor excision in the extremities. Selection of a ME versus an allograft or an APC is largely surgeon dependent, often based on surgeon preference as much as on specific concerns for a given case. A recent review of the literature by our group found 521 distinct skeletally immature patients who underwent limb salvage surgery for lower extremity bone tumor; 393 received a ME; 105 patients had allograft; and 23 had an APC.[41] Although clearly limited by the nature of the literature, this study suggests that ME is the most common reconstruction in this population. Average age of those undergoing limb salvage surgery in

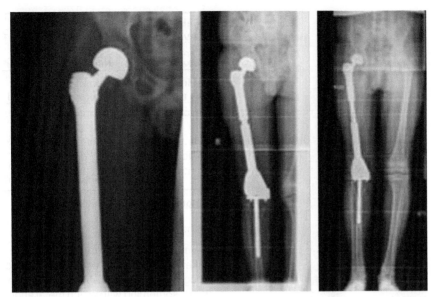

Fig. 4. Stanmore total femur reconstruction expansion progression.

the endoprosthesis group was 10.8 years, whereas the allograft and APC ages averaged 12.4 and 13.9 years, respectively. The younger age in the endoprosthesis group likely reflects the use of expandable constructs in the subpopulation of patients who are far from skeletal maturity. The youngest reported patient was a 2-year-old who received a total femur after resection for Ewing sarcoma.

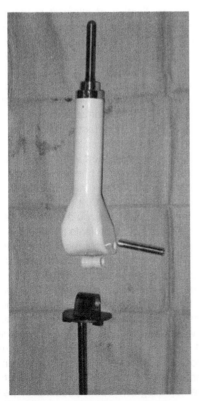

Fig. 5. The Phenix expandable prosthesis.

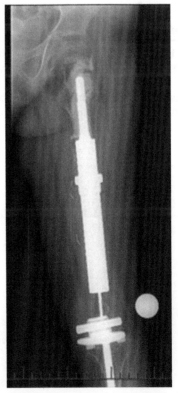

Fig. 6. Radiograph of an implanted Phenix distal femur reconstruction.

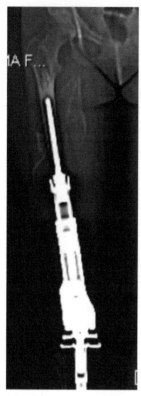

Fig. 7. Stryker distal femur expandable endoprosthesis.

Allograft

Osteoarticular allograft reconstruction after wide excision of bone tumor has a rich history in limb salvage surgery. When a sized matched allograft can be applied, the inherent appeal of reconstructing a joint with an allograft is obvious. The complex

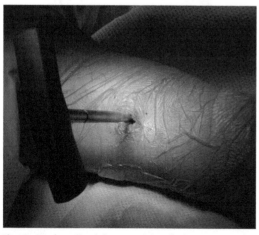

Fig. 8. Stryker distal femur minimally invasive intraoperative expansion.

Table 1
Available expandable prostheses, 2015

Expansion Type	Name, Manufacturer
Minimally invasive	Biomet, Warsaw, IN Stryker, Mahwah, NJ
Noninvasive	Stanmore, Elstree, United Kingdom Repiphysis, Wright Medical, Arlington, TX MUTARS Xpand[a], Implantcast, Buxtehunde, Germany

[a] Not available in the United States.

morphology of the joint is, by the nature of allograft, taken into account. Perhaps most importantly, the allograft provides sites for reattachment of soft tissues, something with which metal endoprostheses have struggled. In this way, function should be maximized with the allograft reconstruction, providing such advantages of reconstructing the abductor mechanism in proximal femur replacements and the extensor mechanism after proximal tibia replacements. Despite the theoretic appeal, the surgical outcomes of allograft reconstructions have been hampered by high complication and failure rates.[74–77]

Specific application of allograft reconstruction to the pediatric limb salvage population has been tempered, perhaps because an allograft is not a growing prosthesis. Case series have been reported, but they suffer from the issues affecting the pediatric limb salvage literature in general: small number of patients, overinclusion of patients based on age and site of reconstruction, limited follow-up, and nonstandardized functional outcome measures. Muscolo and colleagues[76] published the largest cohort with distinctly identifiable pediatric patients. In this series of osteoarticular allografts of the proximal tibia spanning the 20 years from 1982 to 2002, 20 distinct patients aged 10 to 17 years old could be identified from their larger series of 52 patients (range 10–54 years old). Nine of the 20 pediatric reconstructions failed (45%): 7 for infection and 1 each for structural failure and local recurrence.

When the entirety of the English literature was culled for pediatric patients treated with allograft reconstruction after extremity tumor excision, 1 study was found on proximal femur replacement (n = 1 patient), 7 studies on distal femur reconstructions (n = 34 patients), and 7 studies on proximal tibia reconstructions (n = 70 patients). No total femur allograft reconstructions in pediatric patients have been described in the literature.[41]

Autograft

Autograft represents a special subset of reconstruction within the biological umbrella. In this technique, the affected bone is resected, subjected to a treatment aimed at eradicating any viable tumor cells, and subsequently reimplanted. In this manner, the bone functions as a perfectly size-matched graft, without the need for maintaining a bone bank or extensive preoperative planning. Treatment is variable and has been described in pediatric patients to include irradiation or heat pasteurization. Three studies with identifiable pediatric patients have described this technique for osteoarticular reconstruction in the lower extremity: 2 autograft studies and 1 autograft-prosthesis composite report, without incidence of recurrence.[78–80] All of the centers that published the studies were in Asia, suggesting a possible geographic preference for this surgical option. The total number of patients between the series was 8, which is too limited to draw any conclusions regarding superiority of the reconstruction versus other options. However, with the few data that are available, autograft seems to be a safe and viable alternative.

Metallic Endoprosthesis

The most widely reported reconstruction method after bone tumor resection of the extremities, for both the pediatric and the adult population, is the ME.[41,81] The strength of the endoprosthesis lies in its versatility, because current designs are often modular, obviating the historical requirement for custom implants. Particularly relevant to the pediatric patient, expandable prostheses are available, allowing noninvasive lengthening of the affected limb that can match the growth of the contralateral side in a controlled manner. With the noninvasive ME expandable prostheses that use a screw mechanism, controlled shortening can be achieved, should the patient develop a neuropraxia or experience loss of joint motion after a lengthening procedure. The main disadvantage of the ME versus the allograft and APC, from a theoretic perspective, is the limited capacity to achieve any reliable soft tissue ingrowth into the metallic prosthesis. In the adult population, attempts have been made to augment the loss of capsular structures and attachment sites with artificial mesh, such as aortograft or Trevira tube, but definitive benefit of these techniques has yet to be proved.[82,83] Furthermore, use of these augments to the ME in the pediatric population is less documented or analyzed.

Expandable endoprostheses have been placed in pediatric patients for proximal femur, total femur, distal femur, proximal tibia, and total humerus reconstructions. The likelihood that an expandable prosthesis will be lengthened ranges from 51% (distal femur) to 81% (total femur); reasons that affect whether an expandable prosthesis is lengthened include lack of anticipated growth of the contralateral side, failure of the prosthesis before expansion, failure of the expansion device, or death from disease before any relevant growth. When expansions were reported in the literature, the average length gained was 29.9 mm for the proximal femur, 84.8 mm for total femur, 46.5 mm for distal femur, and 31.3 mm for the proximal tibia. No clinical leg length discrepancies have been reported in total femur replacements undergoing expansion, although 23.5% of the proximal femur replacements were noted to have a leg length discrepancy at final follow-up.[41]

Allograft-Prosthesis Composite

APC represents an attempt to address the limitations of allografts and MEs. The appeal of this construct lies in the capacity of the allograft portion to provide attachment sites for the capsule and tendons, whereas the prosthesis portion provides mechanical support against subchondral collapse and potentially poor host-graft osteosynthesis. However, the limited number of pediatric patients with APC reconstruction indicates the lack of universal acceptance of this construct. Twenty-three pediatric patients, aged 8 to 17 years, have been clearly reported in the literature, in an age-specific and anatomically specific manner.[41] One factor that may interfere with greater use in the pediatric population is the lack of a described APC construct that can lengthen. If this construct were to be developed, a greater use of APC constructs mighty find use in the pediatric population, especially for the younger subset.

COMPLICATIONS AND FAILURES
General Concerns

The ideal reconstruction after extremity tumor resection in the growing child would satisfy both the surgical as well as the functional requirements of the patient. The surgical outcomes should minimize local recurrence and infection, withstand the stresses inherent to joint mechanics, and provide the capacity to grow with the growing child. Functionally, the reconstruction should restore the range of motion and strength of the joint complex, maintain distal function, and allow the patient to participate in their professional and recreational pursuits without limitation. These goals have yet to be fully realized in extremity sarcoma surgery. In particular, infection and structural failure have plagued large segmental implants, and functional outcomes have only sporadically been investigated. No specific implant has shown a clear superiority to other constructs.

Henderson and colleagues[81] proposed a classification system to specify the modes of failure for MEs in adults. As listed in **Table 2**, this system was later expanded to include issues specific to allograft reconstructions and pediatric patients.[84] In the original classification study, a meta-analysis of the literature was performed and the outcomes of 5 regional cancer centers were collated; among the findings, the investigators noted that failure modes occurred at different rates for different anatomic sites. To this end, they recommended reporting outcomes and failures of extremity tumor reconstructions in an anatomically specific manner. Using this recommendation and the classification system, a review of the literature for pediatric limb salvage patients[41] likewise showed anatomic-site and reconstruction-type differences in failure rates.

Infection

The mode of failure after extremity tumor-wide resection that is common to all implants, in both adult and children, is infection. Infection affects large metallic implants as well as allograft reconstructions. Although all anatomic areas are susceptible to infection, the proximal tibia constructs have particularly high rates of infection, as shown in **Table 3**. The subcutaneous nature of the region has been implicated as a causative factor, and the routine use of medial gastrocnemius flaps has been adopted to improve the soft tissue coverage. The validity of this procedure to decrease infections is still pending. Other innovations to address the high infection rates, in general, include antibiotic-impregnated cement and silver-coated stems. Likewise, these techniques remain unvalidated.

The consequences of infection can be devastating, potentially leading to multiple revisions and even amputation.[85] A reliable method to prevent infection, and reliably treat it once it occurs, would be a boon to orthopedic oncology.

Allografts

In reviewing the literature, collated failure rates after allograft reconstruction in pediatric bone tumor surgery show high rates of failure. Overall, failure occurred in 51% of lower extremity osteoarticular allograft reconstructions in patients younger than 17 years.[41] When subdivided by anatomic site, 38.7% of distal femur and 57.1% of the proximal

---

Table 2
Classification scheme for mode of failure of tumor endoprosthetic reconstruction

2011 Henderson Classification[81]		2014 - Updated International Society of Limb Salvage Classification[84]		
Category	**Mode**	**Category**	**Mode**	**Subcategory**
Mechanical		*Mechanical*		
Type 1	Soft tissue failure	Type 1	Soft tissue failure	A. Functional: insufficient soft tissue function B. Coverage: dehischence
Type 2	Aseptic Loosening	Type 2	Aseptic Loosening	A. Early: <2 y B. Late: >2 y
Type 3	Structural failure	Type 3	Structural failure	A. Implant: including expandable malfunction B. Bone: periprosthetic fracture
Nonmechanical		*Nonmechanical*		
Type 4	Infection	Type 4	Infection	A. Early: <2 y B. Late: >2 y
Type 5	Tumor progression	Type 5	Tumor progression	A. Soft Tissue B. Bone
		Type 6	Pediatric Specific	A. Physeal arrest: longitudinal or angular B. Joint dysplasia

Adapted from Henderson ER, Groundland JS, Pala E, et al. Failure mode classification for tumor endoprostheses: retrospective review of five institutions and a literature review. J Bone Joint Surg Am 2011;93(5):421; and Henderson ER, O'Connor MI, Ruggieri P et al. Classification of failure of limb salvage after reconstructive surgery for bone tumours: a modified system including biological and expandable reconstructions. Bone Joint J 2014;96-B(11):1437.

Table 3
Failure mode

Prosthesis	Anatomic Location	n	Total % Revised	Type 1 Soft Tissue 1 (%)	Type 2 Aseptic Loosening (%)	Type 3 Structural Failure (%)	Type 4 Infection (%)	Type 5 Local Recurrence (%)	Failure of Lengthening Device (%)	Subsequent Amputation (%)
Endoprosthesis	Proximal femur	29	55.0	10.3	13.8	10.3	13.8	3.4	3.4	3.4
	Total femur	26	9.6	0.0	0.0	4.8	4.8	0.0	0.0	3.8
	Distal femur	244	29.2	1.6	13.2	2.5	8.6	1.2	2.1	3.6
	Proximal tibia	72	33.4	1.4	8.3	0.0	18.1	4.2	1.4	10.5
Allograft	Proximal femur	1	0.0	0.0	—	0.0	0.0	0.0	—	0.0
	Total femur	0	—	—	—	—	—	—	—	—
	Distal femur	31	38.7	3.2	0.0	22.6	12.9	0.0	—	0.0
	Proximal tibia	70	57.1	0.0	0.0	32.9	17.1	7.1	—	8.6
APC	Proximal femur	14	28.5	0.0	7.1	7.1	14.3	0.0	—	0.0
	Total femur	0	—	—	—	—	—	—	—	—
	Distal femur	5	40.0	0.0	20.0	0.0	20.0	0.0	—	0.0
	Proximal tibia	4	25.0	0.0	0.0	0.0	25.0	0.0	—	0.0

From Groundland JS, Ambler S, Houskamp D, et al. Surgical and functional outcomes after limb preservation surgery for tumor in pediatric patients: a systematic review. JBJS Reviews, in press; with permission.

tibia replacements were revised for failure. The modes of failure were primarily structural or infectious. Structural failure, including subchondral collapse and osteolysis at the host-graft junction, occurred in 22.6% of all pediatric allograft distal femur replacements and 32.9% of reported proximal tibia replacements. Attempts to reinforce the subchondral region with cement have been made, but the results have been disappointing. The high rate of structural failure was one of the driving forces for the advent of APC reconstructions.

Metallic Endoprosthesis

In their investigation, Henderson and colleagues[81] found an adult failure rate in lower extremity ME reconstructions of 27.7%. The pediatric failure rate for the same constructs has been reported as 30.5%.[41] Separated by anatomic location for the pediatric population, reconstructions of the distal femur and the proximal tibia failed 29.2% and 33.4% of the time, respectively. Proximal femur replacements had the highest failure rate in pediatric ME reconstructions, with a reported 55% failure rate, and total femurs failed the least, with a 9.6% rate. Infection and aseptic loosening were the predominant modes of failure for the pediatric ME population. The issues with aseptic loosening have been addressed with cemented stems, fluted stems, and augmented prosthesis-host compression (Compress); as with other modifications in surgical techniques, the efficacy of each has yet to be validated.

Soft tissue incompetence as a mode of failure was noted in 10.3% of proximal femur reconstructions. This finding reflects the difficulties of reconstituting a resected capsule to prevent recurrent dislocation and the difficulties of maintaining an abductor mechanism. Some surgeons have adopted the use of a synthetic graft (aortograft, Trevira tube), anchored in the acetabular rim and encircling the prosthesis. This technique ostensibly recreates the capsule and provides a potential site for tendinous attachment.[82,83]

The proximal tibia reconstructions failed only 1.4% of the time as a result of soft tissue incompetence, suggesting that incorporating the extensor mechanism in the medial gastrocnemius flap may provide a satisfactory soft tissue repair.

Allograft-Prosthesis Composite

The small number of patients described in the literature limits the ability to find trends in APC failures in the pediatric population. Of the 23 clearly reported pediatric patients who underwent APC reconstruction in the lower extremity after bone tumor excision, 7 failed (30.5%). No failures were the result of soft tissue causes or structural failures.[41] Although too limited in number to draw conclusions, this finding may reflect the underlying strength of this design: an implant that provides soft tissue attachments like an allograft with the durability of a metal endoprosthesis. However, a reliable expandable APC has yet to be described, hindering its adaption to the very young.

FUNCTIONAL OUTCOMES

Ideally, limb salvage surgery should provide the child with a limb that functions as close to normal as possible. Experience with osteoarticular reconstructions in the growing child indicates that some level of disability is common. However, the literature lacks a well-described measure that is consistently used and highly descriptive of these functional limitations.

Questionnaires

Musculoskeletal Tumor Society
The most consistently reported outcome measure is the revised MSTS questionnaire. Presented in 1993 to assess outcomes after extremity tumor surgery, the questionnaire asks patients to rate 6 domains on a 0 to 5 scale; the domains are (1) pain, (2) function, (3) emotional acceptance, (4) use of supports, (5) walking ability, and (6) gait.[86] The score is converted to a percentage, with 0% representing the worst outcome and 100% the best. By this measure, outcomes in pediatric limb salvage for tumor are consistently rated as good, with all constructs averaging around 70%, although the ranges cross the entire spectrum. This homogeneity in mean scores across anatomic sites and reconstruction types has led some investigators to question the validity of the MSTS questionnaire in regards to true functional capacity.[87] Its reliance on patient report and emotional acceptance may reflect a psychosocial phenomenon of adaptation after a major life event more than a true measure of function. Despite this limitation, the MSTS remains the most consistent outcome measure in the pediatric extremity tumor literature, and its use remains warranted because of its historical widespread use.

Pediatric Outcomes Data Collection Instrument
The Pediatric Outcomes Data Collection Instrument (PODCI)[88] is another subjective questionnaire that has been used to assess outcomes after pediatric extremity bone tumor surgery. Developed in 1998, it addresses patient and parent perceptions of body image, social acceptance, physical function, and satisfaction with

orthopedic treatment. Questions are divided into 6 domains:

1. Upper extremity and physical function
2. Transfer and basic mobility
3. Sports and physical functioning
4. Pain and comfort
5. Happiness
6. Global functioning

In a case series of 17 pediatric patients with metallic expandable lower extremity endoprostheses placed after bone tumor excision,[31] PODCI global scores ranged from 71% to 95.5%, averaging 85.8% across all anatomic sites. Sports and physical function rated the lowest, averaging 70.1%, whereas happiness averaged 89.5%. This finding may suggest, again, that function after tumor resection and subsequent reconstruction is impaired, but patients learn to accept the outcomes and come to appreciate the function they do have. As is common for such studies, interpretation must be guarded because of the retrospective nature of the data collection, the limited representation of patients from the original series (17 of 38 patients completed the surveys), and the lack of a control or comparison group. Use of the PODCI after allograft or APC reconstructions in pediatric patients with tumor has not been described in the literature.

Toronto Extremity Salvage Score

Published in 1996, the Toronto Extremity Salvage Score (TESS) was designed specifically for patients with bone and soft tissue sarcoma.[89] This questionnaire has upper and lower extremity sections, with the lower extremity section composed of 30 activity-related questions, such as ability to put on shoes, shower, garden, drive, kneel, and participate in sports. TESS scores have been reported in the pediatric limb salvage literature, but with insufficient frequency to allow comparisons between surgical constructs or anatomic sites. Future use of this more comprehensive questionnaire, especially in an anatomic-specific and reconstruction-specific manner, may provide insight into patients' tolerance for activities of daily living after limb salvage.

Gait Characteristics

Several studies have investigated gait characteristics after limb salvage in the pediatric population. The difficulty in interpreting the results lies in the frequent overinclusion of adult patients with their pediatric counterparts. Clinical experience informs us that some patients excel postoperatively, without gait deviation and return to sport; others

persistently struggle, needing assistive devices and limiting their participation in recreational activities and sport. As it currently stands, the literature is unable to clearly relate what percentage of skeletally immature patients regain function or how complete that functional return may be.

Bekkering and colleagues[90] published one of the more comprehensive activity tolerance investigations. In this multicenter study, patients receiving an ablative surgery were compared with limb salvage patients in functional abilities, as measured subjectively by the TESS and objectively by timed up-and-go tests, timed stair negotiation, and a 6-minute walk. The patients were also observed over 7 days with an activity monitor, measuring peak amplitude and duration of gait at home. Surgical interventions included allograft reconstruction, ME reconstruction, above-knee amputation, and rotationplasty. The 2 limb salvage groups scored better in the timed up-and-go test and the stair negotiation test, but no differences were found between groups in TESS scores, 6-minute walk tests, or home ambulation levels. Although a thorough and admirable study, generalization to the growing child is limited because of incomplete reporting of age and anatomic location. Age was presented only as averages with standard deviations for the 4 groups of 14.5, 16.2, 14.0, and 12.0 years of age for allograft, prosthesis, amputation, and rotationplasty, respectively; the anatomic site was noted to be tumors about the knee, not specifying between distal femur or proximal tibia.

In the future, objective measures of range of motion, strength, gait velocity, and volume should be measured in an age-specific and reconstruction-specific manner, so that true comparisons can be made. These data may lead to improved understanding of the true limitations of the various reconstructions, allowing more specific implant selection as well as aiding in the development of new reconstruction techniques.

SUMMARY

Limb salvage in the growing child with an extremity bone tumor has gained increasing acceptance in the last 40 years since the advent of adjuvant therapies. The state of the literature, reflective of current practice, shows a multitude of reconstructive options, from MEs to allografts and APCs. However, no 1 option has a clear superiority, with the possible exception of the capacity of the metallic expandable prosthesis to treat the very young.

Despite the increasing acceptance of pediatric limb salvage, many shortcomings persist. Failure rates remain high, albeit comparable with their adult counterparts, and postoperative function is generally poorly defined. Studies should report limb salvage outcomes in an age-specific, reconstruction-specific, and anatomic site–specific manner. Objective measures for function are needed as well, such as motion, strength, and gait capacity.

REFERENCES

1. Sweetnam R. Tumours of bone and their management. Ann R Coll Surg Engl 1974;54(2):63–71.
2. Sweetnam R. Osteosarcoma. Ann R Coll Surg Engl 1969;44(1):38–58.
3. Campanacci M, Bacci G, Bertoni F, et al. The treatment of osteosarcoma of the extremities: twenty year's experience at the Istituto Ortopedico Rizzoli. Cancer 1981;48(7):1569–81.
4. McKenna RJ, Schwinn CP, Higinbotham NL. Osteogenic sarcoma in children. Calif Med 1965; 103:165–70.
5. Price CH, Zhuber K, Salzer-Kuntschik M, et al. Osteosarcoma in children. A study of 125 cases. J Bone Joint Surg Br 1975;57(3):341–5.
6. Jaffe N. The potential for an improved prognosis with chemotherapy in osteogenic sarcoma. Clin Orthop Relat Res 1975;(113):111–8.
7. Pomeroy TC, Johnson RE. Combined modality therapy of Ewing's sarcoma. Cancer 1975;35(1):36–47.
8. Sinks LF, Mindell ER. Chemotherapy of osteosarcoma. Clin Orthop Relat Res 1975;(111):101–4.
9. Cohen IJ, Kaplinsky C, Katz K, et al. Improved results in osteogenic sarcoma 1973-79 vs. 1980-86: analysis of results from a single center. Isr J Med Sci 1993;29(1):27–9.
10. Eilber FR, Mirra JJ, Grant TT, et al. Is amputation necessary for sarcomas? A seven-year experience with limb salvage. Ann Surg 1980;192(4):431–8.
11. Mankin HJ, Hornicek FJ, Rosenberg AE, et al. Survival data for 648 patients with osteosarcoma treated at one institution. Clin Orthop Relat Res 2004;(429):286–91.
12. Rosen G, Caparros B, Nirenberg A, et al. Ewing's sarcoma: ten-year experience with adjuvant chemotherapy. Cancer 1981;47(9):2204–13.
13. van Oosterom AT, Voute PA, Taminiau AH, et al. Combination chemotherapy preceding surgery in osteogenic sarcoma. Prog Clin Biol Res 1985;201: 53–7.
14. Copeland MM, Sutow WW. Osteogenic sarcoma: the past, present, and future. Int Adv Surg Oncol 1979; 2:177–200.
15. Simon MA, Aschliman MA, Thomas N, et al. Limb-salvage treatment versus amputation for osteosarcoma of the distal end of the femur. J Bone Joint Surg Am 1986;68(9):1331–7.
16. Aboulafia AJ, Malawer MM. Surgical management of pelvic and extremity osteosarcoma. Cancer 1993; 71(10 Suppl):3358–66.
17. Bielack SS, Kempf-Bielack B, Delling G, et al. Prognostic factors in high-grade osteosarcoma of the extremities or trunk: an analysis of 1,702 patients treated on neoadjuvant cooperative osteosarcoma study group protocols. J Clin Oncol 2002;20(3): 776–90.
18. Mei J, Zhu XZ, Wang ZY, et al. Functional outcomes and quality of life in patients with osteosarcoma treated with amputation versus limb-salvage surgery: a systematic review and meta-analysis. Arch Orthop Trauma Surg 2014;134(11):1507–16.
19. Rougraff BT, Simon MA, Kneisl JS, et al. Limb salvage compared with amputation for osteosarcoma of the distal end of the femur. A long-term oncological, functional, and quality-of-life study. J Bone Joint Surg Am 1994;76(5):649–56.
20. Aboulafia AJ, Wilkerson J. Lower-limb preservation with an expandable endoprosthesis after tumor resection in children: is the cup half full or half empty? Commentary on an article by Eric R. Henderson, MD, et al.: "Outcome of lower-limb preservation with an expandable endoprosthesis after bone tumor resection in children". J Bone Joint Surg Am 2012;94(6):e39.
21. Nachman JB. Controversies in the treatment of osteosarcoma. Med J Aust 1988;148(8):405–10.
22. Stokke J, Sung L, Gupta A, et al. Systematic review and meta-analysis of objective and subjective quality of life among pediatric, adolescent, and young adult bone tumor survivors. Pediatr Blood Cancer 2015;62(9):1616–29.
23. Unwin PS, Cobb JP, Walker PS. Distal femoral arthroplasty using custom-made prostheses. The first 218 cases. J Arthroplasty 1993;8(3):259–68.
24. DiCaprio MR, Friedlaender GE. Malignant bone tumors: limb sparing versus amputation. J Am Acad Orthop Surg 2003;11(1):25–37.
25. Beebe K, Song KJ, Ross E, et al. Functional outcomes after limb-salvage surgery and endoprosthetic reconstruction with an expandable prosthesis: a report of 4 cases. Arch Phys Med Rehabil 2009;90(6):1039–47.
26. Bryant PR, Pandian G. Acquired limb deficiencies. 1. Acquired limb deficiencies in children and young adults. Arch Phys Med Rehabil 2001;82(3 Suppl 1): S3–8.
27. Eckardt JJ, Kabo JM, Kelley CM, et al. Expandable endoprosthesis reconstruction in skeletally immature patients with tumors. Clin Orthop Relat Res 2000;(373):51–61.
28. Eckardt JJ, Safran MR, Eilber FR, et al. Expandable endoprosthetic reconstruction of the skeletally immature after malignant bone tumor resection. Clin Orthop Relat Res 1993;(297):188–202.

29. Finn HA, Simon MA. Limb-salvage surgery in the treatment of osteosarcoma in skeletally immature individuals. Clin Orthop Relat Res 1991;(262):108–18.

30. Grimer RJ. Surgical options for children with osteosarcoma. Lancet Oncol 2005;6(2):85–92.

31. Henderson ER, Pepper AM, Marulanda G, et al. Outcome of lower-limb preservation with an expandable endoprosthesis after bone tumor resection in children. J Bone Joint Surg Am 2012;94(6):537–47.

32. Kenan S, Lewis MM. Limb salvage in pediatric surgery. The use of the expandable prosthesis. Orthop Clin North Am 1991;22(1):121–31.

33. Lindell EB, Carroll NC. Limb salvage tumor surgery in children. Iowa Orthop J 1993;13:124–35.

34. Nagarajan R, Neglia JP, Clohisy DR, et al. Limb salvage and amputation in survivors of pediatric lower-extremity bone tumors: what are the long-term implications? J Clin Oncol 2002;20(22): 4493–501.

35. Neel MD, Wilkins RM, Rao BN, et al. Early multicenter experience with a noninvasive expandable prosthesis. Clin Orthop Relat Res 2003;(415): 72–81.

36. Nystrom LM, Morcuende JA. Expanding endoprosthesis for pediatric musculoskeletal malignancy: current concepts and results. Iowa Orthop J 2010;30: 141–9.

37. Renard AJ, Veth RP, Schreuder HW, et al. Function and complications after ablative and limb-salvage therapy in lower extremity sarcoma of bone. J Surg Oncol 2000;73(4):198–205.

38. Ruggieri P, Mavrogenis AF, Pala E, et al. Outcome of expandable prostheses in children. J Pediatr Orthop 2013;33(3):244–53.

39. Tan PX, Yong BC, Wang J, et al. Analysis of the efficacy and prognosis of limb-salvage surgery for osteosarcoma around the knee. Eur J Surg Oncol 2012;38(12):1171–7.

40. Temple HT, Kuklo TR, Lehman RA Jr, et al. Segmental limb reconstruction after tumor resection. Am J Orthop (Belle Mead NJ) 2000;29(7):524–9.

41. Groundland JS, Ambler S, Houskamp D, et al. Surgical and functional outcomes after limb preservation surgery for tumor in pediatric patients: a systematic review. JBJS Reviews, in press.

42. Mercuri M, Capanna R, Manfrini M, et al. The management of malignant bone tumors in children and adolescents. Clin Orthop Relat Res 1991;(264): 156–68.

43. Schrager J, Patzer RE, Mink PJ, et al. Survival outcomes of pediatric osteosarcoma and Ewing's sarcoma: a comparison of surgery type within the SEER database, 1988-2007. J Registry Manag 2011;38(3):153–61.

44. Worch J, Matthay KK, Neuhaus J, et al. Osteosarcoma in children 5 years of age or younger at initial diagnosis. Pediatr Blood Cancer 2010;55(2):285–9.

45. Fuchs B, Sim FH. Rotationplasty about the knee: surgical technique and anatomical considerations. Clin Anat 2004;17(4):345–53.

46. Kostuik JP, Gillespie R, Hall JE, et al. Van Nes rotational osteotomy for treatment of proximal femoral focal deficiency and congenital short femur. J Bone Joint Surg Am 1975;57(8):1039–46.

47. Kritter AE. Tibial rotation-plasty for proximal femoral focal deficiency. J Bone Joint Surg Am 1977;59(7): 927–34.

48. Bhamra JS, Abdul-Jabar HB, McKenna D, et al. Van Nes rotationplasty as a treatment method for Ewing's sarcoma in a 14-month-old. Int J Surg Case Rep 2013;4(10):893–7.

49. Sawamura C, Hornicek FJ, Gebhardt MC. Complications and risk factors for failure of rotationplasty: review of 25 patients. Clin Orthop Relat Res 2008; 466(6):1302–8.

50. Veenstra KM, Sprangers MA, van der Eyken JW, et al. Quality of life in survivors with a Van Ness-Borggreve rotationplasty after bone tumour resection. J Surg Oncol 2000;73(4):192–7.

51. Forni C, Gaudenzi N, Zoli M, et al. Living with rotationplasty–quality of life in rotationplasty patients from childhood to adulthood. J Surg Oncol 2012; 105(4):331–6.

52. Hillmann A, Hoffmann C, Gosheger G, et al. Malignant tumor of the distal part of the femur or the proximal part of the tibia: endoprosthetic replacement or rotationplasty. Functional outcome and quality-of-life measurements. J Bone Joint Surg Am 1999;81(4): 462–8.

53. Buchman J. Total femur and knee joint replacement with a Vitallium endoprosthesis. Bull Hosp Joint Dis 1965;26:21–34.

54. Hwang JS, Mehta AD, Yoon RS, et al. From amputation to limb salvage reconstruction: evolution and role of the endoprosthesis in musculoskeletal oncology. J Orthop Trauma 2014;15(2):81–6.

55. Salzer M, Knahr K, Locke H, et al. A bioceramic endoprosthesis for the replacement of the proximal humerus. Arch Orthop Trauma Surg 1979;93(3): 169–84.

56. Burrows HJ, Wilson JN, Scales JT. Excision of tumours of humerus and femur, with restoration by internal prostheses. J Bone Joint Surg Br 1975;57(2): 148–59.

57. Tebbi CK, Gaeta J. Osteosarcoma. Pediatr Ann 1988;17(4):285–300.

58. Scales JT. Bone and joint replacement for the preservation of limbs. Br J Hosp Med 1983;30(4): 220–32.

59. Bar-On E, Beckwith JB, Odom LF, et al. Effect of chemotherapy on human growth plate. J Pediatr Orthop 1993;13(2):220–4.

60. Eifel PJ, Donaldson SS, Thomas PR. Response of growing bone to irradiation: a proposed late effects

scoring system. Int J Radiat Oncol Biol Phys 1995; 31(5):1301–7.

61. Fan C, Foster BK, Wallace WH, et al. Pathobiology and prevention of cancer chemotherapy-induced bone growth arrest, bone loss, and osteonecrosis. Curr Mol Med 2011;11(2):140–51.

62. Belthur MV, Grimer RJ, Suneja R, et al. Extensible endoprostheses for bone tumors of the proximal femur in children. J Pediatr Orthop 2003;23(2):230–5.

63. Schindler OS, Cannon SR, Briggs TW, et al. Use of extendable total femoral replacements in children with malignant bone tumors. Clin Orthop Relat Res 1998;(357):157–70.

64. Lozano-Calderon SA, Kenan S. Total condylar unipolar expandable prosthesis for proximal tibia malignant bone tumors in early childhood. Orthopedics 2011;34(12):e899–905.

65. Henderson ER, Gao J, Groundland J, et al. Expandable total humeral replacement in a child with osteosarcoma. Case Rep Orthop 2015;2015:690159.

66. Unwin PS, Walker PS. Extendible endoprostheses for the skeletally immature. Clin Orthop Relat Res 1996;(322):179–93.

67. Schindler OS, Cannon SR, Briggs TW, et al. Stanmore custom-made extendible distal femoral replacements. Clinical experience in children with primary malignant bone tumours. J Bone Joint Surg Br 1997;79(6):927–37.

68. Gupta A, Meswania J, Pollock R, et al. Non-invasive distal femoral expandable endoprosthesis for limb-salvage surgery in paediatric tumours. J Bone Joint Surg Br 2006;88(5):649–54.

69. Wilkins RM, Soubeiran A. The Phenix expandable prosthesis: early American experience. Clin Orthop Relat Res 2001;(382):51–8.

70. Cipriano CA, Gruzinova IS, Frank RM, et al. Frequent complications and severe bone loss associated with the Repiphysis expandable distal femoral prosthesis. Clin Orthop Relat Res 2015;473(3):831–8.

71. Gitelis S, Neel MD, Wilkins RM, et al. The use of a closed expandable prosthesis for pediatric sarcomas. Chir Organi Mov 2003;88(4):327–33.

72. Staals EL, Colangeli M, Ali N, et al. Are complications associated with the Repiphysis expandable distal femoral prosthesis acceptable for its continued use? Clin Orthop Relat Res 2015;473(9):3003–13.

73. Webber NP, Seidel M. Combining advanced technologies: the Compress-Repiphysis prosthesis for pediatric limb salvage. Orthopedics 2010;33(11):823.

74. Aponte-Tinao LA, Ayerza MA, Muscolo DL, et al. What are the risk factors and management options for infection after reconstruction with massive bone allografts? Clin Orthop Relat Res 2015. [Epub ahead of print].

75. Campanacci L, Manfrini M, Colangeli M, et al. Long-term results in children with massive bone osteoarticular allografts of the knee for high-grade osteosarcoma. J Pediatr Orthop 2010;30(8):919–27.

76. Muscolo DL, Ayerza MA, Farfalli G, et al. Proximal tibia osteoarticular allografts in tumor limb salvage surgery. Clin Orthop Relat Res 2010;468(5):1396–404.

77. Ramseier LE, Malinin TI, Temple HT, et al. Allograft reconstruction for bone sarcoma of the tibia in the growing child. J Bone Joint Surg Br 2006;88(1):95–9.

78. Jeon DG, Kim MS, Cho WH, et al. Pasteurized autograft-prosthesis composite for distal femoral osteosarcoma. J Orthop Sci 2007;12(6):542–9.

79. Kim JD, Lee GW, Chung SH. A reconstruction with extracorporeal irradiated autograft in osteosarcoma around the knee. J Surg Oncol 2011;104(2):187–91.

80. Muramatsu K, Ihara K, Hashimoto T, et al. Combined use of free vascularised bone graft and extracorporeally-irradiated autograft for the reconstruction of massive bone defects after resection of malignant tumour. J Plast Reconstr Aesthet Surg 2007;60(9):1013–8.

81. Henderson ER, Groundland JS, Pala E, et al. Failure mode classification for tumor endoprostheses: retrospective review of five institutions and a literature review. J Bone Joint Surg Am 2011;93(5):418–29.

82. Gosheger G, Gebert C, Ahrens H, et al. Endoprosthetic reconstruction in 250 patients with sarcoma. Clin Orthop Relat Res 2006;450:164–71.

83. Henderson ER, Jennings JM, Marulanda GA, et al. Enhancing soft tissue ingrowth in proximal femoral arthroplasty with aortograft sleeve: a novel technique and early results. J arthroplasty 2011;26(1):161–3.

84. Henderson ER, O'Connor MI, Ruggieri P, et al. Classification of failure of limb salvage after reconstructive surgery for bone tumours: a modified system including biological and expandable reconstructions. Bone Joint J 2014;96-B(11):1436–40.

85. Manoso MW, Boland PJ, Healey JH, et al. Limb salvage of infected knee reconstructions for cancer with staged revision and free tissue transfer. Ann Plast Surg 2006;56(5):532–5 [discussion: 535].

86. Enneking WF, Dunham W, Gebhardt MC, et al. A system for the functional evaluation of reconstructive procedures after surgical treatment of tumors of the musculoskeletal system. Clin Orthop Relat Res 1993;(286):241–6.

87. Lee SH, Kim DJ, Oh JH, et al. Validation of a functional evaluation system in patients with musculoskeletal tumors. Clin Orthop Relat Res 2003;(411):217–26.

88. Daltroy LH, Liang MH, Fossel AH, et al. The POSNA pediatric musculoskeletal functional health questionnaire: report on reliability, validity, and sensitivity to change. Pediatric Outcomes Instrument Development Group. Pediatric Orthopaedic

Society of North America. J Pediatr Orthop 1998; 18(5):561–71.

89. Davis AM, Wright JG, Williams JI, et al. Development of a measure of physical function for patients with bone and soft tissue sarcoma. Qual Life Res 1996;5(5):508–16.

90. Bekkering WP, Vliet Vlieland TP, Koopman HM, et al. Functional ability and physical activity in children and young adults after limb-salvage or ablative surgery for lower extremity bone tumors. J Surg Oncol 2011;103(3):276–82.

Update on Survival in Osteosarcoma

Megan E. Anderson, MD[a,b]

KEYWORDS

- Osteosarcoma • Survival • Prognosis • Limb salvage surgery • Systemic chemotherapy
- Late effects

KEY POINTS

- The development of effective chemotherapy for osteosarcoma in the 1980s led to a drastic improvement in survival. This, along with advances in imaging modalities, allowed safe and effective limb salvage surgery to evolve.
- Survival has reached a plateau since the 1990s, while progress in limb salvage surgery continues to be made.
- Following patients for late effects of chemotherapy and surgery for osteosarcoma is critical now that most patients are long-term survivors.
- Future efforts are needed to identify effective systemic therapy and local surgery and reconstruction for patients with osteosarcoma.

INTRODUCTION

Survival in osteosarcoma is a story of success on many fronts. What was once a disease that was rarely curable even with ablative surgery now has a 5-year overall survival approaching 70% to 80%.[1,2] This is uncommon in orphan diseases, and is a result of collaboration among pediatric oncologists, orthopedic oncology surgeons, biologists, their associated teams, and most importantly the children and parents who were willing to participate in clinical trials and forays into limb salvage surgery. Although the improvement in survival in osteosarcoma has been astounding on some levels, it can be deemed only a partial success, as few gains have been made in recent decades.[3,4] This article is a review of survival in osteosarcoma with a focus on background information, advances in chemotherapy and limb salvage surgery, late effects in survivors, and future directions.

HISTORY AND BACKGROUND

Osteosarcoma is a primary malignant tumor that arises in bone, in which the malignant cells produce osteoid (**Fig. 1**). There are many subtypes, but the most common and the focus of this article is high-grade conventional osteosarcoma. It is the most common primary sarcoma of bone, but is still quite rare. Osteosarcomas represent fewer than 1% of cancers overall, with an incidence of 5 per 1,000,000 children age 19 and younger in the United States.[5] It is slightly more common in male than female patients and has a predilection for the metaphyseal regions adjacent to physes with the greatest growth: distal femur, proximal tibia, and proximal humerus.[6]

It was recognized in some of the earliest medical reporting that even if the primary tumor in osteosarcoma was treated appropriately, many children still succumbed to the disease, mostly due to pulmonary metastases.[7] It was determined that hematogenous dissemination of the disease

The author has nothing to disclose.
[a] Boston Children's Hospital, 300 Longwood Ave, Boston, MA 02115, USA; [b] Beth Israel Deaconess Medical Center, 330 Brookline Ave, Boston, MA 02215, USA
E-mail address: manders6@bidmc.harvard.edu

Orthop Clin N Am 47 (2016) 283–292
http://dx.doi.org/10.1016/j.ocl.2015.08.022
0030-5898/16/$ – see front matter © 2016 Elsevier Inc. All rights reserved.

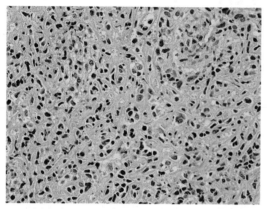

Fig. 1. Photomicrograph of osteosarcoma pathology (hematoxylin-eosin, original magnification ×200). Note the cellular pleomorphism, abnormal mitotic figures, and lacy pink osteoid material.

was to blame, and that although only 20% of patients present with gross evidence of metastatic disease (a number that has not changed over time[8]), the vast majority have micro-metastatic disease.[9] Roughly 80% of metastatic deposits involve the lung,[10] the component of this disease that represents the life-threatening behavior of this cancer.

In the 1970s, some survival successes were achieved initially with methotrexate and then multi-agent regimens, predominantly including doxorubicin, cisplatin, bleomycin, and other agents.[11] Chemotherapy was given postoperatively in these reports with improvements in survival from 20% to 40%. In the 1980s, 2 randomized trials demonstrated improvement in survival to roughly 60% with a combination of agents.[12–15] Thus, within 2 decades, survival improved from 20% to 60% to 70%, truly remarkable advancements. As patients were living longer and chemotherapy was demonstrated to be effective, orthopedic oncology surgeons recognized that there may be opportunities for limb salvage in these patients. Custom prostheses were developed, but required time for fabrication, so surgeons worked with oncologists to demonstrate outcomes were similar if surgery was performed up-front versus after several cycles of chemotherapy first.[16] Thus, the era of limb salvage began and now roughly 80% of patients with osteosarcoma are treated for their primary tumor with limb salvage surgery.[4]

PROGNOSTIC FACTORS

Many of the clinical trials and several large retrospective studies have demonstrated the importance of several factors affecting prognosis in high-grade osteosarcoma.

Metastatic Disease

The presence of metastatic disease has the most impact on prognosis. Patients who present with metastatic disease have overall survival of roughly 20% to 30% compared with 70% to 80% in nonmetastatic patients.[8] The location of the metastatic disease is important: patients with pulmonary-only disease fare better than those with bone metastases or other sites of metastases.[17] Whether the disease is resectable or not also has a large impact on prognosis.[18,19] Timing is important as well: those who present with metastatic disease later, at least 2 years after the end of initial chemotherapy, have a slightly better prognosis, roughly 40% 5-year overall survival.[20]

Chemotherapy Response

The next most important prognostic factor for survival in osteosarcoma is response to chemotherapy. Now that most patients are treated with neoadjuvant chemotherapy, then surgery followed by further adjuvant chemotherapy, there is an opportunity to examine the pathologic specimen to determine the percent necrosis in response to the therapy.[11] Patients with greater than 90% necrosis have improved overall and disease-specific survival compared with those with lower histologic response to chemotherapy.[13,21]

Tumor Characteristics

The size of the primary tumor is an important prognostic factor, and closely tied to it is the location of the tumor. Axial tumors tend to be larger at diagnosis, and thus associated with poorer overall survival than tumors in the appendicular skeleton. However, when larger studies have been able to control for size, axial location often still holds as a significantly worse factor for overall and disease-specific survival.[4,8,22,23]

Histologic subtype can affect prognosis as well. It is linked to chemotherapy response for some subtypes but not all. Fibroblastic and telangiectatic subtypes are associated with higher rates of good response to chemotherapy (>90% necrosis) and in turn better 5-year overall survival compared with osteoblastic and chondroblastic subtypes. However, although better overall survival is associated with good histologic responses in most subtypes, that is not the case for chondroblastic osteosarcomas, in which survival in poor responders is not statistically different from good responders.[24,25]

Patient Characteristics

Age of the patient affects prognosis as well. Older patients tend to have worse outcomes compared with younger patients.[26] This may be in part associated with older patients' inability to tolerate the chemotherapy, but also may be related to the higher number of secondary osteosarcomas and axial location in adult populations compared with children.[27] Osteosarcomas that arise in a preexisting lesions, especially as in Paget disease, are associated with poorer prognoses.[28,29]

CHEMOTHERAPY
Nonmetastatic

The determination of which chemotherapeutic agents to use for patients with osteosarcoma was largely empiric, based on some agents' success in other tumor types. Collaboration across centers and countries has demonstrated the effectiveness of current regimens, although there is no consensus on which medications and what dosing should be used. Most protocols today involve doxorubicin, cisplatin, and high-dose methotrexate, termed MAP (Methotrexate, doxorubicin/Adriamycin, cisPlatin).[30] High-dose methotrexate may not be as effective for adult patients and is associated with greater toxicity in adults,[31,32] so although the 3-drug regimen with MAP is considered standard in most countries for children and young adults, those older than 40 are most commonly treated with doxorubicin and cisplatin only. Controversy exists regarding the addition of ifosfamide alone or in combination with etoposide,[3,30,33] and investigations regarding these agents are ongoing.

It is important to keep in mind that these medications are associated with significant toxicity.[30] Alopecia, mucositis, and nausea and vomiting are not life-threatening, but myelosuppression and doxorubicin-related cardiac failure can be. Renal dysfunction also can be severe in some cases due to both the cisplatin and high-dose methotrexate. With the knowledge that probably 10% to 20% of patients with localized disease could be cured with surgery only and not exposed to these toxic effects of chemotherapy, it would be extremely helpful to determine which osteosarcomas have little metastatic potential and thus be able to stratify treatment. To date, there have been no markers to allow such stratification among high-grade osteosarcomas.

Poor Response

Patients who have less than 90% necrosis in response to preoperative chemotherapy and those with disease progression on chemotherapy have a worse prognosis.[34] Attempts have been made in several trials to "salvage" these patients by adding other agents or changing protocols

entirely with postoperative chemotherapy, the vast majority without any improvement in survival.[3] This is the subject of the recent EURAMOS (European and American Osteosarcoma Study Group)-1 Intergroup collaboration: patients with poor histologic responses were randomized to continuing MAP or MAP with ifosfamide and etoposide.[35] The results of this component of the trial have not been published yet.

Metastatic

Patients with metastatic disease at presentation have a worse prognosis as noted previously. When treated with 3-drug or 4-drug regimens, there are fewer good responders compared with patients presenting without metastases.[34] This lack of response to standard chemotherapy indicates the need to identify other effective medications. Most investigations into new agents involve patients with metastatic disease. For patients not on trials, a standard approach would involve MAP or MAP with ifosfamide ± etoposide along with surgical resection of the primary tumor and all metastatic sites if feasible. If any of the disease is not resectable, the prognosis is grim. Palliative approaches involve systemic therapy along with limited surgery, radiation, and/or percutaneous ablative procedures.[36]

Relapsed

Patients who relapse either at the local site or with distant metastases after an initial disease-free interval have an intermediate survival approaching 30% to 40%.[37,38] As noted previously, timing of the relapse is an important prognostic factor. The longer the disease-free interval, the better the survival. The volume of disease relapse and whether all sites are resectable also greatly affect survival. Treatment approaches thus vary and are individualized based on where the site of relapse is located, whether surgical resection is possible, and what chemotherapy was used previously and how long before the development of the relapse (**Fig. 2**). Most centers will treat patients with relapse with surgery and systemic therapy in some fashion, although patients with a solitary pulmonary relapse that develops over a year off therapy may be treated with surgery alone.[39]

SURGERY

As survival in osteosarcoma has plateaued, the numbers of patients having limb salvage surgery continues to grow.[4] The quality and nature of surgical resection for osteosarcoma has a great

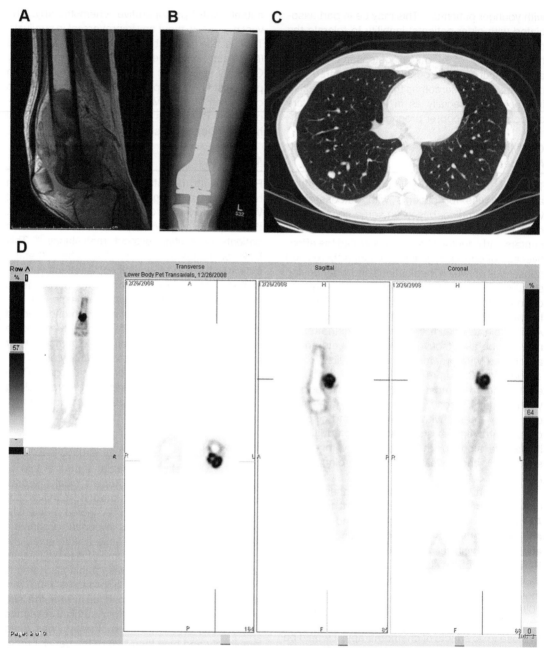

Fig. 2. Nineteen-year-old male patient who presented with localized osteosarcoma of the right distal femur (*A*: sagittal MRI, proton density sequence). He was treated with extra-articular resection of his primary tumor and reconstruction with a megaprosthesis (*B*). His first relapse was a solitary pulmonary nodule (*C*: chest CT), which developed 9 months off therapy and was treated with surgery and inhaled granulocyte-macrophage colony-stimulating factor as part of a research protocol. His second relapse was a local recurrence (*D*: PET imaging of soft tissue recurrence posterior to prosthesis), which developed 3 years later and was treated with above-knee amputation. He has been disease free for 6 years.

impact on survival. Although there are myriad approaches to resection and reconstruction of a bone affected by osteosarcoma, some important requirements hold true for all.

Margins

The goal of surgical resection for osteosarcoma is to achieve a wide margin, as defined by Enneking and colleagues.[40] Over time, the definition of what constitutes a wide margin has changed and cannot be given as an absolute distance. It depends on the nature of the marginal tissue; for example, a wider margin of fat would be necessary compared with fascia due to the quality of the tissue and ability of the tumor to invade such tissue. It can depend on perceived response to chemotherapy; for example, amputation or rotationplasty may be recommended over limb salvage for a patient with disease progression on neoadjuvant chemotherapy (**Fig. 3**). It also depends on the location of the tumor within the bone; for example, tumors that are localized to only a portion of the bone may be resected in an intercalary fashion, thus preserving an articular surface and/or more normal bone in an effort to improve function postoperatively (**Fig. 4**).

Technological advances have made this possible. Advances in MRI in particular have allowed surgeons to clearly identify the margins of marrow involvement and soft tissue extent in osteosarcoma so that all disease can be resected en bloc with more and more focus on preserving as much normal tissue as possible.[41] Newer developments in PET[42] and diffusion-weighted MRI[43] show some promise in predicting response to therapy, but are not in routine use and require further investigation. Intraoperative navigation can be extremely helpful in completing complex bone resections as intended, especially in areas with challenging anatomy, such as the pelvis.[44,45]

Local Recurrence

It should be stressed that none of the technological advancements or preservation of bone and soft tissues should in any way compromise the oncologic goals of surgery. What has come to be accepted in limb salvage surgery is a higher rate of local recurrence compared with amputation (roughly 7%–10% in most studies),[4] without risking overall survival. Close margins are associated with higher rates of local recurrence, but not independently with overall survival from what we can glean from the scientific literature on the topic. What is still unknown and remains controversial is whether local recurrence independently affects overall survival, separately from chemotherapy response.[46,47] There has been conflicting evidence reported in the literature, and this should be an integral part of any outcome investigation of limb salvage surgery.

Pathologic Fracture

Many of the earlier studies on osteosarcoma in the era of chemotherapy and limb salvage reported that pathologic fracture was associated with a poor prognosis and limb salvage should not be attempted in these patients.[48–50] There has recently been more retrospective investigation into this topic that has altered the thinking.[51,52] Most groups now have found that although patients who suffer pathologic fractures may have a worse overall prognosis, likely due to biologic characteristics of the tumor, but, as long as good quality surgical resection is performed with negative margins, limb salvage is not clearly associated with higher risk of poor overall survival compared with amputation. Further investigation in ongoing and may require multicenter collaboration.

Metastasectomy

As discussed previously, if patients present with or develop metastatic disease, prognosis for survival is poor, but improved if all the sites of disease can be resected. Metastasectomy, and in particular, resection of isolated and low-volume pulmonary disease, can be curative in some patients and is thus recommended in most cases.[19,53] Resection of bone metastases may be indicated in some patients as well, depending on the volume and location of the disease, other concomitant metastatic lesions, pace of disease progression, and timing from initial treatment. Although the prognosis is worse for this patient population compared with patients with pulmonary-only metastases, resection of such disease can rarely provide a chance for long-term survival in carefully selected patients.[19,53] Patients with metastases in other locations have a dismal prognosis, and overall care and treatment recommendations must be on a case-by-case basis.[17]

LATE EFFECTS OF THERAPY

Now that roughly two-thirds of patients presenting with nonmetastatic osteosarcoma will be long-term survivors of their disease, it has become apparent that they are at risk for certain late effects of treatment due to the chemotherapy and surgery.

Systemic Therapy

Toxicity
Late toxicity may develop from each of the standard agents used to treat osteosarcoma.[54] These are summarized in **Table 1**. Patients with osteosarcoma thus should ideally be followed for life for these late effects.

Secondary malignant neoplasms
Patients who have had osteosarcoma have a higher risk of developing another malignancy, either as a result of late effects of treatment or due to preexisting genetic predisposition syndromes or both.

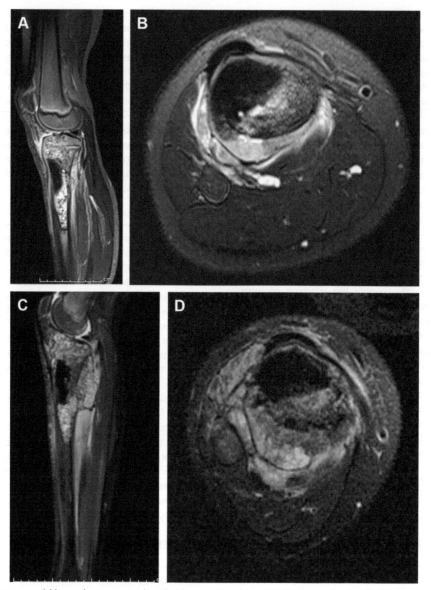

Fig. 3. Eleven-year-old boy who presented with a large osteosarcoma of the proximal tibia (*A*: sagittal MRI, short tau inversion recovery sequence; *B*: axial MRI, T2 with fat-saturation sequence). The tumor was larger in all dimensions after 2 cycles of MAP chemotherapy (*C*: sagittal MRI, short tau inversion recovery sequence; *D*: axial MRI, T2 with fat-saturation sequence), and so he and his parents decided on rotationplasty for local control surgery.

Two recent reviews of population-based cancer databases in the United States[55] and Britain[56] demonstrated 2.7-fold and 4.0-fold increases, respectively, of developing a secondary malignant neoplasm (SMN). This risk was higher in patients treated after 1985, in whom it is assumed most received chemotherapy (4.7 times the risk in the general population) compared with those pre-1985 (1.7 times the risk of the general population). Hematologic malignancies were most common, but patients were also at higher risk of developing breast cancer, thyroid cancer, malignancies of the respiratory system, and of soft tissue. These SMNs can develop at any time after the end of treatment and so patients need to be followed indefinitely for these.

Surgery

No matter whether patients with osteosarcoma have limb salvage surgery, amputation, rotationplasty or other resection/reconstruction options, physical function is almost always affected in

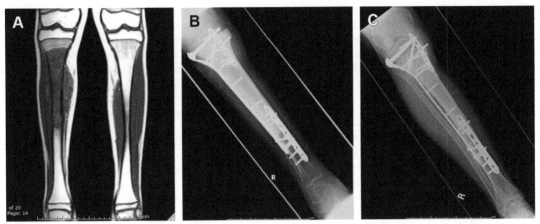

Fig. 4. Eleven-year-old boy who presented with an osteosarcoma of his tibia (*A*: coronal MRI T1 sequence). Local control surgery with negative margins was accomplished with an intercalary resection, sparing the articular surface, and allograft reconstruction (*B*). Nine years after surgery, both allograft-host junctions have healed, and there has been mild graft resorption medially (*C*).

some permanent way by the treatment of their primary tumor. Orthopedic oncology surgeons have been striving to develop accurate ways to assess function and quality of life for the reconstruction options that are available now, but these data are almost always retrospective. Prospective trials focus on systemic therapy and overall survival, which must be top priority in osteosarcoma research until survival takes another leap forward. However, collaboration among centers is improving[57] and so focus on function and quality of life outcomes research will improve.

FUTURE DIRECTIONS
Chemotherapy

There have been almost no promising developments in chemotherapy since the 1980s, and as a result, survival in patients with localized disease has reached a plateau. Two recent and very thorough meta-analyses highlighted this and have brought the discussion to the forefront again.[3,4] The only new agent with any meaningful impact on survival is the immune modulator liposomal muramyl-tripeptide phosphatidyl ethanolamine (L-MTP-PE, mifamurtide), with 8% improvement in overall survival at 6 years.[58] There was a second report from this same trial with some different findings from the first and in the end, the US Food and Drug Administration issued a "not approvable" letter for use of mifamurtide. It is available in Europe and other countries and more data may become available as it is incorporated into clinical trials outside of the United States.

Current efforts in translational biology in osteosarcoma are focused on identifying pathways in normal bone development that can be modulated, specific markers on osteosarcoma cells that would allow for targeted therapy, natural immune

Table 1
Toxicity and late effects of chemotherapy in osteosarcoma

Agent	Toxicity	Incidence %	Timing
Doxorubicin	Cardiac: congestive heart failure	0–4	Lifetime
	Echocardiographic abnormalities	Unknown	Lifetime
Cisplatin	Nephrotoxicity	High	Acute; hypomagnesemia may persist
	Ototoxicity	40	Acute, permanent
High-dose methotrexate	Renal failure	1–2	Usually acute onset
	Neurotoxicity	0.4–5	Acute, transient
Ifosfamide	Neurotoxicity	1–6	Acute, transient
	Nephrotoxicity	7–9	Acute

From Janeway KA, Grier HE. Sequelae of osteosarcoma medical therapy: a review of rare acute toxicities and late effects. Lancet Oncol 2010;11:670–8; with permission.

defenses that can be boosted to target osteosarcoma cells, mechanisms for drug resistance in osteosarcoma cells that can be blocked, and ways to reduce toxicity associated with current standard chemotherapy.[59,60] Again it is collaboration that is critical to success.

Surgery

Many advances have been made in reconstruction options for patients who have had limb salvage surgery and in prosthetic design for patients who have had amputation or rotationplasty, but there is little doubt that these operated limbs have the largest single effect on patients' physical function and quality of life.[56] Current efforts in tissue engineering to construct more normally functioning bones, joints, and muscles provide hope for improvements, but are truly still in their infancy. Defining appropriate margins based on individual tumor response to neoadjuvant chemotherapy will be important, as will developing validated and useful instruments for assessing patient function and quality of life. Surgeons and oncologists will need to continue to work together to improve the quality of research on local control surgery by collecting prospective data in clinical trials going forward.

SUMMARY

Survival in osteosarcoma has improved drastically since the development of effective chemotherapy in the 1970s to 1980s, but has now reached a plateau over several decades. If further gains are to be made, further collaboration is key, and osteosarcoma has been a role model for that in the past. Our goals are to improve survival not only for patients with localized disease, but especially for those with metastatic, relapsed, and/or refractory disease in whom prognosis has remained poor; to improve the quality and function of limbs that can be preserved; and to decrease late effects of treatment in the future.

REFERENCES

1. Meyers PA, Schwartz CL, Krailo M, et al. Osteosarcoma: a randomized, prospective trial of the addition of ifosfamide and/or muramyl tripeptide to cisplatin, doxorubicin, and high-dose methotrexate. J Clin Oncol 2005;23:2004–11.
2. Ferrari S, Meazza C, Palmerini E, et al. Nonmetastatic osteosarcoma of the extremity. Neoadjuvant chemotherapy with methotrexate, cisplatin, doxorubicin and ifosfamide. An Italian Sarcoma Group study (ISG/OS-Oss). Tumori 2014;100:612–9.
3. Anninga JK, Gelderblom H, Fiocco M, et al. Chemotherapeutic adjuvant treatment for osteosarcoma: where do we stand? Eur J Cancer 2011;47:2431–45.
4. Allison DC, Carney SC, Ahlmann ER, et al. A meta-analysis of osteosarcoma outcomes in the modern medical era. Sarcoma 2012;2012:704872.
5. Available at: http://nccd.cdc.gov/USCS/childhood-cancerdetailedbyICCC.aspx. Accessed June 17, 2015.
6. Rosenberg AE, Cleton-Jansen A-M, de Pinieux G, et al. Conventional osteosarcoma. In: Fletcher CDM, Bridge JA, Hogendoorn PCW, et al, editors. WHO classification of tumours of soft tissue and bone. 4th edition. Lyon (France): IARC; 2013. p. 282.
7. Heath FA. Osteo-sarcoma of the femur and lung. Br Med J 1877;2(887):921.
8. Duchman KR, Gao Y, Miller BJ. Prognostic factors for survival in patients with high-grade osteosarcoma using the Surveillance, Epidemiology, and End Results (SEER) Program database. Cancer Epidemiol 2015;39(4):593–9.
9. Bruland OS, Høifødt H, Saeter G, et al. Hematogenous micrometastases in osteosarcoma patients. Clin Cancer Res 2005;11:4666–73.
10. Kager L, Zoubek A, Potschger U, et al. Primary metastatic osteosarcoma: presentation and outcome of patients treated on neoadjuvant Cooperative Osteosarcoma Study Group protocols. J Clin Oncol 2003; 21:2011–8.
11. Rosen G, Marcove RC, Huvos AG. Primary osteogenic sarcoma: eight-year experience with adjuvant chemotherapy. J Cancer Res Clin Oncol 1983; 106(Suppl):55–67.
12. Eilber F, Giuliano A, Eckardt J, et al. Adjuvant chemotherapy for osteosarcoma: a randomized prospective trial. J Clin Oncol 1987;5:21–6.
13. Bernthal NM, Federman N, Eilber FR, et al. Long-term results (>25 years) of a randomized, prospective clinical trial evaluating chemotherapy in patients with high-grade, operable osteosarcoma. Cancer 2012;118:5888–93.
14. Link MP, Goorin AM, Horowitz M, et al. Adjuvant chemotherapy of high-grade osteosarcoma of the extremity. Updated results of the Multi-Institutional Osteosarcoma Study. Clin Orthop Relat Res 1991; 270:8–14.
15. Link MP, Goorin AM, Miser AW, et al. The effect of adjuvant chemotherapy on relapse-free survival in patients with osteosarcoma of the extremity. N Engl J Med 1986;314:1600–6.
16. Rosen G. Preoperative (neoadjuvant) chemotherapy for osteogenic sarcoma: a ten year experience. Orthopedics 1985;8:659–64.
17. Slade AD, Warneke CL, Hughes DP, et al. Effect of concurrent metastatic disease on survival in children and adolescents undergoing lung resection for metastatic osteosarcoma. J Pediatr Surg 2015;50:157–60.

18. Briccoli A, Rocca M, Salone M, et al. High grade osteosarcoma of the extremities metastatic to the lung: long-term results in 323 patients treated combining surgery and chemotherapy, 1985-2005. Surg Oncol 2010;19:193–9.

19. Salah S, Toubasi S. Factors predicting survival following complete surgical remission of pulmonary metastases in osteosarcoma. Mol Clin Oncol 2015; 3:157–62.

20. Gelderblom H, Jinks RC, Sydes M, et al. Survival after recurrent osteosarcoma: data from 3 European Osteosarcoma Intergroup (EOI) randomized controlled trials. Eur J Cancer 2011;47:895–902.

21. Bielack S, Jurgens H, Jundt G, et al. Osteosarcoma: the COSS experience. Cancer Treat Res 2009;152: 289–308.

22. Berner K, Hall KS, Monge OR, et al. Prognostic factors and treatment results of high-grade osteosarcoma in Norway: a scope beyond the "classical" patient. Sarcoma 2015;2015:516843.

23. Bacci G, Bertoni F, Longhi A, et al. Neoadjuvant chemotherapy for high-grade central osteosarcoma of the extremity. Histologic response to preoperative chemotherapy correlates with histologic subtype of the tumor. Cancer 2003;97:3068–75.

24. Hauben EI, Weeden S, Pringle J, et al. Does the histologic subtype of high-grade central osteosarcoma influence the response to treatment with chemotherapy and does it affect overall survival? A study on 570 patients of two consecutive trials of the European Osteosarcoma Intergroup. Eur J Cancer 2002; 38:1218–25.

25. Song WS, Kong CB, Jeon DG, et al. Prognosis of extremity osteosarcoma in patients aged 40-60 years: a cohort/case controlled study at a single institute. Eur J Surg Oncol 2010;36:483–8.

26. Longhi A, Errani C, Gonzales-Arabio D, et al. Osteosarcoma in patients older than 65 years. J Clin Oncol 2008;26:5368–73.

27. Harting MT, Lally KP, Andrassy RJ, et al. Age as a prognostic factor for patients with osteosarcoma: an analysis of 438 patients. J Cancer Res Clin Oncol 2010;136:561–70.

28. Shaylor PJ, Peake D, Grimer RJ, et al. Paget's osteosarcoma—no cure in sight. Sarcoma 1999;3:191–2.

29. Mankin HJ, Hornicek FJ. Paget's sarcoma: a historical and outcome review. Clin Orthop Relat Res 2005;438:97–102.

30. Luetke A, Meyers PA, Lewis I, et al. Osteosarcoma treatment–Where do we stand? A state of the art review. Cancer Treat Rev 2014;40:523–32.

31. Benjamin RS, Patel SR. Pediatric and adult osteosarcoma: comparisons and contrasts in presentation and therapy. Cancer Treat Rev 2009;152:355–63.

32. Collins M, Wilhelm M, Conyers R, et al. Benefits and adverse events in younger versus older patients receiving neoadjuvant chemotherapy for osteosarcoma: findings from a meta-analysis. J Clin Oncol 2013;31:2303–12.

33. Su W, Lai Z, Wu F, et al. Clinical efficacy of preoperative chemotherapy with or without ifosfamide in patients with osteosarcoma of the extremity: meta-analysis of randomized controlled trials. Med Oncol 2015;32:481.

34. Xiao X, Wang W, Wang Z. The role of chemotherapy for metastatic, relapsed, and refractory osteosarcoma. Pediatr Drugs 2014;16:503–12.

35. Whelan JS, Bielack SS, Marina N, et al. EURAMOS-1, an international randomized study for osteosarcoma: results from pre-randomisation treatment. Ann Oncol 2015;26:407–14.

36. Saumet L, Deschamps F, Marec-Berard P, et al. Radiofrequency ablation of metastases from osteosarcoma in patients under 25 years: the SCFE experience. Pediatr Hematol Oncol 2015;32:41–9.

37. Hawkins DS, Arndt CA. Pattern of disease recurrence and prognostic factors in patients with osteosarcoma treated with contemporary chemotherapy. Cancer 2003;98:2447–56.

38. Ferrari S, Briccoli A, Mercuri M, et al. Postrelapse survival in osteosarcoma of the extremities: prognostic factors for long-term survival. J Clin Oncol 2003;21:710–5.

39. Daw NC, Chou AJ, Jaffe N, et al. Recurrent osteosarcoma with a single pulmonary metastasis: a multi-institutional review. Br J Cancer 2015;112:278–82.

40. Enneking WF, Spanier SS, Goodman MA. A system for the surgical staging of musculoskeletal sarcoma. Clin Orthop Relat Res 1980;153:103–20.

41. Bus MP, Bramer JA, Schaap GR, et al. Hemicortical resection and inlay allograft reconstruction for primary bone tumors: a retrospective evaluation in the Netherlands and review of the literature. J Bone Joint Surg Am 2015;97:738–50.

42. Hawkins DS, Conrad EU 3rd, Butrynski JE, et al. [F-18]-flurordeoxy-D-glucose-positron emission tomography response is associated with outcome for extremity osteosarcoma in children and young adults. Cancer 2009;115:3519–25.

43. Byun BH, Kong CB, Lim I, et al. Combination of 18F-FDG PET/CT and diffusion-weighted MR imaging as a predictor of histologic response to neoadjuvant chemotherapy: preliminary results in osteosarcoma. J Nucl Med 2013;54:1053–9.

44. Li J, Wang Z, Guo Z, et al. Precise resection and biological reconstruction under navigation guidance for young patients with juxta-articular bone sarcoma in lower extremity: preliminary report. J Pediatr Orthop 2014;34:101–8.

45. Jeys L, Matharu GS, Nandra RS, et al. Can computer-assisted surgery reduce the risk of an intralesional margin and reduce the rate of local recurrence in patients with a tumour of the pelvis or sacrum? Bone Joint J 2013;95-B:1417–24.

46. Reddy KI, Wafa H, Gaston CL, et al. Does amputation offer any survival benefit over limb salvage in osteosarcoma patients with poor chemonecrosis and close margins? Bone Joint J 2015;97-B:115–20.

47. Bertrand TE, Cruz A, Binitie O, et al. Do surgical margins affect local recurrence and survival in extremity, nonmetastatic, high-grade osteosarcoma? Clin Orthop Relat Res 2015. [Epub ahead of print].

48. Abudu A, Sferopoulous NK, Tillman RM, et al. The surgical treatment and outcome of pathological fractures in localised osteosarcoma. J Bone Joint Surg Br 1996;78:694–8.

49. Jaffe N, Spears R, Eftekhari F, et al. Pathologic fracture in osteosarcoma. Impact of chemotherapy on primary tumor and survival. Cancer 1987;59:701–9.

50. Bacci G, Ferrari S, Longhi A, et al. Nonmetastatic osteosarcoma of the extremity with pathologic fracture at presentation: local and systemic control by amputation or limb salvage after preoperative chemotherapy. Acta Orthop Scand 2003;74:449–54.

51. Salunke AA, Chen Y, Tan JH, et al. Does a pathological fracture affect the prognosis in patients with osteosarcoma of the extremities? Bone Joint J 2014; 96-B:1396–403.

52. Sun L, Li Y, Zhang J, et al. Prognostic value of pathologic fracture in patients with high grade localized osteosarcoma: a systemic review and meta-analysis of cohort studies. J Orthop Res 2015;33: 131–9.

53. Mattei P. Surgery for metastatic disease. Curr Opin Pediatr 2013;25:362–7.

54. Janeway KA, Grier HE. Sequelae of osteosarcoma medical therapy: a review of rare acute toxicities and late effects. Lancet Oncol 2010;11:670–8.

55. Lee JS, DuBois SG, Boscardin WJ, et al. Secondary malignant neoplasms among children, adolescents, and young adults with osteosarcoma. Cancer 2014; 120:3987–93.

56. Fidler MM, Frobisher C, Guha J, et al. Long-term adverse outcomes in survivors of childhood bone sarcoma: the British Childhood Cancer Survivor Study. Br J Cancer 2015;112:1857–65.

57. Ghert M, Deheshi B, Holt G, et al. Prophylactic antibiotic regimens in tumour surgery (PARITY): protocol for a multicentre randomised controlled study. BMJ Open 2012;2 [pii:e002197].

58. Meyers PA, Schwartz CL, Krailo MD, et al. Osteosarcoma: the addition of muramyl tripeptide to chemotherapy improves overall survival–a report from the Children's Oncology Group. J Clin Oncol 2008;26: 633–8.

59. Rivera-Valentin RK, Zhu L, Hughes DPM. Bone sarcomas in pediatrics: progress in our understanding of tumor biology and implications for therapy. Pediatr Drugs 2015;17(4):257–71.

60. Kansara M, Teng MW, Smyth MJ, et al. Translational biology of osteosarcoma. Nat Rev Cancer 2014;14: 722–35.

Index

Note: Page numbers of article titles are in **boldface** type.

Orthop Clin N Am 47 (2016) 293–299
http://dx.doi.org/10.1016/S0030-5898(15)00233-3
0030-5898/16/$ – see front matter © 2016 Elsevier Inc. All rights reserved.

orthopedic.theclinics.com

Moving?

Make sure your subscription moves with you!

To notify us of your new address, find your **Clinics Account Number** (located on your mailing label above your name), and contact customer service at:

Email: journalscustomerservice-usa@elsevier.com

800-654-2452 (subscribers in the U.S. & Canada)
314-447-8871 (subscribers outside of the U.S. & Canada)

Fax number: 314-447-8029

Elsevier Health Sciences Division
Subscription Customer Service
3251 Riverport Lane
Maryland Heights, MO 63043

*To ensure uninterrupted delivery of your subscription, please notify us at least 4 weeks in advance of move.

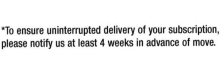
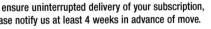